Handbook of Drug Therapy in Reproductive Endocrinology and Infertility

Handbook of Drug Therapy in Reproductive Endocrinology and Infertility

Edited by
Michel E. Rivlin, M.D.
Associate Professor, Department of Obstetrics and Gynecology, University of Mississippi School of Medicine; Director of Ambulatory Gynecology, University of Mississippi Medical Center, Jackson

Foreword by
Winfred L. Wiser, M.D.
Professor and Chairman, Department of Obstetrics and Gynecology, University of Mississippi School of Medicine, Jackson

Little, Brown and Company
Boston/Toronto/London

First Edition

Library of Congress Catalog Card No. 89-63422

ISBN 0-316-74772-6

Printed in the United States of America

RRDVA

To Jane, Sarah, Katy, and David

Contents

Contents

Foreword

Clinical endocrinology represents a search for the golden mean—identification of oversupply or undersupply, then careful manipulation and fine tuning to restore the internal milieu. In this, the last decade of the twentieth century, we have at our disposal accurate measurements of the majority of the hormones that control reproduction. Furthermore, these hormones or chemical messengers are available to us therapeutically either as the native substance or as even more powerful agonists. In addition, antagonists are also frequently available for therapeutic use. These tools also allow for elective manipulation of the reproductive system as in the avoidance or achievement of pregnancy. Complex and sophisticated tools necessitate highly trained and skilled practitioners. As chairman of an academic department of obstetrics and gynecology, I have long noticed a recurring request from students for increased instruction in these areas. The request is usually for more lectures, but reading is five times as fast as speech and a good, short, straightforward text conscientiously studied, to my mind, is more helpful than a lecture series, which frequently benefits only those students who prepare for the lectures, using a text, of course, in the preparation. Michel Rivlin's book is just such a text, concise and easy to follow. Furthermore, while its emphasis is on therapy, in the context of reproductive endocrinology and infertility, it is essential to the understanding of therapy to have the background of physiology, diagnosis, and the clinical picture, all of which are also well covered in this excellent volume. My advice, therefore, is as follows: Continue to accumulate clinical experience, read this excellent little book carefully, and stay out of the chairman's office.

Winfred L. Wiser, M.D.

Preface

The principles of reproductive endocrinology appear deceptively simple. There are, after all, only hypothalamic-releasing hormones, pituitary gonadotropins, and prolactin, together with a few gonadal, thyroid, and adrenal hormones to investigate and manipulate pharmacologically or operatively. In practice, however, the possible combinations and permutations are almost endless. As a result, many clinicians have problems dealing with endocrine abnormalities since their own major interests are often centered on the delivery and operating rooms. Unfortunately, available texts deal primarily with physiology, pathophysiology, and diagnosis. Therapeutics is not considered in any detail. In recent years, one or two publications that have appeared do place their emphasis on therapy, and they have been widely accepted. These texts, however, lack the portability and modest cost of this volume. *Handbook of Drug Therapy in Reproductive Endocrinology and Infertility* is intended for obstetricians, gynecologists, and family practitioners who treat women with endocrine disorders or seek the cause of an elusive pregnancy. However, even subspecialist-trained reproductive endocrinologists should find the information in this book helpful, concise, and readily accessible, since the contributing authors are acknowledged experts in the field.

Following an introductory overview, Part I is devoted to an in-depth description of the major drug classes and their individual agents. Included in these chapters are details of physiology, pharmacology, indications, contraindications, and clinical applications with dosages and protocols. In Part II, selected reviews of special situations are presented and include endocrine therapy of pediatric, male, sexually dysfunctional, and oncologic patients. There is, of course, a great deal of overlap between chapters and the opinions of the various contributors may differ. Since reproductive endocrinology is by no means an exact science, controversy is inevitable. Nevertheless, the practitioner seeking firm guidelines in the management of these often vexing problems will find them in this volume.

I would like to thank Donna White and Jane Searle for their technical expertise in preparing the manuscript, and Susan Pioli of Little, Brown for her invaluable advice. I would also like to acknowledge the contribution of Dr. Dick Worley, who steered me toward several of the outstanding contributors. Special thanks are also due to Dr. Winfred Wiser for writing the foreword and for placing the facilities of his department at our disposal. Preparation of this book was supported in part by the Vicksburg Hospital Medical Foundation, whose contribution is gratefully acknowledged.

M.E.R.

Contributing Authors

Sandra Ann Carson, M.D.
Assistant Professor, Department of Obstetrics and Gynecology, University of Tennessee College of Medicine; Attending Physician, William F. Bowld Hospital, Memphis

Owen K. Davis, M.D.
Assistant Professor of Obstetrics and Gynecology, Cornell University Medical College; Assistant Attending Obstetrician-Gynecologist, The New York Hospital, New York

Gary W. De Vane, M.D.
Clinical Associate Professor, Department of Obstetrics and Gynecology, University of Florida College of Medicine, Gainesville; Director, In Vitro Fertility Program, Center for Infertility and Reproductive Medicine, Orlando, Florida

George A. Hill, M.D.
Assistant Professor, Department of Obstetrics and Gynecology, Division of Reproductive Endocrinology, Vanderbilt University School of Medicine, Nashville

Gary D. Hubert, M.D.
Fellow, Department of Obstetrics and Gynecology, University of Tennessee College of Medicine; Fellow, Division of Reproductive Endocrinology, The University of Tennessee Medical Center, Memphis

Mark L. Jutras, M.D.
Assistant Professor, Department of Obstetrics and Gynecology, Division of Reproductive Endocrinology, University of Mississippi School of Medicine, Jackson

George Rodney Meeks, M.D.
Associate Professor, Department of Obstetrics and Gynecology, University of Mississippi School of Medicine; Director of Gynecology, University of Mississippi Medical Center, Jackson

Domeena C. Renshaw, M.D., F.A.C.P.
Professor and Associate Chairman, Department of Psychiatry, Loyola University of Chicago Stritch School of Medicine, Maywood, Illinois

Michel E. Rivlin, M.D.
Associate Professor, Department of Obstetrics and Gynecology, University of Mississippi School of Medicine; Director of Ambulatory Gynecology, University of Mississippi Medical Center, Jackson

Gregory F. Rosen, M.D., M.S.
Assistant Professor, Department of Obstetrics and Gynecology, University of California, Irvine, California College of Medicine, Irvine; Attending Physician, Section of Reproductive Endocrinology and Infertility, Memorial Medical Center, Long Beach, California

Isaac Schiff, M.D.
Joe Vincent Meigs Professor of Gynecology, Harvard Medical School; Chief, Vincent Memorial Gynecology Service, Massachusetts General Hospital, Boston

Bert Scoccia, M.D.
Assistant Professor of Obstetrics and Gynecology, The University of Chicago Pritzker School of Medicine; Attending Physician, Department of Obstetrics and Gynecology, Michael Reese Hospital and Medical Center, Chicago

Antonio Scommegna, M.D.
Professor and Head of Obstetrics and Gynecology, University of Illinois College of Medicine; Chief, Department of Obstetrics and Gynecology, Michael Reese Hospital and Medical Center, Chicago

Sergio C. Stone, M.D.
Professor, Department of Obstetrics and Gynecology, University of California, Irvine, California College of Medicine, Irvine; Director, Division of Reproductive Endocrinology, University of California, Irvine, Medical Center, Orange, California

Specific Disorders and Clinical Situations

This list provides easy access to major places in the text that discuss the indications for medications in *specific disorders and clinical situations*. The references are given in order of importance rather than order of appearance in the text. The listing does not refer to every citation; that purpose is served by the index.

Hirsutism Estrogen-progestin combinations, pp. 46–47; spironolactone, pp. 124–125; glucocorticoids, pp. 130–131; leuprolide, p. 100

Hyperprolactinemia Bromocriptine, p. 199

Infertility

Cervical factor Clomiphene citrate, p. 4; estrogen, pp. 4–5; hMG, p. 5

Male factor GnRH, pp. 198–199; hCG, pp. 197–198, 199; hMG, pp. 197, 199; bromocriptine, p. 199

Lactation suppression Bromocriptine, p. 118

Luteal phase inadequacy Progesterone, pp. 4, 33–34; clomiphene citrate, pp. 4, 90; gonadotropins, pp. 79–80

Male hypogonadism Testosterone, pp. 63, 187–189; hCG, pp. 187, 197–198; hMG, pp. 187, 197, 198; GnRH, pp. 187, 198

Mastodynia (mastopathy, fibrocystic breast disorder) Bromocriptine, p. 160; danazol, pp. 64, 68, 160–161; tamoxifen, p. 161; progestins, p. 161; estrogen-progestin combinations, pp. 57, 161

Menopause Estrogen, pp. 17, 27–28; MPA, pp. 40–41; estrogen-progestin combinations, p. 56

Oligozoospermia GnRH, p. 187; hCG, pp. 187, 199; hMG, pp. 187, 199

Ovarian failure Estrogen, p. 167; oxandrolone, pp. 167–168; MPA, p. 168

Ovulation induction Clomiphene citrate, pp. 88–90; hMG, pp. 76–79; hFSH, pp. 76–79; hCG, p. 79; GnRH, pp. 97–98; dexamethasone, p. 131; bromocriptine, p. 112

Pituitary adenoma (prolactinoma) Bromocriptine, pp. 112–113

Polycystic ovary syndrome Clomiphene citrate, p. 77; hFSH, p. 77; estrogen-progestin combinations, p. 172; spironolactone, pp. 123, 172; leuprolide, pp. 77, 98, 172; dexamethasone, pp. 130–131, 172; bromocriptine, p. 113

Premenstrual syndrome Estrogen-progestin combinations, p. 158; danazol, p. 158; GnRH, p. 158; progesterone, pp. 41, 158

Puberty

Delayed Estrogen, pp. 18, 167, 168; oxandrolone, pp. 167–168; MPA, p. 168

Precocious MPA, p. 164; leuprolide, pp. 98, 165

Repeated pregnancy loss Progesterone, p. 41

Thyroid

Hyperthyroidism Propylthiouracil, p. 143; methimazole, p. 143

Hypothyroidism Levothyroxine, p. 148; liothyronine, pp. 148–149; liotrix, p. 149

Storm Propylthiouracil, pp. 144–145, 147; sodium iodine, pp. 145, 147; propranolol, pp. 145, 147

Handbook of Drug Therapy in Reproductive Endocrinology and Infertility

Notice

1

Drug Therapy in Reproductive Endocrinology and Infertility: An Overview

George A. Hill

Medical therapy is important in the management of the patient with a reproductive endocrine disorder or infertility. A thorough understanding of the mechanisms of action of each of these drugs as well as their indications and contraindications is essential in the treatment of these patients. This chapter provides a brief review of the major disorders encountered, indicating the place of drugs in their management. For specific facts about any particular medication, the reader is referred to the chapter in this text related to that particular medication.

DISORDERS OF SEXUAL DEVELOPMENT AND PUBERTY

Abnormalities of puberty may include precocious development of puberty as well as delayed development of puberty. In all patients with an abnormality of pubertal development a thorough investigation should be performed to establish a cause and the specific mechanism to be treated.

In the patient with central precocious puberty several modes of therapy are available. *Medroxyprogesterone acetate* or *danazol* may be utilized and will arrest the development of secondary sexual characteristics in these patients. In addition, both these drugs will stop menstrual bleeding; however, neither will delay the advanced bone development that leads these patients to being tall children and short adults. *Gonadotropin-releasing hormone* (*GnRH*) *agonists* offer an attractive alternative in the treatment of central precocious puberty. These agonists will downregulate and desensitize the pituitary gland and lead to an arrest of the development of secondary sexual characteristics and menses. In addition, GnRH agonists arrest the advancement of bone growth seen in these children and preserve final adult height.

In the patient with delayed pubertal development, a thorough investigation is also important. If the patient is found to have premature ovarian failure or some other disorder of ovarian development leading to hypogonadism, estrogen replacement therapy can be used to initiate puberty. *Estrogen* should be administered in a low dose to lead to a slow development of secondary sexual characteristics. This is generally accomplished over 6 to 12 months. If the patient has an intact uterus, cyclic therapy with *progestins* should also be administered.

STEROID CONTRACEPTION

Oral contraceptives have been in use for more than 25 years. In addition to oral contraceptives, various other modes of administration of steroids for contraceptive purposes have been developed. These compounds appear to be very safe when used according to established indications and contraindications.

An estrogen and progestin are used in the different types of oral contraceptives available today. These may be formulated with constant doses (monophasic) or with varying doses (biphasic or triphasic). *Mestranol* and *ethinyl estradiol* are the only two estrogens used in oral contraceptives. All oral contraceptives with more than 50 μg of estrogen are being removed from the market. There are several progestins currently used in oral contraceptives: *ethynodiol diacetate, levonorgestrel, norethindrone, norethynodrel, norethindrone acetate, norgestrel, gestodene, norgestimate,* and *desogestrel.* A progestin-only oral contraceptive or "minipill" is in limited use today. Noncontraceptive benefits also result from the use of the oral contraceptives. All of these, as well as indications and contraindications, should be considered prior to the administration of an oral contraceptive to any patient.

Another utilization of the oral contraceptive pill has been to place it in the vagina. The steroids are well absorbed and this seems to be an efficacious method of steroid contraception. This appears to work as well as other steroid delivery systems used in the vagina without the drawbacks associated with the use of a vaginal ring.

Injectable forms of steroid contraception have been investigated in several countries. Combinations of estrogen and progestin such as *dihydroprogesterone acetophemide* plus *estradiol enanthate* and *medroxyprogesterone acetate* plus *estradiol cypionate* have shown some promise. A new preparation containing *norethindrone (norethisterone) enanthate* plus *estradiol valerate* has also shown promise in early clinical trials. Progesterone-only preparations for injection have also been used. The greatest experience with these has been with *depot-medroxyprogesterone acetate* (*DMPA*) and *norethindrone enanthate.* Because of the occurrence of breast tumors in beagle dogs, the long-term safety of DMPA has been questioned. However, the studies have come under close scrutiny recently as toxicologists question the relevance of pathologic findings observed in the beagle at dose levels 50 times that used in the human.

Various other modes of administration of steroids have been developed. A low-dose *levonorgestrel*-releasing vaginal ring has been found useful in women who cannot or will not use currently available contraceptive methods. Vaginal rings may cause erosion of the vaginal walls, may interfere with intercourse, and may occasionally develop an unpleasant odor.

Subdermal placement of *levonorgestrel*-releasing implants has been studied and found to be efficacious. In addition, levonorgestrel-containing implants seem to be effective for at least 4 years. Biodegradable implants of *norethindrone*-utilizing microcapsules have also been used and found to be effective as a contraceptive. The biodegraded forms are absorbed and therefore do not have to be removed.

Progestin-releasing intrauterine devices (IUD) have been developed. Early experience with a *progesterone*-releasing IUD found it to be effective for approximately 1 year. Recent investigation utilizing a *levonorgestrel*-containing IUD has found it to have an effective lifetime of 5 to 7 years.

Steroids may also be utilized as a postcoital contraceptive in females who have been raped if no other means of contraception was used. Intravenous *conjugated estrogen* as well as *ethinyl estradiol* may be administered within 72 hours after unprotected intercourse. In addition, combinations of *ethinyl estradiol* and *norgestrel* may be used. These therapies are generally effective; however, the patient should understand the risks and options should postcoital contraception fail.

Steroid contraception will continue to be needed and utilized throughout the world as attempts are made to control rapid population growth. Further development of alternative delivery systems is ongoing and will lead to the utilization of multiple modalities of administration.

OVULATORY DYSFUNCTION

Prior to the utilization of any agent for ovulation induction, the patient should undergo a complete pretreatment evaluation. This should include the documentation of oligo-ovulation or anovulation; exclusion of pregnancy or ovarian failure; and exclusion of other disorders such as hyperprolactinemia, thyroid or adrenal dysfunction, or hepatic disorders. All other infertility factors should be completely evaluated. In the patient with hyperestrogenism, an endometrial biopsy should be performed to exclude endometrial hyperplasia. After the pretreatment evaluation has been completed, the treatment of ovulatory dysfunction can be based on the diagnosis.

Clomiphene citrate is a triphenylethylene derivative generally used as the first line of management in patients with normoprolactinemic ovulatory dysfunction. This may include patients who are anovulatory or oligo-ovulatory, or patients with luteal phase inadequacy resulting from poor follicular development. Clomiphene citrate is indicated in patients with normal, low, or inappropriate secretion of gonadotropins.

For patients with pituitary disorders, or in patients who do not respond to clomiphene treatment, the next step in therapy includes the use of *human menopausal gonadotropins* (hMG). hMG contains both follicle-stimulating hormone (FSH) and luteinizing hormone (LH). hMG directly stimulates follicular development within the ovary and is indicated in patients who have failed to respond to clomiphene citrate or in patients with hypothalamic or pituitary disorders. In patients who fail to conceive with clomiphene therapy, hMG may be utilized after other infertility factors have been completely evaluated. Pure *FSH* is also available and may be utilized for induction of ovulation. FSH may be useful in the patient with an elevated LH/FSH ratio. hMG and FSH have more risks involved with their use and therefore, require close monitoring of follicular development with ultrasonography and determinations of serum estradiol levels.

When hMG or FSH are administered to induce follicular development, the majority of patients will not initiate a LH surge in spite of elevated serum levels of estradiol. These patients require the administration of *human chorionic gonadotropin* (hCG) to serve as a surrogate LH surge to induce the physical act of ovulation.

In patients who have pure hypothalamic dysfunction as the cause for anovulation, the use of GnRH is the most appropriate medication. GnRH may be administered either by subcutaneous injection or by an intravenous route utilizing an infusion pump. Patients with polycystic ovarian syndrome or anovulation due to causes other than hypothalamic dysfunction may respond to GnRH; however, the results are not as satisfactory in these groups of patients.

Prolactin secretion from the anterior pituitary is controlled by a prolactin inhibitory factor that is believed to be dopamine. Increased levels of prolactin may suppress GnRH and lead to ovulatory dysfunction. In patients with hyperprolactinemia and ovulatory dysfunction, *bromocriptine* is the agent of choice. Bromocriptine is a dopamine agonist and will suppress prolactin secretion by the lactotroph of the anterior pituitary.

In the patient with anovulation or oligo-ovulation who is found to have an elevation in the adrenal secretion of dehydroepiandrosterone sulfate (DHEA-S), the nightly utilization of *glucocorticoids* such as dexamethasone may lead to a decrease in DHEA-S levels and an increase in the ovulation rate and pregnancy rate after administration of clomiphene citrate. Dexamethasone is useful in patients whose serum level of DHEA-S is greater than 200 μg%.

Mild abnormalities in ovulatory function may be evident only as luteal phase inadequacy (LPI). LPI is a rare cause of infertility in the patient with regular menstrual cycles; however, it can frequently be seen in patients with oligomenorrhea or in patients with recurrent spontaneous abortions as well as in the older infertile patient (>35 years old). In fact, one-third of patients evaluated for recurrent spontaneous abortions will have LPI as the cause. LPI is diagnosed by examination of endometrial biopsy specimens taken during the late luteal phase and dated according to the onset of the next menses. Patients with LPI who have regular cycles and whose biopsy specimens show good glandular development with a lack of stromal decidualization can be treated with progesterone supplementation during the luteal phase in the form of *progesterone vaginal suppositories*. It is important to begin these after ovulation has occurred because progesterone administered prior to ovulation will effectively block the LH surge and block ovulation. In patients who have been diagnosed with LPI who have oligomenorrhea, *clomiphene citrate* is the treatment of choice. Once therapy has been instituted for LPI, a repeat biopsy should be performed to ensure that the LPI has been corrected.

CERVICAL FACTOR INFERTILITY

Very few patients have cervical factor causes of their infertility. In patients who are found to have poor mucus at the time of postcoital examination, the physician should first be sure that the test was performed at the appropriate time. An error in timing is the most frequent cause of a poor result on the postcoital test. Patients who have had surgery on their cervix, such as cold knife conization, are at increased risk for having a cervical factor as the cause of infertility. In these patients, intrauterine insemination of washed spermatozoa may be beneficial. Patients may also have poor cervical mucus during the periovulatory period as a result of an infection. In these cases the mucus should be cultured and the patient treated with an appropriate antibiotic. Patients treated with clomiphene citrate may also develop poor cervical mucus. In this group of patients, if poor follicular development is the cause of the poor cervical mucus, then the dose of clomiphene citrate may be increased or some other therapy instituted for ovulation induction. If, however, follicular development is adequate as judged by serum levels of estradiol and ultrasonography, then intrauterine insemination may be utilized or another drug to induce ovulation may be utilized. Exogenous *estrogens* have been utilized in patients with poor cervical mucus; however, estrogen administered in the follicular phase of the cycle generally results in abnormalities of follicular development and is generally not beneficial in helping the patient achieve a conception. Patients with poor cervical mucus who were treated with clomiphene citrate and who do not achieve a pregnancy may be treated with hMG for induction of ovulation. This generally results in excellent cervical mucus.

ENDOMETRIOSIS

Endometriosis is one of the more difficult diseases to treat for the gynecologist. Both a medical and surgical approach may be necessary in some patients. Various medications are available for the treatment of patients with endometriosis. The mode of treatment is dependent on the patient's desires.

In the young patient with suspected endometriosis who has dysmenorrhea and normal findings on pelvic examination, *oral contraceptives* may be administered if no contraindications exist. In the majority of patients this will afford relief of dysmenorrhea and no further therapy will be needed. *Antiprostaglandins* may also be utilized in addition to oral contraceptives in this group of patients for the treatment of dysmenorrhea.

In the patient with documented endometriosis who desires fertility, other modes of therapy must be considered. At the time of laparoscopy documenting the endometriosis, implants may be vaporized with the laser or cauterized. If medical therapy is deemed necessary, several drugs are available. Currently, *danazol,* a 17α-ethinyl testosterone derivative, is approved by the Food and Drug Administration (FDA) for treatment of endometriosis and may be utilized in these patients. In addition, *GnRH agonists* are being investigated for use in patients with endometriosis; however, they are not approved by the FDA for use in treating endometriosis at this time. GnRH agonists are beneficial in the treatment of endometriosis and have fewer side effects than danazol. Since they are already approved for use in the treatment of prostate cancer, approval for use in treating endometriosis should be forthcoming.

In the patient who cannot tolerate danazol or a GnRH agonist, *progestins* in the form of medroxyprogesterone acetate or DMPA may be used. Caution should be exercised in the use of DMPA because systemic levels may be present for 6 to 9 months after administration.

HIRSUTISM

In the patient with hyperandrogenism and increased hair growth, the cause must be established. After ovarian and adrenal tumors have been excluded, medical therapy can be begun. In patients who do not desire conception, and who have ovarian secretion of androgen as the cause of the hyperandrogenism, *oral contraceptive agents* are useful. Oral contraceptives contain both an estrogen and a progestin. Administration of an oral contraceptive results in increased production by the liver of sex hormone–binding globulin (SHBG) and therefore leads to decreased levels of free hormone (specifically androgens), thereby attaining their beneficial effect. In addition, ovarian production of androgen is suppressed, leading to decreased levels of total androgens. Because of the life cycle of the hair, no change in hirsutism may be apparent for 6 months. If little or no response is evident at the end of 6 months of therapy with an oral contraceptive, or if the hirsutism is severe, *spironolactone* can be considered for its antiandrogen effect. Spironolactone binds to the peripheral androgen receptor and blocks peripheral androgen action. However, in the patient who is being treated with spironolactone, it is imperative that contraception be utilized because of the possibility of teratogenesis. In the patient who has increased adrenal secretion of androgen as the cause of hirsutism, as measured by an increased serum level of DHEA-S, suppression with *glucocorticoids* should be utilized. A dose of dexamethasone at night may be all that is needed.

THYROID DYSFUNCTION

Thyroid homeostasis is modulated by a complex set of interrelated mechanisms. Thyroxine (T_4) secretion from the thyroid gland is stimulated by thyroid-stimulating hormone (TSH) secretion from the anterior pituitary. TSH secretion is under the influence of thyrotropin-releasing hormone (TRH) which is secreted from the anterior hypothalamus and transported through the pituitary portal circulation to the anterior pituitary gland. Both T_4 and triiodothyronine (T_3) feed back at the level of the pituitary to influence TSH secretion; however, the relationship between TSH, T_4, and T_3 is complex and not totally understood.

Hyperthyroidism is a syndrome that develops when body tissues are exposed to above normal concentrations of T_4 or T_3, or both. Graves' disease is the most common cause of hyperthyroidism and is 8 times more common in women than in men. The absence of a normal rise of TSH levels in response to the administration of TRH indicates suppression of the hypothalamic-pituitary axis and is the most sensitive test for hyperthyroidism.

Oligomenorrhea, amenorrhea, and reduced fertility may be seen in patients with hyperthyroidism. The cause of these syndromes is unclear; however, it may be related to increased plasma estrogen levels. In hyperthyroid women, plasma estrogen levels may be twofold to threefold higher than in normal women during all phases of the menstrual cycle. In addition, hyperthyroidism results in an increase in SHBG. Because testosterone is more tightly bound to SHBG than estradiol, as the SHBG concentration increases, more testosterone than estradiol will be bound and, therefore, estrogen action will be increased. The metabolic clearance rate of 17β-estradiol is also decreased in patients with hyperthyroidism. LH during the follicular and luteal phases of the menstrual cycle is twofold to threefold higher in hyperthyroid women when compared with euthyroid women. The peak values of LH may be decreased in thyrotoxic women with minimal bleeding during regular menstrual cycles and may be absent in thyrotoxic patients with amenorrhea. These changes in LH, estrogens, and androgens suggest abnormalities in hypothalamic function. In addition, there seems to be an increased contribution of testosterone and androstenedione to estrogen production in thyrotoxic women. All of these changes in gonadotropins, estrogens, and androgens suggest a cause for the menstrual abnormalities in patients with hyperthyroidism.

The clinician must decide whether to treat the patient with hyperthyroidism with long-term antithyroid medication or with some form of ablative thyroid therapy. Antithyroid medication includes *propylthiouracil* (PTU) and *methimazole* (Tapazole) which are thionamides and function to inhibit biosynthesis of thyroid hormone. In addition, *inorganic iodine* may also be utilized to block synthesis and release of thyroid hormone. Ablative thyroid therapy includes surgery or radioactive iodine therapy.

Thyroid storm is characterized by unregulated hypermetabolism and accounts for much of the mortality associated with hyperthyroidism. Treatment is directed at decreasing the synthesis and release of thyroid hormones and blocking the increased adrenergic activity. *Thionamides* and *iodine* may be utilized. In addition, beta-blockade with drugs such as *propranolol* rapidly reverse the adrenergic effects seen in thyroid storm.

When there is an inadequate effect of thyroid hormone on body tissues, *hypothyroidism* results. The diagnosis is confirmed by finding low serum levels of T_4 and T_3 resin uptake. Hypothyroidism may be rarely seen in patients presenting with infertility. Normal thyroid function is thought to be necessary for fertility. Women with hypothyroidism may be anovulatory and this can lead to infertility. In this situation, treatment of the primary disorder is indicated prior to any therapy with agents that induce ovulation. Thyroid hormone replacement therapy is not indicated in infertile patients who are euthyroid.

Levothyroxine is the treatment of choice because it is inexpensive, can be administered in a single daily dose, and leads to constant levels of serum T_4. T_3 is not routinely used in the treatment of hypothyroidism because the peaks of T_3 following absorption in the gastrointestinal tract are much higher than normal, it must be taken 3 times a day, it is considerably more expensive, and one cannot use the serum T_4 levels to assess replacement therapy when T_3 is utilized for replacement.

ADRENAL DYSFUNCTION

Adrenal insufficiency may result from insufficient secretion of corticotropin or complete or partial destruction of the adrenal glands. In acute adrenal insufficiency, 200 to 300 mg of *hydrocortisone* immediately should be administered intravenously. This should be followed with hydrocortisone, 100 mg, administered intravenously every 8 hours until the patient is stable. In chronic adrenal insufficiency, administration of hydrocortisone, 20 mg each morning and 10 mg each evening, is usually effective. Most patients will also require *fludrocortisone,* 0.05 to 0.10 mg, each day.

In patients with adrenal insufficiency who undergo surgical procedures, *cortisone acetate,* 50 to 75 mg intramuscularly, should be administered the night prior to surgery. One hundred milligrams of hydrocortisone should be administered intravenously on call to the operating room. During surgery, 100 mg of hydrocortisone should be infused continuously as needed, and postoperatively 100 mg of hydrocortisone with dextrose or normal saline solution, or both, should be infused continuously every 8 hours until the patient is stable. The dose of steroid can then be decreased to maintenance levels. Steroid requirements also increase during pregnancy and should be increased appropriately.

Glucocorticoid excess is generally treated surgically once the underlying cause is determined. This may include transphenoidal pituitary surgery or adrenalectomy. Irradiation of the pituitary gland may also be utilized. Administration of neuropharmacotherapeutic drugs may be partially successful. These include serotonin antagonists such as *cyproheptadine,* dopamine agonists such as *bromocriptine,* norepinephrine depletion such as *reserpine,* or gamma-aminobutyric acid antagonists such as *valproate sodium*. The role of the adrenal gland in hirsutism has already been described.

PREMENSTRUAL SYNDROME

The first description of "premenstrual tension" was published by Frank in 1931. It was not until the late 1970s that premenstrual syndrome (PMS) began to be reevaluated and popularized. PMS is defined as any combination of emotional or physical signs or symptoms that occur cyclicly prior to menstruation and regress or disappear after menstruation. PMS may affect 15 to 100 percent of women of reproductive age and peaks during the third and fourth decades of life. Multiple hypotheses have been proposed for the cause of PMS including aberrations in ovarian hormones, decreases in endogenous opiates, vitamin and mineral deficiencies, mineralocorticoid excess, psychologic problems, as well as changes in monoamine neurotransmitters and prostaglandin levels and allergies to various substances. The diagnosis of PMS is based on subjectively documenting exacerbation of symptoms prior to the menses with regression after the menses.

Multiple treatment modalities exist for PMS. Initially the patient should be treated with exercise and nutritional changes, which may lead to significant improvement. Pharmacologic modes of therapy are difficult to evaluate because even placebos will result in improved symptoms in up to 60 percent of subjects. *Progesterone* may be utilized in the treatment of patients with PMS; however, no well-designed study has conclusively demonstrated a beneficial effect of progesterone on PMS. Synthetic progestins should not be used in the treatment of PMS as they may exacerbate these symptoms. Patients may also be treated with ovulation suppressants such as *GnRH agonists, danazol,* or *oral contraceptives*. The side effects of these drugs may be similar to the symptoms seen in patients with PMS and therefore may not be helpful. A diuretic such as *spironolactone* may be used in the treatment of PMS when the patient's main symptoms are related to fluid retention. *Pyridoxine* (vitamin B_6) has also been utilized in the treatment of women with PMS and has been shown to be beneficial in uncontrolled studies. However, controlled studies have failed to demonstrate any efficacy of pyridoxine in these patients. *Prostaglandin antagonists and precursors* have been utilized with varying success. In conclusion, no single treatment has proved to be effective for the management of PMS. Counselling in diet and exercise will generally result in improvement for most women and should be the first step in therapy. Frequent follow-up and counselling are required in all these patients and therapy may be directed to the major complaint.

MENOPAUSE

Hormone replacement therapy is one small part of the total care required in the menopausal patient. In the development of a treatment plan for the menopausal patient, risk factors must be evaluated and indications as well as relative and absolute contraindications to various forms of therapy must be reviewed.

Estrogen replacement therapy (ERT) is beneficial in treating vasomotor symptoms and genitourinary atrophy, as well as the prevention of osteoporosis. The patient may note decreased tiredness and fatigue because of improvement in sleep from the decreasing number of nocturnal hot flashes, and there may be benefits on atherosclerotic heart disease in the menopausal patient treated with ERT. Relative as well as absolute contraindications to ERT must be considered in all patients. These are covered in detail in Chapter 2. Most patients will, however, benefit from some form of ERT. *Oral conjugated estrogens* are probably the most common form of ERT; however, oral *micronized estradiol* or *transdermal estradiol* as well as other forms of estrogen may be utilized.

Progesterone or a synthetic *progestin* should be utilized in all menopausal patients treated with ERT who have a uterus. The progestin is indicated to prevent endometrial hyperplasia and neoplasia which is known to result from continuous exposure of the endometrium to estrogen. Progestins that are currently available include *norethindrone, norgestrel,* and *medroxyprogesterone acetate.* In addition, *oral micronized progesterone* may soon be available for the treatment of the postmenopausal patient.

Estrogens and *progestins* may be administered either on a cyclic or on a continuous basis and must be individualized to the particular patient. In addition to estrogen and progesterone replacement, the postmenopausal patient may benefit from an increased intake of *calcium.* Calcium does not appear to be beneficial in the prevention of osteoporosis when it is administered without estrogen. Whether or not vitamin D or fluoride should be administered is still a controversial point.

HORMONAL THERAPY IN MALE INFERTILITY

Limited modes of therapy are available for the infertile man who is found to be azoospermic or oligospermic. Hypothalamic disorders leading to azoospermia may be treated with *GnRH* administered in a pulsatile fashion to stimulate the pituitary gland and in turn lead to the release of FSH and LH and subsequent spermatogenesis. This requires long-term therapy because of the time required for spermatogenesis. In the patient with azoospermia due to pituitary disorders, *hMG* and *hCG* may be administered to initiate and maintain spermatogenesis; however, this therapy must also be maintained for a long period of time because of the time required for spermatogenesis.

Men may also be noted to have oligospermia that may be due to multiple factors. If the serum FSH level is markedly elevated, suggesting end organ failure, no therapy will be beneficial. In the patient with oligospermia and a normal FSH level, consideration of antiestrogen therapy with *clomiphene citrate* or *tamoxifen* may be indicated. However, no results from good double-blind studies suggest a benefit to this therapy in the infertile man.

CONCLUSION

Numerous medications are utilized in the treatment of the gynecologic patient with endocrine or infertility problems. A thorough understanding of these medications is necessary if one is to use them to the benefit of the patient. The various medications available, their mechanism of action, and their indications and contraindications will be outlined in the chapters that follow.

BIBLIOGRAPHY

Overview

Speroff, L., Glass, R. H., and Kase, N. G. *Clinical Gynecologic Endocrinology and Infertility* (3rd ed.). Baltimore: Williams and Wilkins, 1983.

Wentz, A. C., Herbert, C. M., and Hill, G. A. *Gynecologic Endocrinology for the House Officer*. Baltimore: Williams and Wilkins, 1988.

Yen, S. S. C., and Jaffe, R. B. *Reproductive Endocrinology, Physiology, Pathophysiology, and Clinical Management* (2nd ed.). Philadelphia: W. B. Saunders, 1986.

Disorders of Sexual Development and Puberty

Boepple, P. A., et al. Use of a potent, long-acting agonist of gonadotropin-releasing hormone in the treatment of precocious puberty. *Endocr. Rev.* 7:24, 1986.

Steroid Contraception

ACOG Technical Bulletin #106. Oral contraception. Washington, DC: American College of Obstetrics and Gynecology, July 1987.

Cook, C. L., Wiist, L. J., and Kraft, S. L. Pregnancy prophylaxis: parenteral postcoital estrogen. *Obstet. Gynecol.* 67:331, 1986.

Ginsburg, K. A., and Moghissi, K. S. Alternate delivery systems for contraceptive progestogens. *Fertil. Steril.* 49[Suppl.]:16S, 1988.

Speidel, J. J. Steroidal contraception in the eighties. The role of current and new products. *J. Reprod. Med.* 28:759, 1983.

Van Santen, M. R., and Haspels, A. A. A comparison of high-dose estrogens versus low-dose ethinyl estradiol or norgestrel combination in postcoital interception: a study of 493 women. *Fertil. Steril.* 43:206, 1985.

Ovulatory Dysfunction

Adashi, E. Y. Clomiphene citrate: mechanism(s) and site(s) of action—a hypothesis revisited. *Fertil. Steril.* 42:331, 1984.

Asch, R. H., and Greenblatt, R. B. Update on the safety and efficacy of clomiphene citrate as a therapeutic agent. *J. Reprod. Med.* 17:175, 1976.

Daly, D. C., et al. A randomized study of dexamethasone in ovulation induction with clomiphene citrate. *Fertil. Steril.* 41:844, 1984.

Ory, S. J., et al. Ovulation induction with pulsatile gonadotropin-releasing hormone administration in patients with polycystic ovarian syndrome. *Fertil. Steril.* 43:20, 1985.

Santoro, N., et al. Intravenous administration of pulsatile gonadotropin-releasing hormone in hypothalamic amenorrhea: effects of dosage. *J. Clin. Endocrinol. Metab.* 62:109, 1986.

Schwartz, M., and Jewelewicz, R. The use of gonadotropins for induction of ovulation. *Fertil. Steril.* 35:3, 1981.

Zacur, H. A. Ovulation induction with gonadotropin releasing hormone. *Fertil. Steril.* 44:435, 1985.

Endometriosis

Barbieri, R. L., and Ryan, K. J. Medical therapy for endometriosis: endocrine pharmacology. *Semin. Reprod. Endocrinol.* 3:339, 1985.

Buttram, V. C., Jr., Reiter, R. C., and Ward, S. Treatment of endometriosis with danazol: report of a six year prospective study. *Fertil. Steril.* 43:353, 1985.

Hull, M. E., et al. Comparison of different treatment modalities of endometriosis in infertile women. *Fertil. Steril.* 47:40, 1987.

Schriock, E., et al. Treatment of endometriosis with a potent agonist of gonadotropin-releasing hormone (Nafarelin). *Fertil. Steril.* 44:583, 1985.

Hirsutism

Abuzeid, M. I., and Wiebe, R. H. Clinical evaluation of androgen excess. *Semin. Reprod. Endocrinol.* 4:197, 1986.

Aksel, S. Therapeutic approaches to androgen excess. *Semin. Reprod. Endocrinol.* 4:211, 1986.

Thyroid Dysfunction

Brennan, M. D. Thyroid hormones. *Mayo Clin. Proc.* 55:33, 1980.

Klein, I., and Levey, G. S. Thyroid storm. *Hosp. Med.* 18(March):34a, 1982.

Trooper, D. S. Antithyroid drugs. *N. Engl. J. Med.* 311:1353, 1984.

Adrenal Dysfunction

Carpenter, P. C. Cushing's syndrome: update of diagnosis and management. *Mayo Clin. Proc.* 61:49, 1986.

Chamberlin, P., and Meyer, W. J. Management of pituitary-adrenal suppression secondary to corticosteroid therapy. *Pediatrics* 67:245, 1981.

Hamburger, S., and Rush, D. Series on endocrine metabolic emergencies: II. acute adrenal insufficiency. *J. Am. Med. Wom. Assoc.* 36:199, 1981.

Hormone Therapy in Male Infertility

AinMelk, Y., et al. Tamoxifen citrate therapy in male infertility. *Fertil. Steril.* 48:113, 1987.

LaNasa, J. A., Jr., and Urry, R. L. Evaluation and treatment of the infertile male. *Semin. Reprod. Endocrinol.* 3:113, 1985.

Swerdloff, R. S., Overstreet, J. W., Sokol, R. Z., and Rajfer, J. Infertility in the male. *Ann. Intern. Med.* 103:906, 1985.

I

Hormonal Agents

2

Estrogens

Michel E. Rivlin

Compounds exhibiting estrogenic activity stimulate growth and maintain female sexual characteristics at a genital and a systemic level. The *genital effects* include the development of the vagina with proliferation of vaginal mucosa; the growth and function of the cervix, uterus, and fallopian tubes; ovarian growth and sexual development; and proliferation of breast tissue. The *extragenital effects* include the development and maintenance of the secondary sex characteristics, including body fat and hair distribution; bone maturation and structure; increased liver synthesis of certain hormones, in particular steroid-binding globulin; and effects on mineral metabolism with retention of sodium and water and excretion of potassium.

PHYSIOLOGY

All steroidal estrogens are derived from the hydrocarbon estrane (18 carbons). *Estradiol-17β*, the major estrogen of the reproductive years, is produced by the ovary in both the follicular and luteal phases of the menstrual cycle. The ovary also secretes androstenedione, which is then converted to testosterone (both are androgens). Testosterone is then converted to estradiol-17β. Androstenedione may also be converted to estrone, an estrogen with about half the biologic activity of estradiol-17β. Estrone and estradiol-17β are readily and extensively interconverted.

Estrone is also produced by peripheral conversion of androstenedione in many tissues. In the reproductive years, androstenedione is derived in equal amounts from ovary and adrenal glands and after the menopause, principally from the adrenal glands. Following the menopause, therefore, ovarian production of estradiol-17β essentially ceases, and estrone produced from peripheral conversion of androstenedione is the principal source of estrogenic activity. *Estriol*, an estrogen with only about 10 percent of the activity of estradiol-17β, is formed by peripheral metabolism of ovarian estrogens. Estriol is present in very large amounts during pregnancy.

Much of the circulating estrogen is bound to a beta-globulin protein transport carrier, sex hormone–binding globulin, which also binds to testosterone and albumin. There is only a very small amount of unbound, freely circulating hormone; however, this is the only fraction that is biologically active. Estrogens are inactivated in the liver chiefly by conjugation in the form of sulfates and glucuronates. These conjugates are then excreted in urine and bile.

PHARMACOLOGY

Most estrogens for therapeutic use are naturally occurring or synthetic analogues of endogenous hormones. A variety of preparations exist for oral, parenteral, or topical administration. Natural estrogens are not used orally because of rapid first-pass deactivation in the liver, but they are effective when administered by the parenteral route. An exception is micronized estradiol-17β (Estrace), in which small particle size results in larger surface area with increased absorption and therefore satisfactory oral therapy. The natural estro-

Table 2-1. Estrogen equivalents

Estrogen	Clinically Equivalent Dose
Conjugated estrogen (Premarin, etc.)	0.625
Estrone (Theelin, etc.)	0.9 mg
Estradiol (Estrace)	1.0 mg
Estradiol (Estraderm)	50.0 μg/day
Esterified estrogens (Estratab, Menest, etc.)	0.625 mg
Ethinyl estradiol (Estinyl, etc.)	0.02 mg
Estropipate (Ogen, etc.)	1.25 mg—Ogen 1.5 mg—estropipate
Diethylstilbestrol	0.25 mg

gens include estradiol-17β, estrone, and conjugated equine estrogens (Premarin, Ogen) usually derived from the urine of pregnant mares. Oral preparations result in higher levels of estrogen in the hepatic-portal circulation than what occurs physiologically. Estradiol-17β is readily absorbed vaginally without conversion to estrone, whereas oral administration appears to result in initial conversion to estrone with resulting levels of circulating estrone higher than those of estradiol-17β.

All natural estrogens are steroidal. Synthetic estrogens may be steroidal or nonsteroidal. The addition of a 17α-ethinyl group to estradiol-17β enhances oral activity and potency by impeding hepatic degradation. Ethinyl estradiol (Estinyl, Feminone) is one of two estrogens used in oral contraceptive preparations. Quinestrol (Estrovis), closely related to ethinyl estradiol, is stored in adipose tissue and therefore has a prolonged action. Estradiol esters (benzoate, cypionate, valerate) in oily or aqueous suspensions provide a prolonged action for intramuscular administration.

Nonsteroidal estrogens are usually related to stilbenes. Diethylstilbestrol (DES), a stilbene, is very potent. Further modifications include dienestrol and chlorotrianisene (TACE) which have varying potencies. Clomiphene, derived from TACE, possesses both estrogenic and antiestrogenic properties. The biologic properties of the synthetic preparations are similar but not identical to those of the natural hormones. The potency and side effects vary with structure and route of administration.

Tests of estrogenicity in humans are difficult. They include changes in vaginal mucosa, decreased level of gonadotropins, increased levels of certain proteins, and the buildup of proliferative endometrium in postmenopausal women or women who have had an ovariectomy. As a result, even the comparison between the two estrogens used in oral contraceptives, ethinyl estradiol and mestranol, is a subject of dispute, especially as mestranol is converted to ethinyl estradiol following ingestion. No particular estrogen has been proved to be better than others as regards estrogen replacement therapy (ERT).

INDICATIONS

Estrogens are used to mimic or accentuate inadequate production of endogenous hormone as in the menopausal patient, to correct hormone imbalance as in the woman with dysfunctional uterine bleeding, or to reverse abnormal processes as in endometriosis or hirsutism. Probably the most common indication is for contraception.

ERT for symptomatic menopausal patients reliably reverses vasomotor symptoms (hot flashes), night waking, and atrophic vaginitis. The lower urinary tract contains estrogen receptors and many bladder and urethral symptoms of the climacteric respond to ERT. It is difficult to prove that the emotional symptoms of the climacteric respond to estrogens, although many clinicians believe that they do, at least in some women. Changes in vaginal physiologic parameters related to age may also be reversed with estrogens. A major benefit of ERT is in the prophylaxis of osteoporosis. At greatest risk for this are smokers, white women, and those of low body weight. Estrogens are also used in the therapy of established osteoporosis in order to prevent further bone loss.

ERT for vasomotor symptoms or atrophic vaginitis may be tapered off or discontinued after 3 to 6 months of therapy; however, when employed to arrest the loss of calcium from bone that is associated with the cessation of ovarian function, ERT is continued indefinitely. ERT in women who have not had a hysterectomy should be given together with a progestin in order to prevent endometrial hyperplasia and cancer. Many clinicians include a progestin even if the uterus has been removed, in order to lessen the risk of breast cancer. However, ERT has not been shown to increase the incidence of this neoplasm. Commonly employed regimens supply estrogens from day 1 to day 25 plus progestin from day 16 to day 25 of the menstrual cycle. Should symptoms supervene during the interval, however, ERT may continue on a daily basis. The smallest dose of estrogen required for symptom control and osteoporosis prophylaxis should be used. Bleeding resulting from withdrawal from estrogen and progestin will occur in about half of the treated females and only requires investigation if it occurs during therapy and not in the interval between courses.

Dysfunctional uterine bleeding, a common indication for hormonal treatment, is a diagnosis of exclusion. Organic causes of abnormal flow include pregnancy-related complications, pelvic cancer, fibroids, endometrial polyps, thyroid dysfunction, and rarely, disorders of coagulation. Once these are excluded, dysfunctional uterine bleeding is ascribed to an estrogen-progesterone imbalance usually associated with anovulation. Commonly there is estrogen dominance with a hyperplastic, fragile endometrium and a relatively constant supply of estrogen. Progesterone dominance, generally encountered with the use of oral contraceptives, is associated with an atrophic endometrium. If the endometrium is proliferative or hyperplastic drug therapy generally involves the administration of a progestin. If the endometrium has been denuded, initial control requires the administration of estrogen to build up a stable endometrium, progestin is then added, both are then stopped, and a withdrawal bleed, which is usually heavy and painful (medical curettage), follows. Thereafter, either a birth control pill or intermittent doses of progestin should be prescribed. If bleeding is very heavy, usually encountered in either the adolescent or the perimenopausal patient, intravenous estrogen may be necessary. Rarely, this fails and curettage is then indicated.

Delayed puberty may be due to hypogonadal hypogonadism or simple constitutional delay. The diagnosis may be difficult to make, although in the latter, height is generally appropriate for bone age. Sometimes brief (3–6 months) courses of estrogen may be tried for simple constitutional delay in an attempt to stimulate development without advancing bone age. If pubertal development has not occurred by age 17, gonadotropin deficiency exists and replacement therapy is indicated. In sexual infantilism from any cause, puberty may be mimicked with hormone replacement. Generally commenced at about age 12, estrogen is given for 21 to 25 days monthly; the dosage starts low and is titrated as to results up to double dosage, if required, to induce secondary sexual characteristics. When breakthrough bleeding occurs, progestin is added for the last 10 days of each cycle. If growth hormone is deficient, that medication should first be used for several years in order for the patient to reach maximum height.

The differential diagnosis of *amenorrhea* may be facilitated by the use of estrogen and progesterone challenges. Initially, progesterone is administered, and absence of bleeding on withdrawal indicates a low level of endogenous estrogen. If bleeding does not follow joint administration of estrogen and progesterone, uterine problems such as Asherman's syndrome are probably involved. Women with *ovarian failure* due to gonadal dysgenesis (Turner's syndrome) require hormonal replacement. Small doses that stimulate growth yet avoid early epiphyseal closure should be used. The management of a variety of *hypothalamic-pituitary-ovarian* dysfunctions depends on the patient's wishes and will differ, for instance, if pregnancy is desired. If replacement therapy is all that is required, oral contraceptives that supply pharmacologic rather than physiologic quantities should probably be avoided. Standard regimens of ERT should be administered to maintain secondary sex characteristics and prevent osteoporosis. If sufficient amounts of endogenous estrogen are present, intermittent progestin will protect against endometrial hyperplasia. If contraception is a factor, the birth control pill may be prescribed.

Excessive height in young girls may be prevented with estrogens. If growth tables indicate a final height of more than 6 feet, the administration of large doses of estrogen at bone age 11 or 12 (early puberty to midpuberty) may diminish final stature by 2 to 3 inches. Best results are obtained when therapy commences at age 8 or 9 but precocious puberty will result. The risks of therapy may outweigh the benefits and other medications (e.g., bromocriptine mesylate [Parlodel] which diminishes growth hormone response) may be superior. The *suppression of lactation* was once an indication for estrogen therapy, but results are better with bromocriptine mesylate and estrogen increases the risk of postpartum thrombosis. *Hirsutism and endometriosis* may be treated with estrogens, however; these are then administered together with progestin in the form of birth control pills. The same probably applies to the management of *dysmenorrhea* and the *premenstrual syndrome*. Estrogens have been used as a *postcoital contraceptive*. Given within 72 hours after unprotected intercourse, large doses result in an endometrium that is nonreceptive to implantation. However, small doses of the oral contraceptive Ovral are as successful and have fewer side effects. Estrogens may be given in the therapy of *breast, endometrial*, and *prostatic cancers* as outlined in Chapter 14.

CONTRAINDICATIONS, PRECAUTIONS, AND WARNINGS

Contraindications include known or suspected pregnancy, lactation, known or suspected breast cancer, other estrogen-dependent neoplasias including endometrial carcinoma (exceptions are appropriately chosen patients with metastatic disease), active thrombophlebitis, thrombosis, thromboembolism or a history of these diseases, and undiagnosed abnormal genital bleeding. Precautions and close observation are required when administering estrogens to women with benign breast disease including fibrocystic changes or fibroadenomas, with abnormal findings on mammograms, or with a family history of breast cancer. Patients with hypertension, impaired glucose tolerance, hyperlipidemia, fibroids, migraine headaches, asthma, or epilepsy also require careful follow-up because all of these conditions may be adversely affected by estrogens. Patients with hepatic, renal, or cardiac disease are at extra risk, as are those with metabolic bone disease associated with increases in serum calcium levels. In such women, thoughtful assessment of the risk-benefit ratio is essential.

METABOLIC EFFECTS, ALTERED LABORATORY VALUES, AND DRUG INTERACTIONS

ERT usually does not alter glucose tolerance. The effect on lipids is variable depending on the preparation and route of administration. In general, triglyceride levels are elevated and cholesterol levels are lower. Oral estrogens increase high-density lipoprotein (HDL) levels and decrease low-density lipoprotein (LDL) levels. This effect is lost with other modes of administration. Since the HDL and LDL alterations are protective against atherosclerotic heart disease, they are beneficial. Progestins derived from 19-nortestosterone have an opposite effect, but medroxyprogesterone does not appear to abolish the beneficial effect of estrogens on lipid metabolism. In clinical terms, the long-term effect of ERT on cardiovascular disease has not really been elucidated. The levels of several coagulation factors are elevated by estrogens, but with ERT the risk of thromboembolism and stroke is not elevated; however, estrogens should nevertheless be avoided in patients with a history of these disorders. ERT increases cholesterol saturation of bile with a resultant 2.5 times increase in the incidence of cholelithiasis. Estrogens should be avoided in patients with severe active or chronic active liver disease or with a history of gestational jaundice.

Levels of alkaline phosphatase, bilirubin, and prothrombin clotting factors VII to X are elevated. Antithrombin III levels are depressed. Thyroxine-binding globulin (TBG), protein-bound iodine (PBI), and thyroxine levels are elevated. Resin triiodothyronine uptake is depressed. Thyroid index is unchanged. Serum levels of glucose, cortisol, transcortin, triglycerides, and phospholipids are elevated. Levels of folates and pyridoxine are depressed. Urinary levels of pregnanediol fall.

Drug groups with which interactions may result in therapeutic compromise are similar to those noted with oral contraceptives and include anticonvulsants, barbiturates, and rifampin. Certain antibiotics may decrease enterohepatic circulation of hormones, thus decreasing hormonal function. Further interactions, also more closely associated with the birth control pill, include decreased activity of anticoagulants and increased effectiveness of antidepressive agents.

ADVERSE REACTIONS

Adverse reactions resemble those encountered with oral contraceptives. However, with ERT, doses are lower and therefore both the incidence and the severity of these reactions are diminished. Gastrointestinal symptoms include nausea, vomiting, and bloating. Cholestatic jaundice may occur. Genitourinary problems include candidiasis, cervical ectopy with excessive vaginal secretion, increased growth of fibroids, amenorrhea, or breakthrough bleeding. Fluid retention may result in edema, weight gain, tender breasts, or abdominal or leg pain. Contact lenses may no longer fit. Cerebral changes include headache, migraine, depression, and dizziness. In children, when ERT is used prior to completion of bone growth, it may result in early epiphyseal closure with ultimate loss of height achieved.

Estrogens are contraindicated during *pregnancy* because of an increased incidence of congenital heart and limb reduction anomalies associated with their use. Furthermore, following the administration of DES, as well as many other estrogens, to pregnant females, an increase of genital anomalies and vaginal or cervical cancers has been found in their female offspring and genital anomalies in the male offspring. Estrogens are excreted in breast milk and should therefore not be used in lactating women. If these medications are taken during early gestation, women should be counseled regarding the potential risks and the advisability of continuing the pregnancy.

Estrogens are *carcinogenic* as evidenced by an increased incidence of atypical endometrial hyperplasia and endometrial cancer in women receiving unopposed ERT. The risk is increased when duration of therapy exceeds 3 years and when higher doses are employed. Disease states characterized by long-standing unopposed estrogen excess are also associated with an increased incidence of endometrial cancer as in the obese diabetic, the patient with polycystic ovary syndrome, or women with granulosa cell tumors of the ovary. The tumors associated with ERT have usually been early cancers with a uniformly good prognosis. The carcinogenic effects of ERT appear to be preventable by the addition of a progestin during the latter half of the treatment cycle and this should be standard policy in patients who have not had a hysterectomy. There is no proof that ERT has an adverse effect on the incidence of breast cancer.

ADMINISTRATION

The pretreatment history and physical examination must pay particular attention to personal and family history, examination of the breasts and pelvis, and blood pressure. Pap smear is essential, but a routine endometrial biopsy is probably unnecessary and should be reserved for patients with abnormal uterine bleeding. Determinations of serum lipid levels are desirable as part of screening, but are expensive and are not routinely ordered by most physicians. The same is true of bone densitometry for early evidence of calcium loss from bone. Serial mammography as recommended by the American

Cancer Society has also not been universally accepted, once again, because of costs. Patients should be carefully counseled as regards the potential side effects and should report instances of abnormal bleeding in particular. History, physical examination, and pap smear should be repeated on at least an annual basis or more frequently as necessary.

ESTROGEN PREPARATIONS

Steroidal Estrogens

Estradiol—Estrace (Mead Johnson)

TABLETS (MICRONIZED), 1 OR 2 MG. Micronized estradiol is well absorbed orally. The standard ERT dose (1–2 mg daily) supplies 5 to 10 times the amount of estradiol produced by the normal premenopausal ovary. It is not known whether this dosage might cause any problem in the long term. Estrace contains the dye tartrazine. In rare instances, skin allergic reactions to this drug may occur, especially in aspirin-allergic individuals.

The oral dosage is 1 to 2 mg per day, given in 28-day cycles with 3 weeks on and 1 week off; dosage is adjusted as necessary to control symptoms. If the patient has not undergone hysterectomy, a progestin should be added to the estrogen for the last 10 days of the course.

VAGINAL CREAM, 0.01% (42.5 GM) (0.1 MG/GM IN 42.5-GM CONTAINER). The intravaginal dosage is 2 to 4 gm per day, given for 1 to 2 weeks, followed by a gradual reduction to 1 to 2 gm/day, given for 1 to 2 weeks. For maintenance, 1 gm may be given 1 to 3 times per week after vaginal mucosal integrity has been restored.

Vaginal absorption of estrogen yields systemic levels comparable to those obtained with oral administration; therefore, if vaginal therapy is used for long periods of time, a progestin should be added to prevent endometrial hyperplasia.

PARENTERAL USE. Estradiol is available for parenteral use in aqueous or oily suspension in patients with poor tolerance or compliance or when there has been lack of response to other methods of administration. Depot injections generally yield a variable onset of effect with a variable duration of action of 14 to 28 days. Pain at the site of injection is a not infrequent complaint. If used on a long-term basis, progestin is necessary if the uterus is present.

Preparations. These include:

Estradiol benzoate. Generic. Powder 1 and 5 mg.
Estradiol cypionate. Generic. Solution 5 mg/ml (in oil) in 10-ml containers.
Estradiol cypionate. Depo-estradiol (Upjohn). Vials: 1 mg/ml (10 ml), 5 mg/ml (5 ml).
Estradiol-ionate PA. (Reid-Provident). Solution (in oil) 5 mg/ml in 10-ml containers.
Estradiol valerate. (1) Generic. Solution (in oil) 10, 20, 40 mg/ml in 10-ml containers. (2) Delestrogen (Squibb). Solution (in oil) 10, 20, 40 mg/ml in 5-ml containers.
Polyestradiol Phosphate. Estradurin (Ayerst). 20 mg/ml (2 ml diluent).
Additional Trademarks: Estraval (Reid-Provident), Gynogen LA (Forest).

Dosage. The following are dosages for parenteral estradiol:

Estradiol cypionate. Depo-estradiol (Upjohn). For moderate to severe menopausal vasomotor symptoms, 1 to 5 mg is given intramuscularly every 3 to 4 weeks; for female hypogonadism, give 1.5 to 2.0 mg intramuscularly once a month.
Estradiol benzoate. The duration of action is 2 to 3 days. For ERT, administer 0.5 to 1.5 mg, 2 to 3 times per week.
Estradiol valerate. The duration of action is 14 to 21 days. For ERT, administer 20 mg intramuscularly immediately, then 5 mg every 2 to 4 weeks. For DUB, administer 20 mg immediately, then 5 mg every 2 weeks along with progestin. For lactation suppression, give a 10 to 30-mg single dose soon after delivery.

TOPICAL TRANSDERMAL SYSTEMS. The following preparations comprise topical transdermal systems for estradiol.

Estraderm (with alcohol) (Ciba). 0.05 mg/24 hours (4 mg/10 sq cm).
Estraderm (with alcohol) (Ciba). 0.1 mg/24 hours (8 mg/20 sq cm).

Dosage and Administration. For ERT in the menopause, female hypogonadism, castration, or primary ovarian failure the usual initial dose of transdermal estradiol is one system delivering 0.05 mg per 24 hours applied twice weekly in a 3-week cyclic regimen (one week with no therapy; progestin is added if the uterus is present during last 10 days of estrogen administration). In women already receiving oral estrogen, transdermal administration should be commenced 1 week after discontinuation of oral medication. Subsequent dosage is adjusted according to therapeutic response. Transdermal systems should be applied with at least a 1-week interval between applications at the same site. Breasts and waistline sites should be avoided. If the system detaches, it may be replaced. Clean, dry, nonhairy sites are preferable and the system should be applied immediately after removal from its protective pouch.

As with all nonoral applications, the protective effect of estrogens on serum lipids appears to be lost with transdermal application, which is also more expensive than oral preparations.

Estrone, Estropipate (Piperazine Estrone Sulfate), Esterified Estrogens

CHEMISTRY. Estrone is a naturally occurring estrogen. Estropipate is estrone as the sulfate stabilized with piperazine. Esterified estrogens are a mixture of the sodium salts of the sulfate esters, principally estrone, of the type excreted in the urine of pregnant mares although they may also be prepared synthetically.

PHARMACOLOGY. Effects are similar to those of other natural and synthetic estrogens. On a weight basis, 1.5 mg of estropipate is approximately equivalent to 0.9 mg of estrone or 1.25 mg of estrone sodium sulfate.

USES. Estrone, estropipate, and esterified estrogens are used for the management of menopausal symptoms, atrophic vaginitis, female hypogonadism, and primary ovarian failure as with other estrogens. The usual cautions, precautions, and contraindications associated with estrogen therapy should be observed.

DOSAGE, ADMINISTRATION, AND PREPARATIONS. Estrone is administered intramuscularly; estropipate, orally or intravaginally; and esterified estrogens, orally. Dosage is individualized according to the condition treated and the tolerance and therapeutic response. Therapy is usually given cyclically, once daily for 3 weeks, followed by

1 week drug free. Addition of progestins for 7 or more days of each cycle is indicated if the uterus is present, to decrease the incidence of endometrial hyperplasia and neoplasia.

Estrone	For vasomotor symptoms or atrophic vaginitis, 0.1 to 0.5 mg is given 2 or 3 times weekly. For female hypogonadism, castration, or primary ovarian failure, 0.1 to 1.0 mg is given weekly in single or divided doses. Further dosage adjusted according to response.
Estropipate	For vasomotor symptoms or atrophic vaginitis, the dose is 0.75 to 6.0 mg daily, in a cyclic oral regimen. Alternatively, prescribe 2 to 4 gm of 0.15% vaginal cream once daily. For female hypogonadism, castration, or primary ovarian failure, 1.5 to 9.0 mg is given daily for 21 days, then 8 to 10 days are drug free, and then the cycle is repeated. The number of courses required to induce menstruation varies. An oral progestin may be given concomitantly during the third week of therapy.
Esterified estrogens	For vasomotor symptoms 0.3 to 1.25 mg is given daily in a cyclic regimen. The dosage may be increased to 2.5 or 3.75 mg daily if necessary. For atrophic vaginitis, the usual dose is 0.3 to 1.25 mg daily in a cyclic regimen. If breakthrough bleeding occurs, dosage should be increased as necessary. For female hypogonadism, castration, or ovarian failure, give 2.5 to 7.5 mg daily in divided doses, in a cyclic regimen. Oral progestin should be administered during the last 5 days. If menses begins before the regimen is completed, stop and restart on fifth menstrual day.

Available preparations are as follows:

Estrone	Parenteral. Suspension 2 mg/ml. Estrogenic substance (Ayerst), Estronol (Central), Theelin Aqueous (Parke-Davis). Suspension 5 mg/ml. Estrone 5 (Keene), Kestrone 5 (Hyrex).
Estropipate	Oral tablets 0.75 mg (equivalent estrone sodium sulfate, 0.625 mg). Ogen 0.625 Divide-Tab (Abbott). 1.5 mg (equivalent estrone sodium sulfate, 1.25 mg). Ogen 1.25 Divide-Tab (Abbott). Orapate, Major 3 mg. Ogen 2.5 Divide-Tab (Abbott). Vaginal cream. 0.15% Ogen (Abbott).
Esterified estrogens	Oral tablets. 0.3 mg, 0.625 mg, 1.25 mg, 2.5 mg. Estratab (Reid-Rowell), Menest (Beecham).

Conjugated Estrogens, U.S.P.

CHEMISTRY. This is a combination of the sodium salts of the sulfate esters of estrogenic substances. Preparations generally contain 50 to 65% estrone sodium sulfate and 20 to 35% equilin sodium sulfate. They are effective orally, parenterally, and vaginally. They may be prepared synthetically or from equine urine.

INDICATIONS, DOSAGE, AND PREPARATIONS. For menopausal symptoms or atrophic vaginitis, the usual oral dosage is 0.3 to 1.25 mg daily in a cyclic regimen; higher doses may be required. Generally given 3 weeks on, 1 week off, and repeated as necessary. If the woman still menstruates, the drug is started on the fifth day of the cycle. If the woman is amenorrheic, the drug is started arbitrarily. A progestin may be added the last 10 days. Alternatively, in atrophic vaginitis, 2 to 4 gm of cream may be administered once daily in the usual cyclic fashion.

For female hypogonadism, the usual oral dose is 2.5 to 7.5 mg daily in divided doses for 25 days each month. If menses does not occur, the course should be repeated. Once menses commences, an estrogen-progestin regimen should be initiated with an oral progestin during the last 10 days of estrogen therapy. In the management of castration, primary ovarian failure, and osteoporosis, the usual initial dose is 1.25 mg daily in a cyclic regimen. For dysfunctional uterine bleeding due to atrophic endometrium, administer 2.5 to 5.0 mg daily in divided doses for 1 week with a progestin added to the regimen (medroxyprogesterone acetate, 10 mg, or norethindrone acetate, 5 mg daily) the last 5 days. The patient should be ready for heavy, painful withdrawal bleeding following treatment for 1 to 3 days and should then be regulated with oral contraceptives or progestins. For emergency treatment of dysfunctional uterine bleeding with a denuded endometrium, administer 25 mg IV or IM for 3 doses; oral treatment is then initiated as above or with an oral contraceptive. Nonresponse to the hormonal therapy for dysfunctional uterine bleeding is an indication for curettage.

The following are available preparations:

Oral tablets: 0.3 mg, 0.625 mg, 0.9 mg, 1.25 mg, 2.5 mg; Premarin (Ayerst), Progens (Major).
Parenteral: Premarin IV, 25 mg (Ayerst).
Vaginal: Premarin, Cream 0.625 mg/gm in 42.5-gm containers (Ayerst).

Ethinyl Estradiol (Estinyl, Feminone)

CHEMISTRY. A semisynthetic estrogen, the ethinyl group prevents enzymatic degradation of the estradiol molecule and results in an orally active compound. It is used alone and as a component of some oral contraceptives. It is suggested that in ERT, 5 μg may be equivalent to 0.625 mg of conjugated estrogens with respect to bone and vaginal epithelial effects.

INDICATIONS AND DOSAGE. For menopausal symptoms, administer 0.02 to 0.05 mg daily, cyclically. A progestin may be added the last 10 days. As an initial dosage for severe symptoms, 0.05 mg twice daily may be used. Once clinical improvement has occurred, usually within a few weeks, dosage is reduced to the lowest possible effective maintenance dosage.

For replacement therapy in female hypogonadism, the usual dose is 0.05 mg 1 to 3 times daily during the first 2 weeks of the cycle, followed by concomitant administration of progestin during the last half of the projected cycle. Continue this regimen for 3 to 6 months. If spontaneous menses does not occur for 2 months thereafter, continue artificial cycling. For dysfunctional uterine bleeding 0.05 to 0.1 mg can be given with a progestin for 7 to 10 days; thereafter maintenance with an oral contraceptive or progestin alone can be instituted.

Nonsteroidal Estrogens

Chlorotrianisene—TACE (Merrell Dow)

PHARMACOLOGY. Chlorotrianisene is a synthetic, orally active derivative of DES with weak estrogenic properties, stored in fat tissues resulting in slow onset and prolonged duration of action. TACE is a proestrogen, and estrogenic activity has been found in adipose tissue up to 1 month after cessation of therapy. The long duration of therapy makes TACE unsuitable for the treatment of menstrual disorders and for replacement when cyclic therapy is desired. The drug is used most frequently in the palliative treatment of prostatic carcinoma. TACE capsules contain the dye tartrazine to which some individuals, especially those who are sensitive to aspirin, may evidence allergic reactions.

DOSAGE. Capsules contain 12 mg, 25 mg, or 72 mg of chlorotrianisene. Dose for menopausal symptoms and replacement therapy is 12 to 25 mg daily in a cyclic regimen. A progestin may be added the last 10 days.

Dienestrol

PHARMACOLOGY. Dienestrol is related chemically to DES. It is administered intravaginally as a cream primarily in the treatment of atrophic vaginitis. Since it may be absorbed through the vaginal mucosa, breast tenderness, vaginal hypersecretion, and uterine bleeding may be induced with excessive dosage.

DOSAGE AND PREPARATION. Initial dosage is 6 or 12 gm daily for 1 to 2 weeks, then alternate days for a further 1 to 2 weeks. After restoration of vaginal mucosa, a maintenance dose of 6 gm (1 applicator full) 1 to 3 times weekly may be used. Attempts to reduce dosage should be made at 3- to 6-month intervals. If bleeding occurs, estrogen-induced bleeding must be confirmed by excluding endometrial cancer with endometrial biopsy or curettage. A progestin may be added if necessary as with oral estrogen.

The preparation is a vaginal cream: (1) DV (Merrell Dow), cream 0.01% in 90-gm container; (2) Estraguard, (Reid-Rowell); (3) Ortho Dienestrol (Ortho).

Diethylstilbestrol—DES, Stilbestrol (Lilly), Diethylstilbestrol Diphosphate—Stilphostrol (Miles)

CHEMISTRY. These are the most potent nonsteroidal estrogens; they are active orally, topically, and intravenously. They are inactivated slowly so even if large amounts are required, it can be given in single daily doses. One milligram of DES is equivalent to 1.6 mg of diethylstilbestrol diphosphate. The drug is rapidly absorbed, slowly inactivated in the liver, and excreted in urine and feces as the glucuronide.

PHARMACOLOGY AND PREPARATIONS. Both nausea and pigmentation appear to be more frequent with DES treatment than with some other estrogen preparations. As with all estrogens it is contraindicated in pregnant women, especially during the first 16 weeks, for vaginal adenosis has occurred in 30 to 90% of postpubertal females whose mothers received DES or similar medications during pregnancy. Rare cases of clear cell vaginal adenocarcinoma have also been reported in this group. Epididymal cysts and infertility have been reported in the male offspring. These patients should therefore be closely followed by physicians who are knowledgeable in regard to DES-induced adverse effects. At one time DES was used as a postcoital contraceptive administered within 72 hours after unprotected intercourse in an effort to inhibit nidation. This use has declined in view of the potential adverse effects should pregnancy continue and because simpler techniques are now available.

The usual dose of DES for menopausal symptoms or replacement therapy is 0.2 to 0.5 mg daily for 21 days followed by 7 days without medication. Adding a progestin for the last 10 days of therapy decreased the incidence of endometrial hyperplasia. Up to 2.0 mg daily may be needed in the initial therapy of atrophic vaginitis. As a postcoital contraceptive, oral DES is given 25.0 mg twice daily for 5 days, preferably commenced within 24 hours after coitus.

For intravenous infusion, the dose of diethylstilbestrol diphosphate sodium should be diluted in 300 ml of D_5W or normal saline solution and given slowly such that the entire dose is given over 1 hour.

For the vaginal route for replacement therapy, maximum dose is 7 mg weekly.

Available preparations are as follows:

DES	Tablets, 1-mg, 5-mg Diethylstilbestrol tablets (Lilly).
	Tablets enteric coated, 0.1-mg, 1.0-mg, 5.0-mg Diethylstilbestrol Enseals (Lilly).
	Topical (vaginal) suppositories, 0.1 and 0.5 mg, generic.
Diethylstilbestrol diphosphate	Tablets, 50 mg Stilphostrol (Miles).
Diethylstilbestrol diphosphate sodium	Parenteral injection, 50 mg/ml, Stilphostrol (Miles).

Quinestrol—Estrovis (Parke-Davis)

PHARMACOLOGY. This drug is a synthetic derivative of ethinyl estradiol. After gastrointestinal absorption it is stored in adipose tissue and slowly released such that once weekly administration is possible after an initial priming regimen. There are no data on the effect of concurrent progestin therapy to avoid endometrial hyperstimulation in view of the depot nature of the drug.

DOSAGE AND PREPARATION. For oral replacement therapy, 100 μg is given once daily for 7 days, followed by 100 μg weekly beginning 2 weeks after therapy is started.

Estrovis (Parke-Davis), tablets, 100 μg.

Estrogens Combined with Other Drugs

Estrogens and Androgens

Prolonged androgen administration may cause masculinization and so should be avoided. In small doses and for short-term administration, the combination may decrease estrogenic breast and endometrial stimulation and may enhance libido in postmenopausal women. This use is empirical and the use of fixed-dose combinations should not be encouraged. There is also no evidence that the combination relieves or delays any of the symptoms related to aging. Combination therapy has also been used for suppression of postpartum lactation, but this use has been largely replaced by bromocriptine (Parlodel).

The following are available oral preparations:

Estratest Oral Tablets (Reid-Rowell): Esterified estrogens, 1.25 mg; methyltestosterone, 2.5 mg.
Estratest H.S. (half-strength): Esterified estrogens, 0.625 mg; methyltestosterone, 1.25 mg.
Premarin with methyltestosterone (Ayerst).
Conjugated estrogens, 0.625 mg or 1.25 mg, and methyltestosterone, 5 or 10 mg. Halodrin (Upjohn).
Ethinyl estradiol, 0.02 mg, with fluoxymesetrone, 1 mg.
DES combinations, Tylosterone (Lilly).
DES, 0.25 mg, with methyltestosterone, 5 mg.

The following are parenteral preparations:

Estradiol valerate combinations in oil: 4 mg/ml with testosterone enanthate, 90 mg/ml.—Androgyn L.A. (Forest), Deladumone (Squibb), Estra-Testrin (Pasadena), Teev (Keene), Testaval 90/4 (Legere), Valertest No. 1 (Hyrex); 8 mg/ml with testosterone enanthate, 180 mg/ml—Deladumone OB (Squibb) (lactation suppression), Valertest No. 2 (Hyrex).
Estradiol cypionate combinations in oil: 2 mg/ml with testosterone cypionate 50 mg/ml—Andro/Fem (Pasadena), depAndrogyn (Forest), Depo-Testadiol (Upjohn), Depotestogen (Hyrex), Duo-Cyp (Keene), Duratestrin (Hauck), Menoject-LA (Mayrand), T-E-Cypionate (Legere).

Estrogens with Anxiolytics

Combinations of estrogens with antianxiety agents are used by some when anxiety at perimenopause or menopause has persisted following relief of vasomotor and vaginal symptoms with estrogen therapy. However, most would prefer to administer the components separately. The mixture should be suitable in terms of quality and quantity of each constituent for the individual patient and should be used for a limited period only.

Available preparations are as follows:

Menrium (Roche). Tablet, esterified estrogens, 0.2 or 0.4 mg, and chlordiazepoxide, 5 mg, or esterified estrogens, 0.4 mg, and chlordiazepoxide, 10 mg.
Milprem (Wallace). Tablet, conjugated estrogens, 0.45 mg, and meprobomate, 200 or 400 mg.

PROTOCOLS

For estrogen replacement therapy in the menopause (with or without uterus present) administer conjugated estrogens (Premarin, Ayerst) 0.625 to 1.25 mg for days 1 to 25 each month. Medroxyprogesterone acetate (Provera, Upjohn) is also given 5 to 10 mg daily on days 16 to 25. (Many physicians do not give a progestin if the uterus has been surgically removed.) In addition advise the patient to exercise 10 to 30 minutes daily 3 to 4 times per week, and to take a calcium supplement, 1000 mg daily (5 "Tums" per day). The duration of therapy is indefinite.

For intravenous emergency treatment of dysfunctional uterine bleeding, administer conjugated estrogens (Premarin, Ayerst), 25 mg every 6 hours until the bleeding stops. Then give Premarin, 2.5 mg daily, with Provera, 10 mg daily, for 7 days. After withdrawal bleed, continue therapy with a combination oral contraceptive. In addition correct the anemia. Dilatation and curettage is necessary if medical therapy is unsuccessful.

For Asherman's syndrome, endometrial regeneration following hysteroscopic division of intrauterine adhesions and placement of an intrauterine device for 1 month is aided by the following hormonal schedule for 3 months: Premarin, 2.5 mg, for 3 weeks, and Provera, 10 mg daily, for last 10 days of Premarin course.

Standard replacement therapy for Turner's syndrome entails the problem of a biphasic estrogen effect on bone, with an initial growth stimulation followed by early epiphyseal closure. Replacement at puberty, therefore, should employ low doses with a gradual increase thereafter.

BIBLIOGRAPHY

Reviews

American Medical Association Department of Drugs, Division of Drugs and Technology. *Drug Evaluations* (6th ed.). Philadelphia: W. B. Saunders, 1986. Chap. 39 Pp. 689–705.

Estrogen Replacement Therapy Symposium. *Obstet. Gynecol.* 72 [Suppl.], 1988.

Knoben, J. E., and Anderson, P. O. *Handbook of Clinical Drug Data* (5th ed.). Hamilton, IL: Hamilton Press, 1983. Sec. 68, Pp. 570–576.

McEvoy, G. K. Estrogens. *American Hospital Formulary Service: Drug Information.* American Society of Hospital Pharmacists. 68:1751, 1988.

Pharmacology

DeLignieres, B., et al. Biological effects of estradiol-17 beta in postmenopausal women: oral versus percutaneous administration. *J. Clin. Endocrinol. Metab.* 62:536, 1986.

Gorski, J., et al. Evolution of a model of estrogen action. *Recent Prog. Horm. Res.* 42:297, 1986.

Jensen, J., et al. Long-term effects of percutaneous estrogens and oral progesterone on serum lipoproteins in postmenopausal women. *Am. J. Obstet. Gynecol.* 156:66, 1987.

Padwick, M. W., Pryse-Davies, J., and Whitehead, M. I. A simple method for determining the optimal dosage of progestin in post-menopausal women receiving estrogens. *N. Engl. J. Med.* 315:930, 1986.

Powers, M. S., et al. Pharmacokinetics and pharmacodynamics of transdermal dosage forms of 17β-estradiol: comparison with conventional oral estrogens used for hormone replacement. *Am. J. Obstet. Gynecol.* 152:1099, 1985.

Administration

Berger, H. G., et al. The management of persistent menopausal symptoms with oestradiol-testosterone implants: clinical lipid and hormonal results. *Maturitas* 6:351, 1984.

Burnier, A. M., et al. Sublingual absorption of micronized 17β-estradiol. *Am. J. Obstet. Gynecol.* 140:147, 1981.
Jensen, J., et al. Continuous oestrogen-progestogen treatment and serum lipoproteins in postmenopausal women. *Br. J. Obstet. Gynaecol.* 94:130, 1987.
Magos, A. L., et al. Amenorrhea and endometrial atrophy with continuous oral estrogen and progestogen therapy in postmenopausal women. *Obstet. Gynecol.* 65:496, 1985.
Mattson, L., Cullberg, G., and Samsioe, G. A continuous estrogen-progestogen regimen for climacteric complaints. *Acta Obstet. Gynecol. Scand.* 63:673, 1984.
Place, V. A., et al. Double-blind comparative study of Estraderm and Premarin in amelioration of postmenopausal symptoms. *Am. J. Obstet. Gynecol.* 152:1092, 1985.

Osteoporosis

Aloia, J. F. Estrogen and exercise prevention and treatment of osteoporosis. *Geriatrics* 37:81, 1982.
Consensus Development Conference. Prophylaxis and treatment of osteoporosis. *Br. Med. J.* 295:914, 1987.
Ettinger, B., Genant, H. K., and Cann, C. E. Long-term estrogen replacement therapy prevents bone loss and fractures. *Ann. Intern. Med.* 102:319, 1985.
Ettinger, B., Genant, H. K., and Cann, C. E. Postmenopausal bone loss is prevented by treatment with low-dosage estrogen with calcium. *Ann. Intern. Med.* 106:40, 1987.
Hillner, B. E., Hollenberg, J. P., and Pauker, S. G. Postmenopausal estrogens in prevention of osteoporosis. Benefit virtually without risk if cardiovascular effects are considered. *Am. J. Med.* 80:1115, 1986.
Lindsey, R., Hart, D. M., and Clark, D. M. The minimum effective dose of estrogen for prevention of postmenopausal bone loss. *Obstet. Gynecol.* 63:759, 1984.
Riis, B., Thomsen, K., and Christiansen, C. Does calcium supplementation prevent postmenopausal bone loss. A double-blind, controlled study. *N. Engl. J. Med.* 316:173, 1987.

Cardiovascular Effects

Centerwall, B. S. Premenopausal hysterectomy and cardiovascular disease. *Am. J. Obstet. Gynecol.* 139:58, 1981.
Henderson, B. E., et al. Estrogen replacement therapy and protection from acute myocardial infarction. *Am. J. Obstet. Gynecol.* 159:312, 1988.
Ross, R. K., et al. Estrogen Use and Cardiovascular Disease. In D. R. Mishell (ed.). *Menopause: Physiology and Pharmacology*. Chicago: Year Book Medical, 1986.
Sullivan, J. M., et al. Postmenopausal estrogen use and coronary atherosclerosis. *Ann. Intern. Med.* 108:358, 1988.

Genital Effects

Hilton, P., and Stanton, S. L. The use of intravaginal oestrogen cream in genuine stress incontinence. *Br. J. Obstet. Gynaecol.* 90:940, 1983.
Rud, T. The effect of estrogens and gestagens on the urethral pressure profile in urinary continent and stress incontinent women. *Acta Obstet. Gynecol. Scand.* 59:265, 1980.
Semmens, J. P., and Wagner, G. Estrogen deprivation and vaginal function in postmenopausal women. *J.A.M.A.* 248:445, 1982.

Sherwin, B. B., and Gelfand, M. M. The role of androgen in the maintenance of sexual function in oophorectomized women. *Psychosom. Med.* 49:397, 1987.

Neoplasia

Gambrell, R. D., Bagnell, C. A., and Greenblatt, R. B. Role of estrogens and progesterone in the etiology and prevention of endometrial cancer: a review. *Am. J. Obstet. Gynecol.* 146:696, 1983.

Hammond, C. B., et al. Effects of long-term estrogen replacement therapy. II. Neoplasia. *Am. J. Obstet. Gynecol.* 133:537, 1979.

Nachtigall, L. E., et al. Estrogen replacement therapy. II: A prospective study in the relationship to carcinoma and cardiovascular and metabolic problems. *Obstet. Gynecol.* 54:74, 1979.

Wingo, P. A., et al. The risk of breast cancer in postmenopausal women who have used estrogen replacement therapy. *J.A.M.A.* 257:209, 1987.

Diethylstilbestrol

Leary, F. J., et al. Males exposed in utero to diethylstilbestrol. *J.A.M.A.* 252:2984, 1984.

Robboy, S. J., et al. Pathologic findings in young women enrolled in National Cooperative Diethylstilbestrol Adenosis (DESAD) Project. *Obstet. Gynecol.* 53:309, 1979.

Veridiano, N. P., et al. Delayed onset of clear cell adenocarcinoma of vagina in DES-exposed progeny. *Obstet. Gynecol.* 57:395, 1981.

Other Indications

Biomback, M., et al. Estrogen treatment of tall girls: risk of thrombosis. *Pediatrics* 72:416, 1983.

Ross, J. L., et al. Preliminary study of effect of estrogen dose on growth in Turner's syndrome. *N. Engl. J. Med.* 309:1104, 1983.

Strickler, R. C. Dysfunctional uterine bleeding in ovulatory women. *Postgrad. Med.* 77:235, 1985.

3

Progesterone and Progestins

George Rodney Meeks

Progesterone, also known as corpus luteum hormone, was isolated independently by Corner and Allen and four other groups of researchers in 1934. For some years after its discovery the small amounts of hormone available hampered experimental work and therapeutic applications. The first pure progesterone required processing the ovaries of 50,000 sows. While it can be extracted from animal ovaries, progesterone is now usually prepared synthetically from stigmasterol or diosgenin which is extracted from *Dioscorea mexicana,* a Mexican yam.

Progesterone is rapidly metabolized when given orally in pure form. In the early 1950s, progesterone was chemically modified to enhance its oral effectiveness and prolong its duration of action. These oral alternatives are known as progestogens or progestins and share actions of progesterone. As with other steroid hormones, progesterone and progestins may alter protein, carbohydrate, and lipid metabolism and influence fluid and electrolyte balance.

PHYSIOLOGY

This 21-carbon sex steroid is secreted mainly by the ovulatory ovary, although secretion actually begins just prior to ovulation by the dominant follicle. Progesterone is secreted in small amounts by the adrenal cortex and testes, and progesterone concentrations in preovulatory females are roughly equal to those in males. The placenta produces huge amounts of progesterone to support the fetus.

Progesterone modifies the effect of estrogen on tissues to control growth, development, and physiology of the reproductive tract and other organs such as the breast. Estrogen-induced endometrial proliferation is inhibited by progesterone and proliferative endometrium and is then converted to a secretory type. In the presence of estrogen, withdrawal of progesterone leads to endometrial bleeding. Progesterone stimulates decidua formation in the endometrium, prepares the endometrium for nidation, and maintains pregnancy, at least in part by smooth muscle relaxation. Progesterone increases basal body temperature (thermogenic effect), inhibits pituitary production of follicle-stimulating hormone (FSH) and luteinizing hormone (LH), and produces characteristic histologic changes in vaginal epithelium. Cervical mucus is converted from a thin, clear, watery consistency to a thick, opaque, tenacious consistency. This change alters the penetrability of sperm. In high doses, progesterone inhibits ovulation. Progesterone stimulates the growth of mammary alveolar tissue and has anesthetic properties when administered in high doses or intrathecally.

PHARMACOLOGY

A variety of preparations are now available for oral, parenteral, subdermal, and vaginal administration. Natural progesterone can be administered parenterally and is absorbed by mucous membranes of the mouth, vagina, and rectum. Progesterone is inactivated by the liver and has not been given orally in the past. Recent developments including micronization have improved the activity of orally administered progesterone. The addition of a 17α-ethinyl group to progesterone enhances oral activity by slowing metabolism in the liver. All synthetic progestins are steroidal.

Progesterone demonstrates minimal estrogenic and androgenic activity. Pregnanediol, the main metabolite, is produced in the liver and also is conjugated with glucuronic acid. Urine is the predominant route of excretion. Plasma half-life is only several minutes.

Because orally administered progesterone is rapidly metabolized and because intramuscular injection sometimes produced pain and local reactions, orally active compounds were developed. These compounds are the progestins. The synthesis of progestins was directed at producing compounds that are orally active, more potent, more specific in action, and longer in duration of action. In varying degrees the progestins share the pharmacologic actions of progesterone. They may also demonstrate androgenic, estrogenic, anabolic, mineralocorticoid, and even antiprogestational activity.

Synthetic progestins are derived from two general classes of compounds—pregnanes and estranes. The addition of an ethinyl group at the 17 position of progesterone bestows oral activity by reducing the metabolic clearance rate of these compounds in the liver. Ethisterone was the first progestin to be synthesized but is no longer available. Substitutions and deletions of chemical radicals at various positions produce compounds with interesting structural and pharmacologic properties. Common changes are produced at the 19, 17, and 6 positions. Removing a methyl group at position 19 (19-nor derivatives) produces compounds that demonstrate both estrogenic and androgenic activity. Anabolic side effects including nitrogen retention and weight gain are common. The 17-acetyloxy derivatives elicit responses almost identical to progesterone, and demonstrate little androgenic or estrogenic activity. Catabolic effects are minimal and a slight diuretic effect may be produced. The 19-nor derivatives are more effective in postponing the onset of a normal menstrual cycle. Substitution, especially of methyl groups, at the 6 position increases potency.

Five synthetic progestins are found in oral contraceptives. These are members of the estrane family and are 19-nor progestins. Norethindrone acetate, norethynodrel, and ethynodiol diacetate are converted to norethindrone (norethisterone) in vivo. Norgestrel differs from norethindrone only by the substitution of an ethyl group at position 13. This allows a stereo isomer but only levonorgestrel is active.

Medroxyprogesterone acetate (MPA) and hydroxyprogesterone are compounds with substitutions at the 17 position. Both are suitable for injection, and MPA is also active orally. Other compounds, such as danazol, gestrinone (R2323), and RU-486 may have pronounced antiprogesterone effects.

Tests of potency in humans are difficult to assess because compounds may have estrogen and androgen activity. In rabbits potency is assessed by the Clauberg test. Immature female rabbits are primed with estrogen for 6 days and receive a test progestin for 5 days. The uterus is then evaluated by histologic grading. Norgestrel is the most potent based on results of the Clauberg test, but this may not be true in all species. Attempts to correlate potency in women based on delay of menses and histologic evaluation of endometrial glycogen are difficult. This is because the studies addressing this issue have utilized different estrogen dosage regimens prior to the administration of a test progestin.

INDICATIONS

Dysfunctional uterine bleeding is most commonly due to unopposed estrogen effect on the endometrium. This allows the endometrium to outgrow its hormone support. Also, the corpus luteum may produce progesterone for too short a time or in too low a concentration. Therefore, the endometrium never becomes secretory or fails to undergo uniform secretory conversion. The endometrium does not simultaneously slough to produce withdrawal bleeding, but bleeds irregularly and often heavily. Administration of progesterone or progestin can produce a secretory endometrium and discontinuing therapy will produce uniform withdrawal bleeding. If active bleeding is present, progesterone may stabilize the endometrium and thereby stop bleeding. However, if the bleeding has been present for many days, the remaining endometrium may not respond to progesterone alone.

Amenorrhea may be primary or secondary and is most commonly the result of anovulation. Administration of progestin allows one to determine if estrogen is present or not. Withdrawal bleeding will occur if estrogen is present. Failure to withdraw mandates further evaluation of this sometimes complex problem.

Cessation of menses, vaginal dryness, and hot flashes herald menopause. Estrogen therapy alleviates these symptoms. Hot flashes also can be relieved by progestin therapy. Those women who receive estrogen therapy should receive a progestational compound to protect against endometrial hyperstimulation. Progestins may also help prevent osteoporosis by competing with cortisol receptors. The relationship of progestin therapy to the incidence of breast cancer has not been fully elucidated and continues to stir controversy. All progestins may have an adverse effect on serum lipids by lowering high-density lipoprotein (HDL) concentration, thus estrogen's beneficial effect of increasing HDL concentration may be negated.

Synthetic progestins have contraceptive effects, and this characteristic has allowed oral contraceptives to be developed. Combination (estrogen and progestin) oral contraceptive pills prevent pregnancy by inhibiting ovulation and changing the characteristics of the reproductive tract, which prevents implantation or growth of the blastocyst. Progestin-only oral contraceptives (minipill) are much less effective than combination pills. Progestins can be impregnated into intrauterine devices (IUDs). The progestin enhances contraceptive efficacy and also reduces the menstrual blood loss that would otherwise be increased by IUD use. Progestin may be administered parenterally in depot form, intramuscularly, or as a subdermal implant for contraceptive purposes. Some progestational agents are so weak they function as antiprogestins. Others, while having a formula of progestins, are physiologically antiprogestins. These compounds may interfere with the effect of progesterone to the point of producing abortion.

One cause of habitual abortion is luteal phase defect (too little progesterone). In those women who have habitual abortion secondary to reduced progesterone levels, supplementation may prevent abortion. It will not alleviate other causes of spontaneous abortions and may even prevent spontaneous abortion of a blighted ovum. Therapy should begin as soon as these women suspect pregnancy and continue until approximately 10 to 14 weeks in gestation when the placenta is capable of producing adequate progesterone.

Premenstrual syndrome (PMS) is a poorly defined syndrome that is associated with the premenstrual phase of an ovulatory cycle. Symptoms may range from mild physical symptoms to severe psychiatric disturbance. Commonly, abdominal bloating, breast soreness, food cravings, emotional lability, depression, a sense of being out of control, a sense of not being able to cope, and a sense of not being able to think are presenting symptoms. One accepted theory is that a hormonal imbalance produces symptoms. Therapy is directed at correcting a hormonal imbalance, which some believe is due to insufficient progesterone levels. This can be treated by administration of natural progesterone. Almost always this is administered vaginally. Classically, progesterone is compounded in a glycerin base suppository that melts in the vagina or rectum. An oral troche is also available. Other therapies are available and have varying degrees of success.

Endometriosis is estrogen dependent. Because of the reduced estrogen effect produced when progestins are administered, endometriosis often regresses. Also, oral contraceptive pills may be effective in suppressing endometriosis. Very weak progestins or antiprogestins (such as danazol) may suppress symptoms.

Hirsutism is secondary to an excess of androgen or from an increased response at the end organ (i.e., hair follicle). Most commonly, excess androgen is produced by the ovary as part of a syndrome such as polycystic ovarian syndrome. Progestins are capable of suppressing ovarian function, although suppression is more complete with combination estrogen and progesterone therapy. Progestins may also compete for androgen-binding sites and therefore interfere with androgenic effect on the hair follicle. One must be cautious to avoid those progestins with an androgenic effect that may worsen the problem.

Because sexual drive and fantasy seem to be related to androgen production, progestin therapy may lower sexual feelings. This is likely mediated by suppression of LH, which in turn lowers androgen production in both men and women. Progestins have therefore been used to manage various sexual paraphilias, including homosexual, heterosexual, or bisexual pedophilia; voyeurism; sexual sadism; exhibitionism; and transvestism. Progestins have been advocated as a form of medical castration in men who have repetitively committed rape or other sociopathic forms of sexual expression.

One characteristic of progestins is to increase pulmonary minute ventilation. This property has lead to its use in patients with various hypoventilation syndromes, such as obesity-hypoventilation syndrome (pickwickian syndrome), and more recently in patients with sleep apnea. It should ordinarily be used as adjunctive therapy.

Precocious sexual development often has no specific cause, but seems to be related to elevation of LH levels. Progestins inhibit LH and therefore may suppress further sexual development. Newer drugs including analogues of gonadotropin-releasing hormone (GnRH) have proved to be more effective in managing this problem and have largely replaced progestin therapy.

MPA may have some benefit in sickle-cell disease. In vitro studies show less tendency for red corpuscles with hemoglobin S to sickle, while patient studies show increased red blood cell mass, decreased irreversible sickling, and shorter duration of pain during crisis.

Therefore, there may be a direct benefit to patients with sickle-cell disease when they receive MPA. Because depo-medroxprogesterone acetate (DMPA) may also function as a contraceptive, this may be an appropriate choice for these individuals.

Vulvar dystrophies may respond to topical progesterone applied in gel form. Symptoms of itching and burning may be relieved while the side effects of topical testosterone including clitoral hypertrophy and hypertrichosis are avoided. Patients in whom progesterone therapy fails remain candidates for testosterone therapy.

ADVERSE EFFECTS, CONTRAINDICATIONS, MUTAGENICITY, AND CARCINOGENICITY

Progesterone shares the toxic potentials of other progestins. Because oral contraceptive combination pills contain progestins, the precautions associated with oral contraceptive pills should generally be extended to patients receiving progestins. Patients receiving progesterone or progestin therapy must be thoroughly evaluated before any therapy is prescribed. A general history should be obtained with specific regard to the internal and external genitalia and breasts. These steroids may impact on carbohydrate, lipid, and protein metabolism as well as modify fluid and electrolyte balance. Therefore the history regarding these potential problems must be obtained. Physical examination with emphasis on the pelvis and breasts should be directed at finding contraindications to therapy. A Papanicolaou smear (Pap test) should be obtained. Many would recommend an evaluation of liver function because of the known impact of oral sex steroids on liver function.

Progesterone and progestin may be associated with disturbance of the menstrual cycle. While these agents are commonly used to induce cyclic bleeding, in those women with regular cycles, an increased incidence of breakthough bleeding, changes in the quantity of menstrual flow, and onset of amenorrhea may occur. Therapy changes the consistency of cervical secretions to a tenacious, sticky material and vaginal secretions may be decreased. Edema often associated with weight gain may be seen. Changes in skin pigment including melasma and chloasma, rashes, and pruritus have been reported. Very rarely, allergic-type reactions associated with tight chest, dyspnea, cough, and other allergic manifestations have occurred.

Cardiovascular changes have the most immediate impact. Some individuals are susceptible to elevation of blood pressure, which may be secondary to the aldosterone effect of these compounds. Thrombophlebitis, pulmonary embolus, cerebral thrombosis, and cerebral embolism have an increased incidence in women taking oral contraceptives. Blood clotting factors VII, VIII, IX, and X are also elevated in users of oral contraceptive pills. Whether or not these are associated with progesterone and progestins alone is not well documented, but certainly the possibility of thromboembolic disorders must be considered.

Other documented side effects include premenstrual-like syndrome, changes in libido and appetite, fatigue, and loss of scalp hair. Asthma, seizures, migraine headaches, cardiac dysfunction, and renal dysfunction may be aggravated by progestogen therapy because of its fluid retention properties. Patients with a history of depression should be observed closely for recurrence. If significant symptoms recur, the progestin should be discontinued.

Progestins have been associated with the occurrence of mammary nodules in beagle dogs. Some of these were malignant. Relevance of these findings in humans has not been established. One study in black women reported no increase in risk of breast, uterine, or ovarian cancer associated with progestin therapy.

Progestins have been advocated in therapy of first-trimester recurrent (habitual) abortion. No well-controlled studies are available to support such treatment. Therapy may delay spontaneous abortion of a blighted ovum. Potential adverse reactions may occur in the first 4 months. Masculinization, clitoral hypertrophy, cardiac defects, and smaller limbs have been documented in infants whose mothers received progestins during early pregnancy. Progestins have been administered to women with amenorrhea as a test of pregnancy. In light of the data just mentioned this practice should be abandoned. In those women receiving therapy for suspected luteal phase defect as a cause of recurrent abortion, only natural progesterone should be utilized. Progesterone has been administered to stop preterm labor in the third trimester and no complications have been documented. Progestins are distributed in breast milk of lactating women and progestin effects may be seen in the infant. Additionally, progestins may alter the chemical constituency of breast milk, thereby changing its nutrient values.

LABORATORY INTERFERENCE AND DRUG INTERACTIONS

Some laboratory tests are potentially altered by use of progestin. Hepatic microsomal enzyme induction occurs secondary to both estrogen and progestin. This may be similar in mechanism to other known liver inducers. Because of the risk of contraceptive failures when other enzyme inducers are taken, one must consider additional contraceptive measures. Antibiotics that reduce the intestinal flora may reduce the enterohepatic circulation of drugs; thus, a higher dose of drugs may be required to produce a desired effect. One may see breakthrough bleeding for instance. Oral contraceptive pills may block metabolism of some drugs or in some way enhance effectiveness. Oral contraceptive pills delay oxidative metabolism of benzodiazepines, while at the same time enhance glucuronide metabolism. First-pass metabolism may also be decreased for beta-adrenergic blockers and a decreased dose of these drugs may be needed for the desired therapeutic effect. A similar enhancement may be seen with corticosteroids. Manufacturers caution that analgesics, isoniazid, antimigraine compounds, and minor tranquilizers may lower the efficacy of oral contraceptive pills. The effects of oral anticoagulants, anticonvulsants, hypotensive agents (guanethidine), vitamins, and antidiabetic agents may be significantly altered.

Metyrapone tests show a diminished response. This seems to be a specific interaction since the adrenals still respond to corticotropin. Altered results on liver function tests may be present. Tests using sulfobromophthalein show increased retention. Less frequently, levels of transaminases and alkaline phosphatase are elevated.

Decreased glucose tolerance occurs in a significant number of women. Both prediabetic and diabetic women must be monitored for elevations of glucose levels. Progesterone and progestins decrease HDL cholesterol concentrations. The amount of decrease varies with each compound. Thyroid test results may be misinterpreted in patients receiving therapy. Thyroid-binding globulin (TBG) is increased, thereby increasing total circulating thyroid hormone as measured by protein-bound iodine (PBI), thyroxine (T_4), and butanol-extractable iodine. Decreased triiodothyronine (T_3) resin uptake reflecting elevated levels of TBG occurs, while free T_4 is unaltered. Basal metabolic rate, uptake of iodine 131, and free T_4 index remain unchanged, indicating that thyroid function is not changed.

Variable effects on immunoglobulins have been reported. Levels of cholinesterase and haptoglobulins decrease. Transferrin, plasminogen, α_2-macroglobulin, testosterone-binding globulin, and estradiol-binding globulin (sex steroid–binding globulin) levels are increased. Cryofibrinogenemia also has been reported. Pregnanediol excretion may be reduced. Renin substrate is increased and aldosterone excretion rate is elevated. Serum magnesium, copper, zinc, and iron concentrations may be increased, but clinical significance has not yet been determined. Folate deficiency may occur, possibly by interfering with absorption of dietary intake. Reduced cyanocobalamin (vitamin B_{12}) and pyridoxine (vitamin B_6) absorption occurs but seems to have minimal impact.

PREPARATIONS

This list of progestational agents is not inclusive. It does give representative compounds as well as compounds used in clinical practice. For very specific therapies, other specific compounds may be appropriate.

Progesterone

Injection—Gesterol "50" in Oil (Forest), Progestaject-50 in Oil (Mayrand)

These compounds are generally available in concentrations of 25 to 100 mg/ml and are commonly supplied in vegetable oil. Progesterone is unique among the steroids in that local irritation is produced at the site of injection, and no more than 100 mg can be given in a single injection. Aqueous sterile suspensions are particularly painful and are no longer commercially available.

Powder—Micronized or Microcrystalline for Compounding (Millgood, Paddock, Pharma-Tek, Upjohn); Capsules—Progestoral (Delk Pharmaceutical)

Progesterone powder may be compounded in a suppository for vaginal or rectal administration. Absorption seems to be equal from both mucosal epithelial surfaces. Vaginal administration may worsen candidiasis and rectal administration is contraindicated in patients who have colitis. It may also be compounded as a troche for buccal or sublingual administration. These products are not commercially available. They must be compounded by a pharmacist. Progesterone concentration varies from 25 to 400 mg.

Oral administration of progesterone has had limited utility in the past because of rapid inactivation. Recently, micronized progesterone with mean diameter of particle size being 11 microns has been shown to provide sustained serum progesterone concentrations. Originally, plain gelatin capsules were used as the administration vehicle, but dissolving micronized progesterone in oil enhances its availability. Progestoral is the only commercially available preparation. It is supplied in 100-mg, 75-mg, 50-mg, and 25-mg concentrations. Progestoral may be administered up to 4 times daily.

Serum progesterone concentration peaks at 6 hours and remains above baseline for 24 hours after oral administration.

Intrauterine Contraceptive Device

The Projestasert IUD (Alza) is impregnated with 38 mg of progesterone. Progesterone enhances the contraceptive effect of the inert IUD itself. The IUD must be replaced yearly when the medication is fully absorbed.

Hydroxyprogesterone Caproate (Hexanoate)—Delalutin (Squibb), Duralutin (Hauck)

17α-hydroxyprogesterone is a natural weak progestin isolated originally from the adrenal gland. When esterified with caproate at the 17 position, it has substantial progestational effects and prolonged duration of action. It must be administered deep intramuscularly. It is supplied in 125-mg and 250-mg/ml concentrations in a castor oil and benzyl alcohol vehicle. Because the duration of action is 7 to 14 days and because it is more potent than progesterone, therapy is indicated when longer duration is needed or when an inadequate response is seen to progesterone.

Medroxyprogesterone Acetate (Acetyloxymethylprogesterone)

Oral—Provera (Upjohn), Amen (Carnrick), Curretab (Reid-Rowell), Cycrin (Ayerst)

MPA is a derivative of 17α-hydroxy-progesterone with the addition of a 6α-methyl group and 17α-acetate group. The compound is active both orally and intramuscularly.

Oral tablets are supplied in 2.5-mg, 5.0-mg, and 10.0-mg strengths by Upjohn. Nonproprietary 10-mg tablets are also available. The drugs are indicated when progesterone effect is needed and oral administration is preferred. While all progestins affect the lipid profile, MPA seems to have the least adverse effect. It may therefore be appropriate for long-term use in hope of reducing potential consequences of lower HDL cholesterol levels.

Injectable—Depo-Provera (Upjohn)

Intramuscular solutions are formulated for sustained release. Because of the insoluble nature of MPA and because the rate of metabolism varies from individual to individual, duration of 90 days is not uncommon and the duration of effect may last much longer than anticipated. Indications include those conditions where prolonged effect and infrequent therapy are desired. This compound should be used cautiously in those individuals desiring additional fertility. While this product is available for contraception outside the United States, it is not currently approved for contraception in the United States. Concentrations of 100 mg/ml and 400 mg/ml are available. It must be vigorously shaken to ensure complete suspension before injection.

Norethindrone (Norethisterone)—Aygestin (Ayerst), Norlutate (Parke-Davis); Norethindrone Acetate (Norethisterone Acetate)—Norlutin (Parke-Davis), Micronor (Ortho)

This is the 17α-ethinyl derivative of 19-nortestosterone. Norethindrone acetate, the acetic acid ester of the parent compound, is roughly twice as potent. It has estrogenic, androgenic, and anabolic activity. The equivalent dose of norethindrone is twice that of norethindrone acetate. Both are administered orally. Norethindrone is available as a progestin-only oral contraceptive pill.

Norgestrel—Ovrette (Wyeth), Norplant (Population Council)

Norgestrel is a racemic mixture, the levo isomer of which is pharmacologically active. It differs from norethindrone by the substitution of an ethyl group at the 18 position. It is available in a progestin-only oral contraceptive pill. It contains tartrazine dye (yellow No. 5), and there is therefore a slight chance of an allergic reaction, especially in patients sensitive to aspirin. Recently, levonorgestrel has been placed in vaginal rings and in subdermal implants. Both provide effective contraception for up to 5 years, but are not available in the United States.

Estrogen-Progesterone Combinations

These compounds make up the various oral contraceptive preparations. The formulations are numerous and include various concentrations of estrogen and progestin. A full report follows in another section of this text. These compounds are administered orally.

Antiprogestins—Mifepristone (RU-486) (Roussell), Gestrinone (R2323)

These compounds are derivatives of the progesterone family, but in effect are antiprogesterones. They are primarily utilized as contraceptives. The mode of action is interference of progesterone effect on the developing secretory endometrium and an anti-implantation effect. Contraception is achieved by taking pills only a few days each month. They are effective postcoital contraceptives, and some have been used as abortifacients. These compounds may also be given by subdermal implant. They are not yet commercially available in the United States.

Danazol—Danocrine (Winthrop-Breon)

This compound is a derivative of 17α-ethinyl testosterone and is supplied in 200-mg capsules. It is administered orally in doses of 400 to 800 mg daily, and primarily is used for treatment of endometriosis. It strongly inhibits pituitary release of gonadotropins, thus reducing estrogenic effect on endometriosis. It also has androgenic effects.

PROTOCOLS

Dysfunctional Bleeding

One must exclude nonendocrine causes of abnormal bleeding. Once this has been done, the majority of patients have absent or inadequate levels of progesterone as the cause of bleeding. The immediate goal is to stop bleeding and progestins are specific. It is generally best to give orally active progesterone in full doses to stop the bleeding. Norethindrone, 5 to 10 mg orally, every 6 hours is usually effective. This can be followed by 5 mg once or twice daily for 1 to 2 weeks. Therapy can then be stopped and a withdrawal period can be expected. This period should have the characteristics of normal menses with cramps and self-limited duration of flow. Other orally active progestins in equivalent doses are effective alternatives. Combination estrogen-progestin therapy may also be effective.

In women with chronic anovulation, regular cyclic therapy will often prevent irregular bleeding. In addition to irregular bleeding, the possibility of endometrial hyperplasia must be considered. While short duration of progestin therapy will provide regular withdrawal bleeding, longer duration of therapy is necessary to prevent hyperplasia. A minimum of 10 days is recommended, and many recommend 14 days of therapy. In recent studies, no hyperplasia has been found in women receiving 14 days of therapy and it appears that duration is equally important to dosage in preventing hyperplasia. Recommended doses include MPA, 10 mg daily (or 5 mg daily), for 14 days. Doses as low as 2.5 mg of MPA on a continuous basis are also effective. Equivalent doses of other progestins can be used.

Contraceptives

Oral—Norethindrone (Micronor [Ortho], Nor-Q.D. [Syntex]), Oral Tablets 0.35 mg; Norgestrel (Ovrette [Wyeth]), Oral Tablets 75 μg

Progestins alone prevent ovulation by inhibiting LH surge. Even if ovulation occurs, progestin changes may interfere with sperm penetration of the cervical mucus and implantation of a fertilized ovum. These medications usually are administered on a continuous daily basis. Since they are less effective than combination pills, a woman should be evaluated if she has amenorrhea of 60 days or if she has missed any pills and has amenorrhea in excess of 45 days. There is a high incidence of breakthrough bleeding, irregular bleeding, and amenorrhea.

Injectable—MPA (Depo-Provera [Upjohn]), Norethindrone (Norethisterone) Enanthate

MPA should be given every 3 months in doses of 150 mg. Because absorption is irregular, a substantial delay in return of fertility may be experienced. Therefore, if the possibility of permanent infertility is not acceptable, this should not be used.

Norethindrone (norethisterone) enanthate is administered every 3 months in doses of 200 mg. Although these long-acting preparations are employed for contraception, such use remains investigational in the United States. The Food and Drug Administration (FDA) has not approved them for contraceptive purposes.

Menopause

Estrogen replacement therapy (ERT) is beneficial to postmenopausal women but unopposed estrogen increases the risk of endometrial hyperplasia and adenocarcinoma. Progesterone therapy protects patients although it will not prevent all abnormalities. The protective effect is related to duration of use and currently a minimum of 10 days is recommended. In a recent controlled study, no hyperplasia was identified in those receiving progesterone therapy for 14 days. Cyclic therapy is associated with menstrual-like bleeding in most women. The incidence of withdrawal bleeding decreases once a woman is beyond age 65. To avoid cyclic bleeding, some authors have recommended continuous daily therapy with reduced dosage. Progestins alone may reduce the number of hot flashes.

MPA (Provera [Upjohn], Cycrin [Ayerst]) which comes in oral tablet of 10 mg or 5 mg should be taken daily for 10 to 14 days. One oral tablet, 2.5 mg, should be taken daily continuously. As an injection MPA (Depo-Provera [Upjohn]) should be administered intramuscularly, 50 to 150 mg every 3 to 12 weeks, to control symptoms of hot flashes.

Premenstrual Syndrome

Natural progesterone in doses as high as 400 mg daily have been advocated to relieve symptoms. Controversy exists as to whether synthetic preparations have any utility.

Progesterone suppositories are for vaginal or rectal use. These suppositories are formulated as a glycerol base and contain doses ranging from 25 to 400 mg. They may be administered once or twice daily. Begin with 25 mg once daily and increase as necessary to control symptoms. The suppositories may be made in concentrations of 25 mg, 50 mg, 100 mg, 200 mg, and 400 mg. Because of these different strengths, dosage may be tailored to provide optimal therapy.

Progesterone oral preparations by buccal administration have been shown to be effective. A troche or lozenge is placed under the tongue. These preparations must be compounded by a pharmacist. Recently, micronized progesterone has been shown to be effective when given orally. This preparation is available in a 100-mg capsule. It can be administered up to 4 times per day to achieve the desired effect.

Habitual Abortion

Habitual abortion may be secondary to low progesterone levels. This can be documented by measuring midluteal serum progesterone levels. A single progesterone level of less than 10 mg/ml or the average of 3 serum progesterone levels of less than 14 mg/ml supports the diagnosis. Natural progesterone can be administered via intramuscular or vaginal routes. Twenty-five-milligram vaginal suppositories are given twice daily or a 50-mg intramuscular injection is given daily. Therapy must be continued for up to 14 weeks. Synthetic compounds should not be used.

Vulvar Dystrophies

Progesterone has been shown to be effective for vulvar dystrophy. Because of fewer side effects, this should be considered as first-line therapy and testosterone proprionate reserved for resistant cases. The progesterone is compounded as a gel so that 1 gm of gel contains 20 mg of steroid. Usual therapy is 1 gm of gel twice daily.

Hypoventilation Syndrome

While weight reduction, specific pulmonary therapy, and surgical correction of anatomic obstruction comprise the primary therapy, progestin with its increased respiratory drive may be therapeutic in some individuals. Usual dosage is 60 to 120 mg per day in 3 divided doses between meals.

Sexual Paraphilia in Males

High-dose progestin lowers LH levels, thereby reducing androgen production. The lowered androgen production is in effect medical castration and reduces sexually deviant behavior. This reduction of deviant behavior is not associated with change of sexual orientation or impotence. Sexual thoughts and fantasy are reduced and the level of tumescence related to visual sexual stimulation is slightly decreased when measured by plethysmographic erectile response.

MPA administered intramuscularly has been used. Initial doses are as high as 200 mg 2 to 3 times daily. Dosage is modified based on patient tolerance and response. A direct measure of effectiveness can be obtained by measuring serum testosterone levels. Serum testosterone concentration is usually reduced 30 to 50 percent with therapy. Once a desired response is achieved, maintenance of 100 mg weekly is usually adequate.

Endometriosis

Whether danazol has its effect directly by interfering with progesterone receptors or whether it works primarily by inhibiting gonadotropins is not clear. Both may be effective. Androgenic side effects are common. Danazol in doses of 400 to 800 mg per day for 4 to 6 months has been employed for endometriosis therapy and in doses of 200 to 400 mg per day has been used for long-term endometriosis therapy and mastodynia.

Abortion

Antiprogestins may function as contraceptives and abortifacients. RU-486 has recently been released in China and France. When administered in doses of 10 mg/kg during the midluteal phase, it consistently induced menses within 72 hours in ovulatory women and was associated with no risk of pregnancy. Because this agent can also induce abortions in women known to be pregnant, it has generated significant controversy. It is not currently available in the United States.

BIBLIOGRAPHY

General

Anfere, M. B., and Benson, H. Progesterone. An overview and recent advances. *J. Pharm. Sci.* 65:783, 1976.

Bardin, C. W., Milgrom, E., and Mauvais-Jarvis, P. (eds.). *Progesterone and Progestins.* New York: Raven Press, 1984.

Metabolism

Barbosa, J., Seal, U. S., and Doe, R. P. Effects of steroids on plasma protein-progestational agents. *J. Clin. Endocrinol. Metab.* 32:547, 1971.

Beck, P. Effects of progestins on glucose and lipid metabolism. *Ann. N.Y. Acad. Sci.* 286:434, 1973.

Burkman, R. T. Lipid and lipoprotein changes in relation to oral contraception and hormone replacement. *Fertil. Steril.* 49:39S, 1988.

Hirronen, E., Malkonen, M., and Manninen, V. Effects of different progestogens on lipoprotein during postmenopausal hormone replacement therapy. *N. Engl. J. Med.* 304:560, 1981.

Knopp, R. H. Cardiovascular effects of endogenous and exogenous sex hormones over a woman's lifetime. *Am. J. Obstet. Gynecol.* 158:1630, 1988.

Meade, T. W. Risks and mechanisms of cardiovascular events in users of oral contraceptives. *Am. J. Obstet. Gynecol.* 158:1646, 1988.

Tseng, L., and Gurpide, E. Effects of progestins on estradiol receptor levels in human endometrium. *J. Clin. Endocrinol. Metab.* 41:402, 1975.

Woods, J. W. Oral contraceptives and hypertension. *Hypertension* 11(Suppl):II-11, 1988.

Therapy

Chihal, H. J. Indications for drug therapy in premenstrual syndrome patients. *J. Reprod. Med.* 32:449, 1987.

Crosignani, P. G. The defective luteal phase. *Hum. Reprod.* 3:157, 1988.

Gambrell, R. D. Hormone replacement therapy and breast cancer. *Maturitas* 9:123, 1987.

Ginsburg, K. A., and Moghiss, K. S. Alternate delivery systems for contraceptive progestogens. *Fertil. Steril.* 49:16S, 1988.

Key, T. J., and Pike, M. C. The role of oestrogens and progestagens in the epidemiology and prevention of breast cancer. *Eur. J. Cancer Clin. Oncol.* 24:29, 1988.

Kovacs, L. Luteal contraception. *Hum. Reprod.* 3:169, 1988.

Lee, C. S. Luteal phase defects. *Obstet. Gynecol. Surv.* 42:267, 1987.

Lindsay, R. Prevention of postmenopausal osteoporosis. *Obstet. Gynecol. Clin. North Am.* 14:63, 1987.

Murray, J. B. Psychopharmacologic therapy of deviant sexual behavior. *J. Gen. Psychol.* 115:101, 1988.

Murray, M. A. F., et al. Endocrine changes in male sexual deviants offered treatment with antiandrogens, estrogens, or tranquilizers. *J. Endocrinol.* 67:179, 1975.

Onnis, A., and Becagli, L. Topical treatment of vulvar dystrophy with progesterone. *Clin. Exp. Obstet. Gynecol.* 13:15, 1986.

Scholten, P. C., Christaens, G. C., and Haspels, A. A. Intrauterine steroid contraception. *Wien. Med. Wochenschr.* 137:479, 1987.

Sitruk-Were, R., Sterkers, N., and Mauvais-Jarvis, P. Benign breast disease. I. Hormonal investigation. *Obstet. Gynecol.* 53:457, 1979.

Strohl, K. P., et al. Progesterone administration and progressive sleep apneas. *J.A.M.A.* 245:1230, 1981.

Ulmann, A. The antiprogestins: a recent advance in fertility regulation. *J. Steroid Biochem.* 27:1009, 1987.

Whitehead, M. I., and Fraser, D. The effects of estrogens and progestogens on the endometrium. *Obstet. Gynecol. Clin. North Am.* 14:299, 1987.

4

Estrogen-Progestin Combinations

Mark L. Jutras

Estrogen-progestin combinations are well known to most primary care physicians through their use as contraceptives. Oral contraceptives (OCs) are currently the most popular form of reversible contraception. Fifty million women worldwide and at least 10 million women in the United States are currently using this form of contraception. It is for that reason that the therapeutic properties and potential side effects of this group of drugs are so important. The discovery of major benefits unrelated to contraception has focused new light on the risk-benefit considerations for OCs. First licensed for use in 1960, the combinations currently used have evolved into a safe and reliable form of therapy.

In this chapter I briefly discuss the use of estrogen-progestin combinations as contraceptives. Since their introduction, many other therapeutic uses have been described. These other uses will be a major focus.

PHYSIOLOGY

An important point to remember about OCs is that they induce a pharmacologic, not a physiologic, state. While many of their actions are typical of estrogens or progestins, the total picture cannot be compared to pregnancy or any part of the normal menstrual cycle.

Estrogen-progestin combinations function as contraceptives primarily by preventing normal luteinizing hormone (LH) and follicle-stimulating hormone (FSH) pulsatility and by inhibiting the LH surge. Their effect is due to suppression at the hypothalamic as well as the pituitary level. The progestin primarily suppresses LH secretion, while the estrogen suppresses FSH secretion. Even the lowest dose pill is at least 95 percent effective in this function.

The estrogenic component is also required to stabilize the endometrium. This is an important concept when addressing bleeding problems associated with OC usage. Estrogens also potentiate the effect of progestins, probably by increasing the intracellular concentration of progestin receptors.

In the few cycles that do result in ovulation, other physiologic effects prevent conception. Progestins act on the cervical mucus to make it thick and impervious to sperm. This change in the cervical mucus is thought to be the explanation for the decreased incidence of pelvic inflammatory disease in users of the pill. Endometrial samples from patients treated with OCs show a decidualized or atrophic pattern that would be inconsistent with implantation. Some theorize that tubal motility is affected, but it is doubtful that this would be important in humans.

PHARMACOLOGY

The two estrogen compounds in use in the United States, ethinyl estradiol and mestranol, can be addressed together when considering physiology since mestranol does not appear to have significant effect until metabolized to ethinyl estradiol by demethylation in the liver. Ethinyl estradiol is one of the most potent estrogens ever synthesized. Comparative estrogenicity of ethinyl estradiol and mestranol in humans indicates that ethinyl estradiol is approximately twice as potent on a per weight scale, but that this difference is of no significance in the range used in combination preparations. The markedly increased potency of these synthetic estrogens as compared to estradiol is primarily due to their enhanced gastrointestinal absorption. Approximately 50 percent of mestranol is demethylated in the liver to ethinyl estradiol. Thirty percent of a given dose is excreted in feces, with the remainder being excreted in conjugated form by the kidney.

As with all orally administered estrogens there are characteristic genital and extragenital effects. The genital effects include proliferation of the endometrium, maturation of the vaginal epithelium, and support of breast tissue. Extragenital effects include development and maintenance of secondary sex characteristics, stimulation of hepatic synthesis of some proteins and suppression of the production of others, decreased bone turnover, and effects on bone maturation.

There are currently five synthetic progestins used in OCs in the United States, all derivatives of 19-nortestosterone. They are norethindrone, norgestrel, ethynodiol diacetate, norethindrone acetate, and norethynodrel (no preparations with <50 μg of ethinyl estradiol or mestranol). Three other progestins in wide use in other countries may be released in the United States. They are desogestrel, gestodene, and norgestimate. The variability in potency between the progestins is much greater than that between ethinyl estradiol and mestranol.

All progestins in the currently available OCs are 19-nortestosterone derivatives. By removing the 19-C carbon, almost all of the androgenic and anabolic properties of testosterone have been removed. The structural differences between these compounds vary their ability to interact with estrogen, androgen, and progestin receptors. Progestins halt endometrial proliferation and induce its maturation. Their primary purpose in the birth control pill is to stabilize the endometrium.

INDICATIONS

Oral contraceptives provided the first truly reliable form of contraception. Since their introduction, several unexpected benefits as well as risks have been defined. One can assure patients that with few exceptions their health will be better with the use of OCs. Important reductions in the incidence of anemia, fibrocystic breast disease, and ovarian and endometrial cancers are now well documented. With the introduction of the triphasic preparations almost all risks have been eliminated.

The starting preparation should be chosen with regard to physician familiarity with the product, beginning at the lowest dose consistent with good control of cycle. There is no justification to begin patients on 50 μg of ethinyl estradiol in the hope that she will be better protected if she misses pills during the learning phase. Patients should be informed of the likelihood of breakthrough bleeding in the initial months of therapy. One of the most common mistakes in prescribing OCs is the frequent change of preparation in the hope that a different product will immediately relieve breakthrough bleeding. An adequate trial requires 3 months of the same preparation to allow time for the pill to establish control.

It was thought previously that a formulation especially well tailored for a particular patient could be selected. Women with acne who needed a more "estrogenic" preparation were given one combination while women with fibrocystic disease who needed a more "androgenic" preparation were given another. As all combination preparations are progestin dominant, it is questionable if there was ever any validity to this concept. With the change to predominantly low-dose preparations any basis for this strategy is now gone.

High-dose OCs can quickly control acute *dysfunctional bleeding*. The status of the endometrium, however, must be considered before choosing OCs over an estrogen. There must be sufficient endometrial depth to allow response to the progestin component. If the patient has had prolonged bleeding, there is a greater chance that this condition will not be met and the patient will not respond.

With the demise of the intrauterine device (IUD) and the reluctance to use diethylstilbestrol (DES) in any pregnant patient, estrogen-progestin combinations have become the only easily obtainable option for *"morning after" contraception*. Effectiveness has been proven with failure rates of less than 2 percent. It is important to take this opportunity to give these patients a reliable contraceptive.

With the wider application of vigorous chemotherapy and the growing utilization of bone marrow transplantation, the gynecologist is more frequently being called on to construct a regimen for prolonged *menstrual suppression* in these females. With the availability of the new gonadotropin-releasing hormone (GnRH) superagonist that can be given subcutaneously, intravenously, intramuscularly, or nasally, or in depot form there are now other options for prolonged menstrual suppression. However, because of the adverse effects these agents have on bone mass, combination estrogen-progestin therapy must be considered the standard choice for the time being.

It has long been observed that *dysmenorrhea* is lessened in most women using OCs. The majority of women presenting with a chief complaint of menstrual pain will have an adequate response to these agents. The mechanism of action is not fully understood but is most likely related to a reduction in prostaglandin production.

Many women with documented *endometriosis* will improve symptomatically while taking combination OCs. This led to the assumption that OCs could prevent or limit the development of endometriosis. More recent evidence has cast doubt on this idea and even suggested that some preparations promote the growth of endometriosis.

These preparations are effective *hormonal replacement* for treating the symptoms of menopause. However, the dose of estrogen provided in OCs is several times that of physiologic replacement. A more appropriate replacement is provided with the standard preparations used for this purpose. Young women with ovarian failure may feel more like their peers if they are taking "the pill." The increased risk over standard replacement is justified for improved mental well-being.

Fibrocystic breast disease will show improvement after several months of therapy. Users of OCs have a much lower incidence of suspicious breast masses.

Some women will notice a reduction in *acne* and *hirsutism* while using OCs. Formerly, great thought was put into "tailoring" the preparation to the patient. It is doubtful that there was ever any validity to the assumptions used in making these decisions. Certainly available preparations do not have enough variance in their relative estrogenicity or androgenicity to make this type of selection necessary. Studies looking at the usefulness of OCs as a treatment for acne have been inconclusive. Elevated androgen levels of ovarian origin can be decreased by the use of OCs. In severe cases there may be greater suppression with a 50-μg preparation, though this is not clear. At least 6 months of therapy is required before noticeable reduction of hirsutism occurs.

OCs provide effective *suppression of ovarian cysts*. It is well documented that all combination preparations reduce the incidence of pathologic cyst formation. In the face of recent reports in the medical and especially in the lay press, this point needs to be emphasized to patients. No combination OC has been shown to increase the risk of cyst formation. There is a suggestion that patients presenting with a cyst have more consistent reduction in cyst size if they are treated with a preparation containing 50 μg of ethinyl estradiol or mestranol. Higher doses of estrogen do not add increased therapeutic benefit.

Premenstrual syndrome (PMS) may respond to OC therapy. As with any treatment for PMS it is difficult to distinguish real improvement from placebo effect. Only time will tell with each individual.

CONTRAINDICATIONS, PRECAUTIONS, AND WARNINGS

Absolute

Any history of or predisposition to *thrombophlebitis, thromboembolism, cerebral vascular disease*, or *atherosclerotic coronary artery disease* should preclude the use of these agents. Since the majority of the increased morbidity and mortality from these complications occurs in smokers, smokers older than 35 years should not receive treatment with these preparations. There is some preliminary evidence that patients with the lupus anticoagulant are at increased risk of thrombotic complications when taking OCs.

Hormonally stimulated tumors are a contraindication to any form of estrogen therapy. A suspicious breast lump would also preclude its use until the nature of the lesion is determined.

Impaired liver function from any cause will interfere with the metabolism of these drugs and therefore is a contraindication to their use. In the patient with acute hepatitis, therapy should be discontinued and then restarted once results of liver function tests return to normal. Liver tumors, either benign or malignant, may respond unfavorably to OCs.

In healthy women low-dose combinations do not appear to induce significant negative changes in lipid profile. This may not be the case for women with *congenital hyperlipidemia*. Current recommendations are that all people should have their cholesterol levels checked. Any woman with an abnormal lipid profile should be counseled to the possible adverse effects of OCs on lipid metabolism. If they choose to use OCs, their lipid profile should be followed and OCs discontinued if the profile is worsened. Changes may not be apparent for several months, necessitating continued surveillance.

A great deal of controversy has arisen in regard to the ability of contraceptives to induce malformations in the developing human fetus. The data are reassuring in that the risk, if present, is at the verge of detectability. Early reports have associated OCs with the VACTERL (vertebral, anal, cardiac, tracheal, esophageal, renal, and limb) syndrome, cardiac defects, and limb hypoplasia. This information was derived from case reports and as such does not appear to reflect a true association. Nevertheless, it is prudent to avoid the use of any steroidal compound during *pregnancy*. Abnormal vaginal bleeding may be associated with pregnancy or neoplasia, and therefore would be a contraindication until the cause of the bleeding was established.

Relative

Women with *diabetes* may have more problems with metabolic control while using OCs. There is some disagreement as to the extent of the abnormalities induced by these agents, but it is apparent that they can induce some degree of glucose intolerance. Some authors have reported elevation in glucose levels during glucose tolerance tests while others have reported normal glucose curves with elevation only in insulin levels. The significance of these changes is not known. A related question is whether or not overt diabetics should be treated with these preparations. In general, this has not presented a problem. However, if a patient who has previously been in good control develops a more brittle pattern, consideration should be given to discontinuing treatment. Patients who have risk factors for adult-onset diabetes should have periodic glucose tolerance testing. The primary message here is that these preparations do not increase the risk that a woman will become overtly diabetic.

There is still more controversy concerning the question of *migraine headaches* and OCs. It would be prudent to inform patients of the increased incidence of stroke in women who have migraine headaches and the possibility that these agents may increase that risk. Some women will report improvement in their headaches while receiving treatment with these agents. If, however, a woman reports increased problems with headaches, scotoma, blurred vision, episodic blindness, or hemiplegia, OC therapy should be discontinued.

Low-dose preparations do not appear to stimulate growth or increase the incidence of *leiomyomas*. There is now evidence that long-term use of the pill reduces the risk of developing fibroids. The usual procedure is to examine the patient every 6 months and to discontinue treatment or lower the dosage if growth is detected. In view of the more recent data, these patients can be followed in routine fashion once it has been determined that their leiomyomas are not growing in response to the OCs.

Traditionally it is said that the frequency of *epileptic seizures* is increased while a patient is taking OCs. In truth, there is no evidence that OCs exacerbate epilepsy. Some women will even improve during therapy. Another consideration, however, is the interaction of the pill and antiseizure medication. Phenytoin, barbiturates, and meprobamate all increase hepatic clearance of OCs and may interfere with their effectiveness. This accelerated metabolism may be a reason for recommending that these patients choose another form of contraception.

Well-controlled *hypertension* does not appear to be a contraindication to OC therapy. However, it is advisable to have patients older than 35 years change to another form of contraception. Uncontrolled hypertension or hypertension exacerbated by OCs should be considered a contraindication.

It is recommended that these agents be discontinued 4 weeks before *surgery*. There is an increased risk of thrombosis for surgeries that may involve prolonged immobilization. Shorter procedures such as tubal ligation are frequently done while the patient continues to take OCs. Ideally these patients should discontinue usage before surgery. Practical considerations may not permit this and the small theoretical risk is acceptable if the patient is properly informed.

Gallbladder disease is often thought to be associated with the use of OCs. Careful analysis indicates that the rate of symptomatic disease is increased during initial therapy but that long-term rates are not increased. Apparently, patients at risk show their disease early. There is no increased risk in patients not predisposed.

Sickle-cell disease has a strong association with thromboembolic disorders. However, there are no data indicating that the risk is increased by OCs. To the contrary, laboratory evidence suggests that progestins may inhibit sickling. Epidemiologic data from the United States and Europe verify the safety of OC use in these patients. The medical legal picture in the United States has clouded the issues. Though the medical safety is clear, the high background rate of stroke (8%) in these patients places the physician at high risk for liability. This is the only reason that sickle-cell disease is listed as a relative contraindication.

The evidence is now clear that most of the increase in mortality is associated with the combined usage of OCs and *tobacco*. In areas where use of smokeless tobacco products is common (including the use of nicotine gum) women should be advised that their risks may be increased by these habits. Women older than 35 who smoke should be directed toward other forms of contraception. Short-term use (e.g., for cyst suppression) is permissible.

METABOLIC EFFECTS, ALTERED LABORATORY VALUES, AND DRUG INTERACTIONS

Metabolic Effects

OCs have been shown to increase cardiac work. This is probably secondary to fluid retention. Preexisting cardiac compromise should be considered a contraindication to OCs. Many, if not most, patients will complain of fluid retention usually in the first few months of therapy. Studies that have specifically looked at weight fluctuation in women beginning OC therapy have not shown an associated weight gain in the population as a whole. Patients expressing this concern should be reassured that any weight gain associated with initiating therapy will resolve in a short time.

Carbohydrate tolerance is reduced with any of these preparations. This rarely presents as a clinical problem. The abnormality most often is reflected as hyperinsulinemia and not as abnormal glucose levels.

There is some difference of opinion as to the effect of these preparations on lipid metabolism. It appears that low-dose preparations do not cause a significant change in lipid profiles. Fifty-microgram preparations have been shown to decrease high-density lipoprotein (HDL) and increase low density lipoprotein (LDL) levels. Norgestrel may have more adverse affects.

Altered Laboratory Values

Levels of prothrombin, fibrinogen, and factors VII, VIII, IX, and X are increased during contraceptive therapy. Levels of antithrombin III are decreased. Reports of changes in platelet function have been inconsistent with the general trend showing no change or a small increase in aggregation and adhesion. Clotting and bleeding times do not change significantly.

Estrogens elevate the level of several binding proteins. It is well known that estrogen-containing compounds elevate thyroxine-binding protein and total thyroxine levels without affecting the free thyroxine levels. Estrogens increase the production of transcortin. This results in elevated total cortisol levels. Free cortisol levels are also elevated. This is thought to be due to both the displacement of cortisol from transcortin and the decreased metabolism of cortisol by the liver.

Drug Interaction

Several drugs are thought to alter the metabolism of OCs. It has been reported that the following agents may lessen OC effectiveness by a nonspecific increase in the hepatic metabolism of drugs: barbiturates, phenylbutazone, phenytoin sodium, griseofulvin, and rifampin. The penicillins decrease the effectiveness of OCs by decreasing enterohepatic circulation of the estrogen component. Tetracyclines may alter estrogen metabolism by the same mechanism.

OCs may affect the actions of other drugs. They may interfere with hepatic metabolism of tricyclic antidepressants and benzodiazepines. The clearance of theophylline is delayed.

ADVERSE REACTIONS

Breakthrough bleeding is normally thought of as a nuisance side effect. Its importance should not be underrated as it is the primary reason that pills containing 50 μg of ethinyl estradiol and mestranol are prescribed. Contraceptive effectiveness is not decreased in women with breakthrough bleeding. Rather than permanently increasing the hormonal dosage in the pill, a short course of supplemental ethinyl estradiol should be given. Most patients will have relief from this symptom for months. A related side effect, pill-induced amenorrhea, should be treated in the same fashion if the patient or health care provider is not comfortable with the amenorrheic state.

Thromboembolism has been a concern since the report of the Royal Academy of General Practitioners on the side effects of oral contraception. Initial reports indicated that OC users had 4 times the risk of deep venous thrombosis and 2 times the risk of superficial venous thrombosis. Since that time data have demonstrated a direct dose-response curve. There is no relationship with the duration of use. The risk does not remain elevated after discontinuation of the pill. Estrogens induce changes in several coagulation factors in such a way as to induce a relatively hypercoagulable state. As the amount of estrogen in the pill has decreased, so have the thrombotic complications. When the dosage is dropped below 50 μg of ethinyl estradiol, coagulation changes and risks all but disappear.

There has been extensive debate on the issue of OC use and the risk for *cerebral vascular accident*. Early reports reported a fourfold increase in the risk of thrombotic stroke and a twofold increase in the risk of hemorrhagic stroke. There is no evidence of an association of thrombotic stroke with the use of low-dose pills. There may be an increase in hemorrhagic stroke in users of the low-dose pills.

Cardiac mortality primarily due to *myocardial infarction* increases with the amount of estrogen in the pill. With the current low-dose preparations, there is little, if any, increased risk in screened patients. Further reassurance comes from recent data indicating that there is no long-term increase in risk for former users. The patients at increased risk are those with documented hyperlipidemia, family history of premature infarction, hypertension, smoking habit, or diabetes. These patients should be guided to other forms of contraception especially when they are older than 35 years.

Hepatic adenoma is associated with steroid therapy. The relationship seems to be influenced by dosage and length of therapy. The incidence of these rare tumors has decreased further as the amount of hormone used in OCs has dropped. There does not appear to be any association with hepatocellular carcinoma.

Much has been said in regard to the potential of these agents to influence induction and growth of tumors. Recent studies have enabled us to make some valid conclusions regarding their influence on various tumors. Large epidemiologic studies have been conducted to evaluate OC's effects on the incidence of ovarian, endometrial, breast, and cervical neoplasias.

It is clear that women taking combination OCs have a reduced incidence of functional ovarian cysts and the complications related to them. This has been documented in several retrospective and prospective studies. Even more significant is recent evidence for a long-term and potentially lifelong decrease in the incidence of epithelial ovarian cancers.

Estrogens by themselves have been shown to increase the risk for endometrial cancer up to fifteenfold. When discussing estrogen-progestin combinations, one must remember that all combinations currently available in the United States are progestin dominant. That is, the typical histologic picture of the endometrium in a woman taking these combinations is one of pseudodecidualization or atrophy. Clinical data that are now available confirm an overall reduced risk of adenomatous and cancerous changes in women treated with OCs when compared with women who have never received such therapy.

Early data indicated that there was an increase in dysplasia and cervical cancer in women using combination OCs. More recent data have convincingly shown that there are no statistical differences when confounding factors are taken into account. The most obvious factor to consider is the probability that a woman using a reliable contraceptive may be more likely to have a higher-than-average number of partners or vice versa. Further consideration reveals a plausible association with this form of hormonal therapy when one remembers the association of cervical glandular hyperplasia and OCs. The increased glandular area on the exocervix may predispose to dysplastic changes. This issue is far from settled. It remains a prudent measure to recommend annual cervical cytologic examination on any sexually active female. There is currently no evidence that active intervention for asymptomatic glandular hyperplasia is warranted.

There has been much discussion in the scientific and lay literature concerning the association of breast cancer and OC usage. Though the final word is not yet in, the current overall picture is reassuring.

Part of the confusion in interpreting this information is the fact that some women have been placed on particular combinations because of the known beneficial effect on fibrocystic breast disease. Though not all women with fibrocystic breast disease are at increased risk for later development of breast cancer, it is clear that those women with biopsy-proved proliferative changes are at increased risk. It was the nonrandom inclusion of these women in specific treatment groups that led to the incorrect conclusion that these combinations promoted the development of breast cancer. Futher studies by both the Centers for Disease Control (CDC) in the United States and the Royal Academy of General Practitioners have provided firm data refuting the association of certain combinations, and OCs in general, with the induction of breast cancer. However, the long lag time between the time of induction of a cancer and its clinical expression mean that continued careful follow-up is necessary before a dogmatic statement can be made.

As with the potential association of cervical cancer and OCs, the association of melanoma and combination OCs appears to be related to life-style. The association is scientifically plausible in that some melanomas appear to respond to sex steroids.

ADMINISTRATION

Drug Preparations

Recommendations have been made to the Food and Drug Administration (FDA) to remove contraception as an indication for preparations containing more than 50 μg of ethinyl estradiol or mestranol. Many, if not all, pharmaceutical companies have made the decision to remove these from the market. This list will include only those drugs that are expected to be of continued availability over the next few years. The divisions will be by the progestational agent and the order will be from the lowest to the highest hormonal content (Tables 4-1 and 4-2).

Norethindrone

Ovcon-35 (Mead Johnson)	Ethinyl estradiol 35 μg	
	Norethindrone 0.4 mg	
Brevicon (Syntex), Modicon (Ortho), Nelova 0.5/35E (Warner Chilcott)	Ethinyl estradiol 35 μg	
	Norethindrone 0.5 mg	
Tri-Norinyl (Syntex)	Ethinyl estradiol 35 μg	
	Norethindrone	
	Day 1 to 7	0.5 mg
	Day 8 to 16	1.0 mg
	Day 17 to 21	0.5 mg
Ortho-Novum 7/7/7 (Ortho)	Ethinyl estradiol 35 μg	
	Norethindrone	
	Day 1 to 7	0.5 mg
	Day 8 to 14	0.75 mg
	Day 15 to 21	1.0 mg
Ortho-Novum 10/11 (Ortho)	Ethinyl estradiol 0.35 mg	
	Norethindrone	
	Day 1 to 10	0.5 mg
	Day 11 to 21	1.0 mg

Table 4-1. Monophasic preparations

Estrogen	Ethynodiol diacetate Trade Name	Ethynodiol diacetate P Content (mg)	Ethynodiol diacetate E Content (μg)	Norethindrone Trade Name	Norethindrone P Content (mg)	Norethindrone E Content (μg)	Norethindrone Acetate Trade Name	Norethindrone Acetate P Content (mg)	Norethindrone Acetate E Content (μg)	Norgestrel Trade Name	Norgestrel P Content (mg)	Norgestrel E Content (μg)
Ethinyl estradiol	Demulen 1/35	1.0	35	Ovcon-35	0.4	35	Loestrin 1/20	1.0	20	Nordette, Levlen	0.15	30
	Demulen 1/50	1.0	50	Brevicon, Modicon, Nelova 0.5/35E	0.5	35	Norlestrin 1/50	1.0	50	Lo/Ovral	0.3	30
				Ortho-Novum 1/35, Norinyl 1+35, Nelova 1/35E, Norethin 1/35E	1.0 1.0	35 50	Loestrin 1.5/30	1.5	30	Ovral	0.5	50
				Ovcon-50	1.0	50	Norlestrin 2.5/50	2.5	50			
Mestranol				Norinyl 1+50, Ortho-Novum 1/50, Nelova 1/50M, Norethin 1/50M	1.0	50						

P = progestin, E = estrogen.

Table 4-2. Multiphasic preparations

	Progestin							
	Norethindrone				Levonorgestrel			
Estrogen	Trade Name	Day of Cycle	P Content (mg)	E Content (μg)	Trade Name	Day of Cycle	P Content (mg)	E Content (μg)
Ethinyl estradiol	Tri-Norinyl	1–7	0.5	35	Triphasil, Tri-Levlen	1–6	0.05	30
		8–16	1.0	35		7–11	0.075	40
		17–21	0.5	35		12–21	0.125	30
	Ortho-Novum 7/7/7	1–7	0.5	35				
		8–14	0.75	35				
		15–21	1.0	35				
	Ortho-Novum 10/11	1–10	0.5	35				
		11–21	1.0	35				

P = progestin, E = estrogen.

Ortho-Novum 1/35 (Ortho), Norinyl 1+35 (Syntex), Nelova 1/35E (Warner Chilcott), Norethin 1/35E (G.D. Searle), N.E.E. 1/35 (Lexis)	Ethinyl estradiol 35 μg Norethindrone 1.0 mg
Ortho-Novum 1/50 (Ortho), Norinyl 1+50 (Syntex), Nelova 1/50 (Warner Chilcott), Norethin 1/50M (G.D. Searle)	Mestranol 50 μg Norethindrone 1.0 mg
Ovcon-50 (Mead Johnson)	Ethinyl estradiol 50 μg Norethindrone 1.0 mg

Norethynodrel

None available

Norgestrel

Triphasil (Wyeth-Ayerst), Tri-Levlen (Berlex)	Ethinyl estradiol Day 1 to 6 30 μg Day 7 to 11 40 μg Day 12 to 21 30 μg Levonorgestrel Day 1 to 6 0.05 mg Day 7 to 11 0.075 mg Day 12 to 21 0.125 mg
Nordette (Wyeth-Ayerst) and Levlen (Berlex)	Ethinyl estradiol 30 μg Levonorgestrel 0.15 mg
Lo/Ovral (Wyeth-Ayerst)	Ethinyl estradiol 30 μg Norgestrel 0.3 mg
Ovral (Wyeth-Ayerst)	Ethinyl estradiol 50 μg Norgestrel 0.5 mg

Ethynodiol Diacetate

Demulen 1/35 (Searle)	Ethinyl estradiol 35 μg Ethynodiol diacetate 1.0 mg
Demulen 1/50 (Searle)	Ethinyl estradiol 50 μg Ethynodiol diacetate 1.0 mg

Norethindrone Acetate

Loestrin 1/20 (Parke-Davis)	Ethinyl estradiol 20 μg Norethindrone acetate 1.0 mg
Loestrin 1.5/30 (Parke-Davis)	Ethinyl estradiol 30 μg Norethindrone acetate 1.5 mg
Norlestrin 1/50 (Parke-Davis)	Ethinyl estradiol 50 μg Norethindrone acetate 1.0 mg
Norlestrin 2.5/50 (Parke-Davis)	Ethinyl estradiol 50 μg Norethindrone acetate 2.5 mg

Protocols

Oral Contraception

The usual recommended start time is day 5 of the cycle or the first Sunday after menstruation. Contraceptive effectiveness during the first cycle is higher when the pill is started on day 1 of the cycle. The trade off is an increased incidence of breakthrough bleeding during the first months of therapy. With the standard start times it is suggested that the patient use another form of contraception as backup during the first 7 days of treatment to prevent the rare first cycle pregnancy.

Therapy should be started with preparations containing 30 to 35 μg of ethinyl estradiol. Triphasic preparations are the preferred choice. Women currently on higher dose pills should be reduced to the lower dose preparations. Higher dose pills should only be considered if cycle control continues to be poor after more than 3 months of therapy. There is no indication for the use of preparations containing greater than 50 μg of ethinyl estradiol or mestranol for contraception.

Recent epidemiologic data indicate that women without risk factors for cardiovascular or thromboembolic disease may safely continue to take OCs up to age 45. The primary risk factor is smoking. Women older than 35 who smoke should not receive OCs. In screening all patients, the practitioner should inquire specifically about a history of cardiac or thromboembolic disorder, hypertension, diabetes, lipid abnormality, and stroke or a family history of premature cardiovascular disease.

Cycle Regulation for Chronic Oligo-Ovulation or Anovulation

Treat as you would for contraception.

Acute Menorrhagia

Oral contraceptives are not an appropriate choice for a patient with prolonged bleeding. There must be sufficient endometrium remaining for the progestins to have an effect. For acute severe bleeding 1 pill is to be taken 4 times a day for 5 to 7 days. Following this, without a break, take 1 pill a day for the duration of one cycle pack. Continue the oral contraceptives for at least 3 months. After 3 cycles reevaluate the need for continued cycle control.

Suppression of Menses in Hematology, Oncology, or Transplant Patients

Two 50-μg pills a day are taken continuously. The preparation most commonly used contains ethinyl estradiol, 50 μg, and norgestrel, 0.5 mg per pill.

Dysmenorrhea

Use as for contraception using lowest dose consistent with relief of symptoms. Some patients may respond better with uninterrupted use.

Suppression of Endometriosis

This is now considered of questionable use. Still, there is no question that many patients are improved symptomatically. Therapy may be more beneficial if used continuously. Prescribe as for contraception.

Hormonal Replacement

Use as for contraception. Use the lowest dose consistent with symptom control.

Fibrocystic Breast Disease

Use as for contraception. Inform patients that it may take several months before a benefit is noted.

Acne

Use as for contraception. If improvement is not seen with a low-dose preparation, increase dose to a preparation containing 50 μg of ethinyl estradiol or mestranol. Some patients will have a paradoxical increase in acne when therapy is first started.

Cyst Suppression

Begin with a 50-μg estrogen pill. Follow with pelvic examinations at monthly intervals until the cyst resolves. This treatment plan is not accepted by all. Some believe that low-dose OCs give equivalent suppression to the 50-μg pills.

Morning-After Pill

Therapy should be initiated before 72 hours after the incident of unprotected intercourse. Patients should also be informed of the possible teratogenic effects to a fetus if the method fails and they choose not to abort the pregnancy. Pretreat with an antiemetic such as 12.5 to 25.0 mg of promethanzine PO followed 30 minutes later by two pills, each containing 50 μg of ethinyl estradiol and 0.5 mg of norgestrel (i.e., 2 Ovrals). Repeat the dose (i.e., 2 Ovrals, 12 hours later).

Protocols for OC Complications

The common OC complications are nuisances from a medical standpoint but are very worrisome from a patient standpoint. The patient must be assured that she is protected from pregnancy despite their occurrence if she is taking her pills as prescribed. In the past these patients were changed to increasingly high-dosage OCs. This is no longer considered appropriate as a first measure. The two most common side effects, *breakthrough bleeding* and *amenorrhea*, are representative of an atrophic endometrium. This can usually be treated with a short course of ethinyl estradiol, 20 μg per day for 7 days. Patients who do not respond or do not wish to try this treatment should be treated with another low-dose combination before being changed to the 50-μg pills.

Breakthrough Bleeding

Ethinyl estradiol, 20 μg/day is taken orally for 7 days along with her usual OCs.

Amenorrhea

The first step is to question the patient regarding missed pills or a late start of her pill pack. If any risk for pregnancy exists, a pregnancy test must be checked. If there is no risk of pregnancy, OCs may be continued. If there is no withdrawal bleeding in the next cycle, a pregnancy test is obtained and the situation must be discussed with patient. If she is accepting of the absence of withdrawal bleeding, no treatment is needed. If she is not comfortable with this, treatment should be directed toward the atrophic nature of the endometrium. Treatment consists of ethinyl estradiol, 20 μg per day, administered orally for 7 days along with her usual OCs. This generally gives the patient several months of light withdrawal bleeding.

Missed Pill

It appears that delayed start of a new pill pack may be the most common forerunner to a conception cycle while the patient is taking OCs. This would argue strongly for prescribing 28-day packs for all patients and to encourage them to take the inactive pills.

If the start is delayed, the patient should use another form of contraception for the first 7 days of the new pack. If 1 pill is missed after the start, a pill should be taken as soon as remembered and the next at the usual time. If 2 pills are missed, the patient should take 2 pills a day until caught up and use another form of contraception as backup for 7 days.

Melasma (Chloasma)

This condition is rarely seen with today's contraceptives. If it becomes a problem, a sunscreen should be used to minimize the changes. Bleaching agents such as 2- to 4-percent hydroquinone in an opaque base may be tried. Expect a slow response.

BIBLIOGRAPHY

Contraceptive Technology

Henzl, M. R. Contraceptive Hormones and Their Clinical Use. In S. S. C. Yen and R. B. Jaffe (eds.), *Reproductive Endocrinology* (2nd ed.). Philadelphia: W. B. Saunders, 1986. Pp. 643–682.

Speroff, L., Glass, R. H., and Kase, N. G. Steroid Contraception. In *Clinical Gynecologic Endocrinology and Infertility* (4th ed.). Baltimore: Williams and Wilkins, 1989. Pp. 461–498.

Metabolic Effects

Beller, F. B., and Ebert, C. Effects of oral contraceptives on blood coagulation. A review. *Obstet. Gynecol. Surv.* 40:425 1985.

Adverse Reactions

Stampfer, M. J., et al. A prospective study of past use of oral contraceptive agents and risk of cardiovascular diseases. *N. Engl. J. Med.* 319:1313, 1988.

Vessey, M., et al. Oral contraceptives and venous thromboembolism: findings in a large prospective study. *Br. Med. J.* 292:526, 1986.

Safety

The Cancer and Steroid Hormone Study of the Centers for Disease Control and the National Institute of Child Health and Human Development. Oral-contraceptive use and the risk of breast cancer. *N. Engl. J. Med.* 315:405, 1986.

The Cancer and Steroid Hormone Study of the Centers for Disease Control and the National Institute of Child Health and Human Development. Combination oral contraceptive use and the risk of endometrial cancer. *J.A.M.A.* 257:796, 1987.

The Cancer and Steroid Hormone Study of the Centers for Disease Control and the National Institute of Child Health and Human Development. The reduction in risk of ovarian cancer associated with oral-contraceptive use. *N. Engl. J. Med.* 316:650, 1987.

Mishell, D. R., Jr. Use of oral contraceptives in women of older reproductive age. *Am. J. Obstet. Gynecol.* 158:1652, 1988.

Paul, C., et al. Oral contraceptives and breast cancer: a national study. *Br. Med. J.* 292:526, 1986.

Porter, J. B., Jick, H., and Walker, A. M. Mortality among oral contraceptive users. *Obstet. Gynecol.* 70:29, 1987.

Ross, R. K., et al. Risk factors for uterine fibroids: reduced risk associated with oral contraceptives. *Br. Med. J.* 293:359, 1986.

Other

Bagshaw, S. N., Edwards, D., and Tucker, A. K. Ethinyl oestradiol and D-Norgestrel is an effective emergency postcoital contraceptive: a report of its use in 1,200 patients in a family planning clinic. *Aust. N.Z. J. Obstet. Gynaecol.* 28:137, 1988.

5

Androgens And Antiandrogens

Gary D. Hubert and Sandra Ann Carson

Androgens are steroids that are capable of stimulating and maintaining male sexual development. Endogenous androgens are 19-carbon steroids synthesized in the testes, ovary, and adrenal cortex. These compounds include dehydroepiandrosterone (DHEA), dehydroepiandrosterone sulfate (DHEA-S), androstenedione, and testosterone, all of which have significantly different biologic potencies.

Androgens are responsible for the formation of male internal and external genitalia, the development of male secondary sex characteristics, and normal spermatogenesis. They also affect behavioral and physiologic functions within the central nervous system, which include male coital and mating behavior, aggressiveness, and libido. Female androgen production is shared by the ovary and adrenal cortex and provides a source of estrogen precursors.

In addition to affecting male development, androgens are capable of inducing several physiologic alterations in both males and females, including an increase in body weight and muscle mass, thickening of the skin and proliferation of sebaceous glands, loss of subcutaneous fat, growth of the larynx leading to a deepening of the voice, and male pattern hair growth. The anabolic effects of androgens, which cause the prepubertal increase in height and skeletal musculature, include a positive protein balance and retention of potassium, sodium, and water. Androgens also increase libido in both sexes, stimulate erythropoiesis, and reverse the loss of bone calcium. Finally, androgens may function as estrogen antagonists, as evidenced by their efficacy in treating endometriosis and carcinoma of the breast.

The most obvious use of exogenous androgens is for replacing deficient androgen production in the male. Other indications include decreased libido in both men and women, endometriosis, suppression of postmenopausal hot flashes, nocturia, and incontinence, Addison's disease, constitutional delay of growth, fibrocystic breast disease, lichen sclerosus, hereditary angioedema, carcinoma of the breast, and certain chronic anemias. Androgen therapy for premenstrual syndrome, osteoporosis, male contraception, and growth hormone deficiency is presently under investigation.

PHYSIOLOGY

Testosterone, the principal androgen secreted in males, is necessary for normal masculine phenotype and physiology. In adult males, more than two-thirds of testosterone precursors are secreted by the adrenal cortex but over 95 percent of testosterone is directly produced by Leydig's cells of the testes, predominantly under the influence of pituitary luteinizing hormone (LH). Before puberty, testosterone concentrations are less than 20 ng/dl but rise to 300 to 1000 ng/dl with production rates of 2.5 to 11 mg per day in men. Normal testosterone concentrations in premenopausal and postmenopausal females are approximately 20 to 80 ng/dl and 10 to 40 ng/dl, respectively. Under normal conditions the production rate is 0.2 to 0.3 mg per day with 50 percent of testosterone produced from peripheral conversion of androstenedione, and the remainder secreted by both the ovary and the adrenal cortex.

In many androgenic target tissues, such as the seminal vesicles, prostate, skin, and seminiferous tubules, testosterone is reduced to 5-α dihydrotestosterone (DHT), which has approximately twice the androgenic potency of testosterone. Serum levels in normal men are approximately 55 ng/dl. Daily production rates of DHT are 300 and 60 μg per day in men and women, respectively. The formation of DHT from testosterone is required for the proper development of the prostate, penis, and scrotum in the fetus.

Testosterone enters the cells of its target tissue passively. A cytoplasmic carrier protein may be involved in transporting the hormone into the nucleus of the cell. Testosterone or DHT then enters the nucleus and binds to a nuclear receptor. The hormone-receptor complex then binds to the DNA to begin the process that leads to their biologic effect.

In men, circulating testosterone is 98 percent protein bound, 60 percent of which is bound to sex hormone–binding globulin (SHBG), and the remainder to albumin. Women have a lower circulating free fraction of testosterone, with approximately 99 percent protein bound. Hepatic synthesis of SHBG is decreased by androgens, and increased by estrogens.

The adrenal cortex is the primary source of testosterone precursors that include DHEA, DHEA-S, and androstenedione, all of which have weak androgenic activity. Over 90 percent of DHEA, which has 0 to 15 percent of the biologic potency of testosterone in vitro, is of adrenal origin in both sexes. DHEA-S has approximately half the potency of DHEA, but its serum concentration is 1000 times greater. DHEA-S is almost entirely secreted by the adrenal cortex. Androstenedione, an immediate precursor to testosterone, is produced by the adrenal and gonad equally. In vitro experiments have shown that the androgenicity of androstenedione is 12 to 20 percent that of testosterone. Nonetheless, in vivo effects are probably mediated either by testosterone or by dihydrotestosterone rather than by the androgenic activity of testosterone precursors.

Androgens are metabolized in the liver by reduction, oxidation, hydroxylation, and conjugation. The kidneys and other target tissues may also metabolize androgens. Physiologically significant androgen metabolites include DHT and estradiol. Inactive urinary metabolites are predominantly androsterone and etiocholanolone, which are the main excretion products following testosterone metabolism by the liver. Testosterone is also excreted in the urine after glucuronide conjugation. Nearly all androgen metabolites are excreted in the urine, with only 6 percent excreted in the feces.

PHARMACOLOGY

Both oral and parenteral testosterone is rapidly absorbed by the portal circulation and degraded by the liver. Free testosterone in the blood has a half-life of 10 to 20 minutes.

Alkylation of testosterone at C-17 interferes with degradation and allows oral effectiveness. Androgenic potency is proportional to the half-life of the compound. The longer the added chain is, the more prolonged the action is. Esterification of the 17β-hydroxyl group decreases the polarity of the steroid, making it more soluble for lipid-based injection preparations. Other modifications of the ring structure act either to retard degradation or to enhance potency at the receptor site.

Synthetic androgens include danazol, an isoxazole derivative of 17-ethinyl testosterone, and gestrinone, a 19-nortestosterone derivative that is not yet approved for use in the United States. Both have mixed progesterone agonist-antagonist and androgen agonist activity.

Androgenic potency was previously determined by a bioassay measuring the growth of the comb of the capon, but has since been replaced by bioassays measuring growth of the seminal vesicles or ventral prostate in castrated rats. Assays determining the ability of the compound to displace testosterone from its receptor or from SHBG are also used.

INDICATIONS

Hypogonadism

Absent testosterone production may be due to either deficient gonadotropin production by the pituitary or testosterone synthesis by the testis. The consequences of deficient testosterone production vary depending on the age of the patient. Before puberty, deficient testosterone production results in tall stature with absent libido, spermatogenesis, and secondary sex characteristics. Hypogonadism after puberty results in decreased libido and erectile dysfunction, as well as atrophy of the prostate and seminal vesicles. Fertility and ejaculate volume are reduced. A variety of clinical disorders (Table 5-1) are associated with decreased or absent production of testosterone.

Patients with hypogonadism require evaluation for hypothalamic, pituitary, or testicular dysfunction. If the disorder is at the level of the hypothalamus or pituitary, the testes have the potential to secrete androgens if stimulated. These individuals may be given testosterone, but exogenous gonadotropins or gonadotropin-releasing hormone (GnRH) may be used to stimulate the testes to secrete tes-

Table 5-1. Clinical disorders associated with decreased or absent testosterone production

Testicular disorders associated with low gonadotropin levels
- Hypopituitarism
- Kallmann's syndrome
- Isolated leuteinizing hormone deficiency (fertile eunuch)
- Alstrom's syndrome
- Prader-Willi syndrome
- Laurence-Moon-Biedl syndrome
- Isolated gonadotropin deficiency (tumor, radiation)

Testicular disorders associated with low testosterone and elevated gonadotropin levels
- Testicular failure (orchidectomy, orchitis, bilateral torsion, tumor, trauma, radiation)
- Vanishing testes syndrome
- Klinefelter's syndrome
- Noonan's syndrome
- Reifenstein's syndrome
- Sertoli-cell-only syndrome
- 46, XX male
- Congenital deficiencies of steroidogenic enzymes

tosterone. This is in contrast to those individuals who have underdeveloped testes and therefore low testosterone and high gonadotropin levels. Further testicular stimulation by even higher levels of gonadotropins will not produce testosterone and these individuals require androgen replacement therapy.

The use of androgens in normal boys with delayed sexual maturation is controversial. Therapy is undertaken to accelerate the growth and pubertal changes that would probably have occurred without treatment. Prepubertal administration of testosterone prior to epiphyseal closure results in an acceleration of linear bone growth, but whether this affects final adult height is not clear as androgens may also stimulate epiphyseal closure. Androgen therapy for pubertal development can be given in courses of 4 to 6 months duration, at which time therapy may be stopped and spontaneous development assessed. Caution must be used in order to avoid premature epiphyseal closure.

With complete testicular failure, prolonged therapy is required. Intramuscular administration of long-acting testosterone preparations such as testosterone cypionate or enanthate may be used. Full sexual development is usually achieved in 3 to 4 years. Parenteral testosterone preparations are preferred for maintenance therapy as well, because they are more potent and less hepatotoxic than the 17-alkyl substituted testosterone derivatives used for oral therapy (discussion to come). The concentrations of testosterone needed by each individual will vary and must be titrated. If therapy is started long after the usual onset of puberty, the degree of virilization that can be achieved is variable, although complete masculinization can usually be achieved. At least 10 mg per day of testosterone is necessary.

Women with hypogonadism, including primary and secondary hypopituitarism, should be treated with replacement doses of estrogen and progesterone. Menses and breast development may be induced using estrogen and progestin therapy, but unless androgen production is normal, sexual hair growth will not occur. Androgens are also required after pubertal development for the maintenance of a normal sexual hair pattern, as evidenced by the diminution of axillary and pubic hair following the withdrawal of androgen replacement therapy in these patients. Similarly, androgen replacement therapy is of benefit in women with Addison's disease in restoring lost sexual hair, muscle mass, strength, and libido.

With decreased gonadal function, androgen therapy may be used to increase libido, although masculinizing side effects may occur in women. Androgens reduce the number of hot flashes, and may be of benefit in treating nocturia as well as mild cases of stress urinary incontinence. Androgens may be used alone if estrogens are contraindicated, or in combination with estrogen should estrogen therapy alone prove unsuccessful.

Chronic Anemia

Androgen therapy increases red blood cell production by directly stimulating erythropoiesis and increasing renal erythropoietin production. This effect is beneficial in treating anemias caused by decreased erythrocyte production (aplastic anemia, sideroblastic anemia, myelofibrosis), hereditary anemias (Fanconi's anemia), and anemias associated with systemic lupus erythematosus and renal failure. Responses vary and depend on the amount of residual functioning marrow when therapy is started. Because improvements are often seen within a few weeks, the drug should be discontinued if no benefit is obtained by 3 months.

In patients with autoimmune hemolytic anemias and thrombocytopenic purpura, administration of danazol may be effective in inducing remissions at doses between 200 and 800 mg per day.

Hereditary Angioedema

Hereditary angioedema is an autosomal dominant disorder in which there is either a nonfunctional C1-esterase inhibitor or decreased concentrations of the inhibitor. Consequently, unopposed activation of the complement system leads to increased vascular permeability and angioedema. The disease is characterized by episodic edema involving the face, skin, larynx, and abdominal viscera, and is potentially fatal. Androgen therapy increases C1-esterase inhibitor activity, thereby restoring complement component concentrations. Danazol and 17-alkylated testosterone derivatives are particularly efficacious for prophylaxis because of their effects on hepatic metabolism to increase plasma inhibitor concentrations. Doses between 400 and 800 mg per day are needed.

Carcinoma of the Breast

Testosterone therapy for carcinoma of the breast is discussed in Chapter 14.

Fibrocystic Breast Disease

Danazol is capable of relieving breast pain, nodularity, and tenderness in most patients with fibrocystic breast disease after oral analgesics and other simple supportive measures have proved unsuccessful. Several months of continuous therapy may be required, but significant improvement is usually noted within 3 months of therapy. Recurrence rates are high if therapy is discontinued. The total daily dosage is 200 to 400 mg per day, and should be titrated to clinical response and side effects.

Endometriosis

Pelvic pain and infertility are the most common indications for using androgen therapy to suppress endometriotic implants. However, their advantage over other therapeutic modalities, including expectant management, in improving fertility rates is still controversial. Danazol causes direct atrophy of endometriotic implants and prevents further stimulation by suppressing midcycle gonadotropin surges as well as estrogen and progesterone production. GnRH agonists, which also lower serum levels of estrogen and induce atrophy of endometriotic implants, are probably as effective as danazol, although they are not yet approved for this indication by the Food and Drug Administration.

The dose of danazol should be titrated to prevent menstruation and significantly lower serum levels of estradiol, and may be reduced following a few weeks of therapy at an initial dose of 800 mg per day, but doses of at least 400 mg per day are required to consistently cause amenorrhea. Ovulation occurs in less than 1 percent of patients when given in doses of 400 to 800 mg per day.

The duration of therapy requires individualization. As a preoperative adjunct to surgery, an 8- to 12-week course of continuous therapy may be appropriate, but longer courses may be necessary if danazol is used without surgical intervention. Fertility rates vary depending on the extent of the disease, but significant pain relief can be expected in over 90 percent of patients treated with at least 600 mg per day. Recurrence rates are fairly high once medical therapy is discontinued, and range from 5 to 36 percent per year.

Lichen Sclerosus

Lichen sclerosus (lichen planus vel atrophicus) is a benign cutaneous vulvar dystrophy, characterized by a thin, atrophic epithelium associated with fissures, ecchymoses, and intense pruritus. Postmenopausal women are most frequently affected. Without treatment the lesion can progress to involve the entire vulva, causing introital stricture and dyspareunia. Relief of pruritus and regression to normal histological features have been demonstrated following the application of topical testosterone ointment. Topical testosterone results in increased levels of DHT, which are decreased in patients with lichen sclerosus lesions. Testosterone ointment (2%) is initially applied 2 or 3 times daily (see Protocols). The dose may be reduced after 6 to 9 months to a weekly application, but lesions often recur if therapy is discontinued. Increased libido and clitoral growth may occur as side effects of therapy, but usually do not preclude further treatment.

CONTRAINDICATIONS, WARNINGS, AND PRECAUTIONS

Contraindications to androgen therapy include carcinoma of the prostate or breast in male patients, carcinoma of the breast in female patients with hypercalcemia, and hypersensitivity to androgens. In addition, androgens should not be administered to pregnant women, as female pseudohermaphroditism may occur with large doses given during the first or second trimesters.

Patients receiving high doses of androgens should be monitored for polycythemia. Women should be observed for signs of virilization. Although hirsutism is often reversible, clitoral enlargement usually is not. Voice changes also may not be reversible after treatment with danazol. In men, priapism, excessive sexual stimulation, oligospermia, and reduced ejaculatory volume may develop. Gynecomastia may paradoxically occur and may persist after therapy is discontinued. Androgens may be excreted in breast milk and should be used with caution in nursing mothers.

Androgens should be used with caution in adolescents. Determinations of bone age should be performed in adolescent patients receiving androgens. Accelerated bone maturation without linear bone growth may occur, as well as the previously mentioned side effects of virilization, priapism, and gynecomastia.

Elderly patients may be at risk for developing prostatic hypertrophy and urinary tract obstruction. Edema with or without congestive heart failure may occur.

Prolonged use of androgens has been associated with the development of peliosis hepatis and hepatic neoplasms, including hepatocellular carcinoma. Cholestatic hepatitis and jaundice may occur when 17-alkylated androgens are administered at a relatively low dose. Periodic liver function tests are necessary for all patients receiving androgens. If symptoms of liver disease appear, or results of liver function tests become abnormal, the drug should be discontinued. The long-term use of 17-alkylated steroids should be avoided.

METABOLIC EFFECTS

Androgens have anabolic effects, causing the retention of nitrogen, potassium, sodium, phosphorus, sulfur, chloride, and water. When administration of androgen is stopped, a rapid loss of sodium, chloride, and water occur, followed by a loss of nitrogen several weeks later. In patients with breast cancer, androgen therapy may cause hypercalcemia by stimulating osteolysis.

Increases in levels of prealbumin, C1-esterase inhibitor, haptoglobin, transferrin, antithrombin III, prothrombin, and plasminogen may occur, and decreases in levels of SHBG, thyroxine-binding globulin (TBG), and pregnancy zone protein may occur. Increased concentrations of low-density lipoprotein (LDL) cholesterol and decreased concentrations of high-density lipoprotein (HDL) cholesterol have been associated with androgen therapy.

DRUG INTERACTIONS

17-Alkylated testosterone derivatives have been reported to decrease the anticoagulant requirements of patients receiving oral anticoagulants, thereby increasing the risk of hemorrhage. Elevated serum levels of oxyphenbutazone may occur during androgen administration. In diabetic patients, blood glucose and insulin requirements may decrease.

ALTERED LABORATORY VALUES

Total thyroxine (T_4) levels may decrease due to decreased TBG, although free T_4 levels remain unchanged. Clinical evidence of thyroid dysfunction rarely occurs. Androgens increase serum hemoglobin, hematocrit, and haptoglobin levels. The administration of testosterone, but not the 17-alkylated derivatives, will increase the measurement of urinary 17-ketosteroids.

ADVERSE REACTIONS

In women, menstrual irregularities and virilization may occur. In men, gynecomastia, oligospermia, and increased libido may occur. (See Contraindications, Warnings, and Precautions.) Side effects include those related to androgen therapy, such as acne, oily skin, hirsutism, and deepening of the voice, which may not be reversible. Other side effects include weight gain, which may occur in as many as 50 percent of patients receiving danazol therapy, as well as the previously mentioned metabolic effects.

Bleeding in patients taking anticoagulant therapy, polycythemia, increased or decreased libido, headache, anxiety, depression, generalized paresthesia, and increased serum cholesterol levels may occur. Stomatitis with buccal preparations may develop.

Compounds containing the dye tartrazine (FD&C yellow No. 5) may cause allergic reactions, including bronchial asthma, in susceptible individuals.

ADMINISTRATION

History and physical examination prior to administration of androgen therapy must focus on ruling out hormonal-dependent and hormone-producing tumors as well as pregnancy. (See Contraindications, Warnings, and Precautions.)

ANDROGEN PREPARATIONS

Testosterone is rapidly degraded and hence has limited practical value for oral or parenteral administration. Androgen preparations for use include esterified testosterone (e.g., testosterone propionate, cypionate, and enanthate), 17-alkylated derivatives (e.g., methyltestosterone, fluoxymesterone), and testosterone analogues (e.g., danazol).

For full androgen replacement, a dose equivalent to 10 mg per day of testosterone should be administered. Due to the hepatotoxic effects of 17-alkylated derivatives, longer acting intramuscular testosterone ester preparations are preferred for long-term use.

Fluoxymesterone. Oral, short-acting preparation (half-life approximately 10 hours). Supplied: Android-F (Brown), tablets, 10 mg. Halotestin (Upjohn), tablets, 2, 5, and 10 mg.

Methyltestosterone. Oral and buccal, short-acting preparation (half-life approximately 2.5 hours). Buccal doses are approximately one-half of oral dosage. Oral preparations, supplied: Android (Brown), Metandren (CIBA), Oreton Methyl (Schering), tablets, 10 and 25 mg; Testred (ICN) capsules, 10 mg. Buccal preparations, supplied: Android (Brown), tablets 5 mg; Metandren (CIBA), tablets, 5 and 10 mg; Oreton Methyl (Schering), tablets, 10 mg.

Testosterone cypionate. Supplied: Testred Cypionate (ICN) solution, 200 mg/ml. Depo-Testosterone (Upjohn) solution, 50, 100, and 200 mg/ml.

Testosterone enanthate. Supplied: Testosterone enanthate (generic), 100 and 200 mg/ml.

Testosterone propionate. Shorter acting intramuscular preparation useful for breast carcinoma in women, but less practical for androgen replacement in boys or men. Supplied: Testosterone propionate (generic), 25, 50, and 100 mg/ml.

Danazol. Supplied: Danocrine (Winthrop-Breon), capsules 50, 100, and 200 mg.

COMBINATION ESTROGEN-ANDROGEN PREPARATIONS

Preparations containing both estrogen and androgen are available for use in postmenopausal women with symptoms of estrogen deficiency and decreased libido. The dose of androgen must be titrated in each patient to attain symptomatic relief without virilizing side effects (see Chap. 2).

PROTOCOLS

Androgen Replacement

For complete androgen replacement of endogenous hormone, fluoxymesterone, 10 mg, or methyltestosterone, 30 mg, is the usual oral starting dose. However, for prolonged replacement (>6 months) parenteral preparations are preferred because of the risk of hepatotoxicity with the oral preparations.

The usual starting intramuscular dosage for replacement is testosterone propionate, 10 to 25 mg 2 or 3 times weekly, or testosterone enanthate, 100 to 200 mg every 2 weeks. Changes in dosage should be made following an evaluation of therapeutic response and patient's side effects. If priapism occurs, therapy should be temporarily discontinued and restarted at a lower dose.

Chronic Anemia

Fluoxymesterone, 0.4 to 1.0 mg/kg, is administered orally everyday. Testosterone enanthate or cypionate, 4 to 7 mg/kg per week, is administered intramuscularly.

Lichen Sclerosus

Testosterone powder can be solubilized in either petroleum jelly or polyethylene glycol to produce a 2 percent ointment. The ointment is initially applied 2 or 3 times daily, and may be reduced after 6 to 9 months to a weekly application.

Pubertal Development

Testosterone cypionate or testosterone enanthate, 25 to 50 mg/sq m per month, is administered intramuscularly for the induction of puberty in boys and should be increased to 100 mg/sq m per month for midpubertal sexual development and growth spurt. Dosage is then gradually increased to adult levels. Usual dosage is 150 to 200 mg every 2 weeks or 400 mg every 4 weeks, intramuscularly.

Fibrocystic Breast Disease

Danazol, 100 to 400 mg per day, is administered in 2 divided oral doses.

Endometriosis

Danazol, 800 mg, in divided doses is the recommended starting dose. The dose should be titrated to prevent menstruation and significant side effects while substantially lowering serum estradiol levels. The dose may be reduced should significant side effects occur, but doses of at least 400 mg per day are required to consistently cause amenorrhea. Average monthly costs are approximately $180 to $240 at a dose of 800 mg per day. Therapy should be initiated either following a negative result on pregnancy test or during menses to avoid use during pregnancy.

The duration of therapy requires individualization. As a preoperative adjunct to surgery, an 8- to 12-week course of continuous therapy may be appropriate, but longer courses (6–9 months) may be necessary if danazol is used without surgical intervention.

BIBLIOGRAPHY

Overview

Murad, F., and Haynes, R. C., Jr. Androgens. In A. G. Gilman and L. S. Goodman (eds.), *The Pharmacological Basis of Therapeutics* (7th ed.). New York: MacMillan, 1985. Pp. 1440–1458.

Steinberger, E. Hormonal control of mammalian spermatogenesis. *Physiol. Rev.* 51:1, 1971.

Physiology

Bardin, C. W., and Mahoudeau, J. A. Dynamics of androgen metabolism in women with hirsutism. *Ann. Clin. Res.* 2:251, 1970.

Brotherton, J. *Sex Hormone Pharmacology*. New York: Academic Press, 1976.

Lipsett, M. B., Wilson, H., Kirschner, M. A., et al. Studies on Leydig cell physiology and pathology: secretion and metabolism of testosterone. *Recent Prog. Horm. Res.* 22:245, 1966.

Rosenfield, R. L. Role of androgens in growth and development of the fetus, child, and adolescent. *Adv. Pediatr.* 19:172, 1972.

Snyder, P. J. Clinical use of androgens. *Ann. Rev. Med.* 35:207, 1984.

Tezon, J. G., Vazquez, M. H., and Blaquier, J. A. Androgen-controlled subcellular distribution of its receptor in the rat epididymis: 5α-dihydrotestosterone-induced translocation is blocked by antiandrogens. *Endocrinology* 111:2039, 1982.

Vermeulen, A., Verdonck, L., Van der Straeten, M., and Orie, N. Capacity of the testosterone-binding globulin in human plasma and influence of specific binding of testosterone on its metabolic clearance rate. *J. Clin. Endocrinol. Metab.* 29:1470, 1969.

Pharmacology

Barbieri, R. L., Lee, H., and Ryan, K. J. Danazol binding to rat androgen, glucocorticoid, progesterone, and estrogen receptors: correlation with biological activity. *Fertil. Steril.* 31:182, 1979.

Brotherton, J. *Sex Hormone Pharmacology.* New York: Academic Press, 1976.

Vermeulen, A., Stoica, T., and Verdonck, L. The apparent free testosterone concentration, an index of androgenicity. *J. Clin. Endocrinol. Metab.* 33:759, 1971.

Wentz, A. C., Jones, G. S., Sapp, K. C., and King, T. M. Progestational activity of danazol in the human female subject. *Am. J. Obstet. Gynecol.* 126:378, 1976.

Indications

Hypogonadism

Greenblatt, R. B. The use of androgens in the menopause and other gynecic disorders. *Obstet. Gynecol. Clin. North Am.* 14:251, 1987.

Sobel, E. H., Raymond, C. S., Quinn, K. V., and Talbot, N. B. The use of methyltestosterone to stimulate growth: relative influence on skeletal maturation and linear growth. *J. Clin. Endocrinol. Metab.* 16:241, 1956.

Chronic Anemia

Ahn, Y. S., Harrington, W. J., Mylvaganam, R., et al. Danazol therapy for autoimmune hemolytic anemia. *Ann. Intern. Med.* 102:298, 1985.

Ahn, Y. S., Harrington, W. J., Simon, S. R., et al. Danazol for the treatment of idiopathic thrombocytopenic purpura. *N. Engl. J. Med.* 308:1396, 1983.

Shahidi, N. T. Androgens and erythropoiesis. *N. Engl. J. Med.* 289:72, 1973.

Fibrocystic Breast Disease

Mansel, R. E., Wisbey, J. R., and Hughes, L. E. Controlled trial of the antigonadotropin danazol in painful nodular benign breast disease. *Lancet* 1:928, 1982.

Endometriosis

Barbieri, R. L., Canick, J. A., Makris, A., et al. Danazol inhibits steroidogenesis. *Fertil. Steril.* 28:809, 1977.

Biberoglu, K. O., and Behrman, S. J. Dosage aspects of danazol therapy in endometriosis: short-term and long-term effectiveness. *Am. J. Obstet. Gynecol.* 139:645, 1981.

Greenblatt, R. B., Dmowski, W. P., Mahesh, V. B., and Scholer, H. F. L. Clinical studies with an antigonadotropin—danazol. *Fertil. Steril.* 22:102, 1971.

Olive, D. L., and Haney, A. F. Endometriosis-associated infertility: a critical review of therapeutic approaches. *Obstet. Gynecol. Surv.* 41:538, 1986.

Seibel, M. M., Berger, M. J., Weinstein, F. G., and Taymor, M. L. The effectiveness of danazol on subsequent fertility in minimal endometriosis. *Fertil. Steril.* 38:534, 1982.

Lichen Sclerosus

Friedrich, E. G., Jr., and Kalra, P. S. Serum levels of sex hormones in vulvar lichen sclerosus, and the effect of topical testosterone. *N. Engl. J. Med.* 310:488, 1984.

Friedrich, E. G., Jr. Lichen sclerosus. *J. Reprod. Med.* 17:147, 1976.

Zelle, K. Treatment of vulvar dystrophies with topical testosterone propionate. *Am. J. Obstet. Gynecol.* 109:570, 1971.

Contraindications and Precautions

Duck, S. C., and Katayama, K. P. Danazol may cause female pseudohermaphroditism. *Fertil. Steril.* 35:230, 1981.

Suchowshy, G. K., Turolla, E., and Arcari, G. Studies of the so-called virilizing effects of steroids in female rat fetuses. *Endocrinology* 80:255, 1967.

Wardle, P. G., Whitehead, M. I., and Mills, R. P. Nonreversible and wide ranging vocal changes after treatment with danazol. *Br. Med. J.* 287:946, 1983.

Adverse Reactions

Barbieri, R. L., Evans, S., and Kistner, R. W. Danazol in the treatment of endometriosis: analysis of 100 cases with a 4-year follow-up. *Fertil. Steril.* 37:737, 1982.

ANTIANDROGENS

Antiandrogens are those compounds that exert androgen antagonism by interfering with the intracellular androgen receptor and blocking the biologic effect of the androgen as discussed already. Cyproterone acetate and cimetidine are examples of antiandrogens that block the end organ androgen receptor. Other groups of drugs that interfere with androgen synthesis may retard androgenic effects by decreasing the levels of androgens available for biologic effect. For example, estrogen will decrease testicular secretion of testosterone and result in decreased virilization and maintenance of secondary sex characteristics.

Antiandrogens are used in patients who display androgen excess. Females manifest high levels of androgens in a spectrum of clinical virilization beginning with hirsutism. As the androgen levels become higher for longer periods of time, temporal balding, voice deepening, decreased breast size, increased muscle mass, loss of female body contours, clitoral enlargement, and amenorrhea become evident. After a careful search to rule out an androgen-producing tumor, therapy with antiandrogens may be initiated to reverse the hirsutism and virilization.

Androgen excess in the male is a more difficult diagnosis to make. Males can have androgen-producing tumors that must be ruled out, but therapy with antiandrogens is seldom necessary and may interfere with normal function. One arguable indication for antiandrogens in the male is in the sex offender. Rapists and other convicted sex offenders have been treated with antiandrogens to alter their sexual obsessions and aggression.

Practically, the only primary indication for antiandrogens is hirsutism. The concomitant treatment of acne is a benefit of such therapy.

PHARMACOLOGY

Androgenic steroids with a modified A or B ring have potent antiandrogenic activity. These compounds displace androgens from their cellular receptors, from human SHBG, and also inhibit 5-α reductase. Despite binding to the androgen receptor, these compounds have no biologic androgen effect. Potent antiandrogens with a phenanthrene nucleus and steroid structure, such as cyproterone acetate, interfere with the translation of the DHT-receptor complex in the nucleus of androgen responsive cells.

Spironolactone, also a synthetic steroid, is a diuretic and specific aldosterone antagonist with antiandrogenic properties. The drug interferes with the action of DHT at the end organ, particularly the pilosebaceous unit on the hair follicle. In addition, spironolactone interferes with androgen production by inhibiting the enzyme, 17-α hydroxylase.

A chemically dissimilar compound, cimetidine, is a specific H_2 antihistamine that also has antiandrogenic properties. The drug blocks androgen action by binding to the androgen receptors at the target tissue.

INDICATIONS

Hirsutism

Spironolactone and cyproterone acetate have been shown to be of benefit in preventing further hair growth in hirsute women by converting terminal to vellus hair and decreasing acne. This effect has been duplicated in several studies and is independent of the concentration of endogenous androgens. Cimetidine has also been used to treat hirsute women with similar success. Most patients require 3 to 6 months of therapy before seeing a diminution in hirsutism. The effect of antiandrogen therapy is reversed once the drug is stopped.

Acne

Essentially all reports that examine the effectiveness of antiandrogens on hirsutism also inquire about the effect on acne. The results are usually parallel. However, other drugs such as antibiotics and topical treatment are used as first-line therapy for acne. Therefore, treatment of acne remains a benefit to antiandrogen therapy rather than a primary indication.

Precocious Puberty

Antiandrogens have also been used to inhibit precocious puberty. Although they may retard the growth of secondary sex characteristics, they have not been shown to alter the adult height significantly. In general, they have been replaced by GnRH analogues for this indication.

Deviant Sexual Behavior

Males who are convicted of rape, incest, and other maladaptive sexual behavior have been treated with cyproterone acetate in an attempt to medically castrate them and perhaps prevent such behavior. The results are difficult to assess because of the intricacies of human behavior and this indication for the use of antiandrogens is widely debated by psychoanalysts.

CONTRAINDICATIONS, PRECAUTIONS, AND WARNINGS

Antiandrogens should not be administered during pregnancy. They may cause male pseudohermaphroditism or ambiguous genitalia in developing fetuses if they are taken in high doses at the time of genital embryogenesis.

Antiandrogens that decrease the production of androgens by interfering with enzymes necessary for the synthesis of androgens will also decrease the production of estrogen. Androgens are an important estrogen precursor, so any decrease in their production will obviously be reflected in a decrease in estrogen production. In the female, this may influence estrogen maintenance functions such as menstruation.

Each antiandrogen has side effects and precautions peculiar to that particular class of drugs. For example, if spironolactone is chosen for use as an antiandrogen, its diuretic effect is then considered a side effect of antiandrogen therapy.

METABOLIC EFFECTS, ALTERED LABORATORY VALUES, AND DRUG INTERACTIONS

The systemic effect of antiandrogens is different for each drug. As a direct aldosterone antagonist, spironolactone may cause electrolyte disturbances, particularly in patients with hepatic or renal disease. Hyperkalemia, hyperchloremic metabolic acidosis, hyponatremia, and transient elevations of blood urea nitrogen can occur in patients with these disorders.

Spironolactone may potentiate the effect of other diuretics and antihypertensives. Reduced vascular responsiveness to norepinephrine caused by spironolactone warrants caution during anesthetic administration. In addition, spironolactone has been shown to prolong the half-life of digoxin.

Cimetidine does not significantly change plasma levels of androgens. The drug has been reported to interfere with the hepatic metabolism of warfarin-type anticoagulants, phenytoin, propranolol, chlordiazepoxide, diazepam, lidocaine, theophylline, and metronidazole, thereby increasing blood levels of these drugs.

Cyproterone acetate does not affect the concentrations of plasma testosterone, DHEA, and androstenedione but has been associated with severe adrenal insufficiency.

ADVERSE REACTIONS

Cyproterone acetate, which is not available in the United States for clinical use, has been shown to cause adrenal insufficiency and loss of libido. Thus, the clinical use of this drug is limited. Adverse reactions that occur soon after starting the drug, such as lethargy, depression, and an increased appetite, diminish with time.

Cimetidine has been associated with transient forgetfulness, dizziness, and nausea. Reversible alopecia is a rare side effect of the drug.

Gynecomastia is a recognized side effect of spironolactone. Agranulocytosis has been reported in patients taking the drug. The drug may also cause cramping and diarrhea, drowsiness, lethargy, headache, urticaria, mental confusion, drug fever, ataxia, impotence, irregular menses, or amenorrhea. Adverse reactions are usually reversible on discontinuation of the drug.

ADMINISTRATION

Pregnancy should be carefully ruled out prior to beginning antiandrogen therapy. History, physical examination, and laboratory tests should be geared to detecting the presence of an androgen-secreting tumor or adrenal dysfunction, including Cushing's syndrome and late-onset congenital adrenal hyperplasia. As part of the initial evaluation, serum levels of testosterone and DHEA-S should be obtained. In general, a serum testosterone level of less than 200 ng/dl and a DHEA-S level of less than 700 μg/dl make the presence of an androgen-secreting tumor unlikely.

Oral contraceptives may be used either alone or in combination with antiandrogens if fertility is not desired. Oral contraceptives have an inherent antiandrogen effect because of the increase in SHBG levels and subsequent decrease in free testosterone levels, and are often used as first-line therapy. Antiandrogens can then be given if oral contraceptives are ineffective. Other options including electrolysis, hair bleaching, and shaving should be discussed with the patient before therapy is administered.

ANTIANDROGEN PREPARATIONS

Cyproterone acetate. Not available in the United States but readily available as DIANE in Mexico.

Spironolactone. Supplied: Spironolactone, U.S.P. (Lerderle, Parke-Davis, Zenith, Generic), 25-mg tablets; Aldactone (Searle), 25-mg, 50-mg, and 100-mg tablets.

Cimetidine. Supplied: Tagament (Smith Kline & French), 200-mg, 300-mg, 400-mg, and 800-mg tablets; 300 mg/5 ml of liquid.

PROTOCOLS

Spironolactone, 100 mg, is administered orally twice daily. Cimetidine, 300 mg, is administered orally five times per day. Cyproterone acetate, 50 to 200 mg per day is administered orally. (When used for hirsutism, the drug is often combined with 10 and 50 μg of ethinyl estradiol to provide adequate contraception.)

BIBLIOGRAPHY

Pharmacology

Funder, J. W., and Mercer, J. E. Cimetidine, a histamine H_2 receptor antagonist occupies androgen receptors. *J. Clin. Endocrinol. Metab.* 48:189, 1979.

Menard, R. H., Stripp, B., and Gillette, J. R. Spironolactone and testicular cytochrome P-450: decreased testosterone formation in several species and changes in hepatic drug metabolism. *Endocrinology* 94:1628, 1974.

Starka, L., Hampl, R., Bicikova, M., et al. Steroids with modified ring A or B: screening for potential antiandrogenic and synandrogenic activity. *J. Steroid Biochem.* 13:455, 1980.

Tezon, J. G., Vazquez, M. H., and Blaquier, J. A. Androgen-controlled subcellular distribution of its receptor in the rat epididymis: 5α-dihydrotestosterone-induced translocation is blocked by antiandrogens. *Endocrinology* 111:2039, 1982.

Indications

Hirsutism

Ebling, F. J., Thomas, A. K., Cooke, I. D., et al. Effect of cyproterone acetate on hair growth sebaceous secretion and endocrine parameters in a hirsute subject. *Br. J. Dermatol.* 97:371, 1977.

Frolich, M., Vader, H. L., Walma, S. T., and De Rooy, H. A. M. The influence of long-term treatment with cyproterone acetate or a cyproterone acetate-ethinyl oestradiol combination on androgen levels in blood of hirsute women. *J. Steroid Biochem.* 12:499, 1980.

Jones, K. R., Katz, M., Keyzer, C., and Gordon, W. Effect of cyproterone acetate on rate of hair growth in hirsute females. *Br. J. Dermatol.* 105:685, 1981.

Peereboom-Wynia, J. D. R., and Boekhorst, J. C. Effect of cyproterone acetate orally on hair density and diameter and endocrine factors in women with idiopathic hirsutism. *Dermatologica* 160:7, 1980.

Shapiro, G., and Evron, S. A novel use of spironolactone: treatment of hirsutism. *J. Clin. Endocrinol. Metab.* 51:429, 1980.

Vigersky, R. A., Mehlman, I., Glass, A. R., and Smith, C. E. Treatment of hirsute women with cimetidine. *N. Engl. J. Med.* 303:1042, 1980.

Adverse Reactions

Hammerstein, J., Meckies, J., Leo-Rossberg, I., et al. Use of cyproterone acetate (CPA) in the treatment of acne, hirsutism and virilism. *J. Steroid Biochem.* 6:827, 1975.

Savage, D. C. L., and Swift, P. G. F. Effect of cyproterone acetate on adrenocortical function in children with precocious puberty. *Arch. Dis. Child.* 56:218, 1981.

6

Gonadotropins and Gonadotropin-Releasing Factors

Bert Scoccia and Antonio Scommegna

GONADOTROPINS

The gonadotropins comprise a class of glycoprotein hormones that originate either in the pituitary (luteinizing hormone [LH] and follicle-stimulating hormone [FSH]) or in the placenta (chorionic gonadotropin [hCG]).

The pituitary gonadotropins are responsible for ovarian follicular recruitment and growth, and for the initiation of ovulation. In the ovary, FSH acts primarily on granulosa cells to stimulate estrogen synthesis and follicular development. The preovulatory surge of LH, on the other hand, is important in follicular rupture and luteinization.

The placental glycoprotein hormone hCG is biologically and immunologically similar to pituitary LH. hCG is used therapeutically in place of LH because of its longer half-life and ease of isolation from the urine of pregnant women.

PHYSIOLOGY

Pituitary secretion of gonadotropin is controlled by the pulsatile release of gonadotropin-releasing hormone (GnRH) from the hypothalamus. Peaks of gonadotropin secretion occur approximately every 60 to 100 minutes. Both LH and FSH are synthesized by the same gonadotropic cell in the pituitary, which has GnRH cell surface receptors.

The release of gonadotropins is modulated by ovarian hormones (steroidal and nonsteroidal) that act on the hypothalamus or the pituitary, or both. In the follicular phase of the menstrual cycle, ovarian follicles produce increasing amounts of estrogen that feedback centrally on the pituitary and hypothalamus, resulting in an increased gonadotropin pulse frequency and decreased pulse amplitude. The midcycle gonadotropin surge is due to a positive feedback effect of estrogens on the pituitary that results in the preovulatory surge of both LH and FSH. During the luteal phase the increased secretion of progesterone from the luteinized granulosa and theca cells of the corpus luteum results in a decreased frequency of gonadotropin pulses and an increased pulse amplitude. These latter changes may be mediated by the endogenous opiate peptides (endorphins) through GnRH control.

Secretion of FSH is also regulated by a separate mechanism that involves inhibin, a peptide produced by the granulosa cell of the ovary. Its effect is mainly on secretion of FSH.

The action of the gonadotropins in the ovary is mediated by cell surface receptors that utilize cyclic adenosine monophosphate (cAMP) as second messenger to stimulate conversion of cholesterol to pregnenolone and induce sex steroid biosynthesis. FSH, by stimulating FSH receptors in granulosa cells, induces granulosa cell aromatase activity and preantral follicle growth. On the other hand, receptors for LH/hCG are present initially only in the theca cells. Later, in the follicular phase, the synergistic action of estradiol and

FSH induces granulosa cell LH/hCG receptors in the preovulatory antral follicles as well. Stimulation of LH/hCG receptors results in the synthesis of androgens utilized as precursors of follicular estrogens. In addition, LH/hCG receptors in the corpus luteum mediate LH-induced progesterone secretion after ovulation.

hCG originates in the embryonic syncytiotrophoblast as early as 7 days after ovulation (i.e., 1 day after implantation). Its production increases rapidly, peaking at 9 to 10 weeks from the last menstrual period (LMP). At that time hCG secretion begins to decrease and remains at low levels for the remainder of pregnancy. The role of hCG in early pregnancy is to prevent the corpus luteum involution and maintain its function until the time of the luteoplacental shift in steroid production (i.e., 8–10 weeks from LMP). The mechanism of action of hCG involves binding to cell surface LH/hCG receptors in the corpus luteum and activating the cAMP second messenger that initiates a cascade of steroid production.

PHARMACOLOGY

The gonadotropins LH, FSH, and hCG, together with thyroid-stimulating hormone (TSH), comprise a family of structurally similar glycosylated hormones. They are all heterodimers of two noncovalently linked subunits. The alpha subunit has a common sequence of 89 (LH and FSH) or 92 (hCG) amino acids. The beta subunit is unique to each hormone and confers receptor-binding specificity. FSH- and LH-beta subunits contain 115 amino acids. The beta subunit of hCG has 145 amino acids. The carbohydrate content of each hormone is inversely related to the metabolic clearance (LH [16%] $<$ FSH [18%] $<$ hCG [31%]). The clearance time for LH, FSH, and hCG from the circulation is 30 minutes, 1 hour, and 8 hours, respectively. The gonadotropic hormones are effective only when given by injection.

INDICATIONS

Gonadotropin therapy is indicated only for the purpose of achieving pregnancy.

Anovulation

Women who are unresponsive to maximum doses of clomiphene citrate or who have severe side effects from use of antiestrogens are candidates for ovulation induction using human menopausal gonadotropins (hMG) or urofollitropin (hFSH). The use of hMG/hFSH should be undertaken only when facilities for daily ultrasonography and rapid estradiol (E_2) radioimmunoassay (RIA) are readily available. Patients should first undergo a thorough endocrine and infertility evaluation, including laparoscopy, to rule out conditions that would not respond to gonadotropin therapy or that should be treated by other modalities.

Overall results of hMG/hFSH therapy in anovulatory patients are: ovulation, 61 to 77 percent; pregnancy, 22 to 24 percent; abortions, 15 to 25 percent; multiple pregnancies, 14 to 28 percent (twins, 9–18%; 3 babies or more, 5–10%); ovarian hyperstimulation syndrome, 2 percent; and fetal abnormalities, 1.7 percent.

Polycystic Ovary Syndrome

The polycystic ovary syndrome is characterized by a fixed elevation of LH and a relative suppression of FSH, which result in an increased ratio of LH to FSH. The altered gonadotropin secretion results in theca-cell hyperplasia and hyperandrogenism, arrested follicular development, and impaired estradiol production, which, over time, leads to multiple ovarian cyst formation and impaired ovulation. In addition, relative insulin resistance and mild hypersecretion of prolactin are common in polycystic ovary syndrome.

Patients with polycystic ovary syndrome who are oligomenorrheic should first undergo a trial of clomiphene citrate to induce ovulation, with careful monitoring because of the increased incidence of hyperstimulation syndrome in these patients. When such a regimen fails, these patients become candidates for ovulation induction with hFSH. Unlike hMG, hFSH should provide a more balanced gonadotropin-induced folliculogenesis under conditions of an increased endogenous LH-FSH ratio. Overall results of hFSH therapy in patients with polycystic ovary syndrome are: ovulation, 88 percent; pregnancy, 30 percent; abortions, 25 percent; multiple pregnancies, 17 percent; and hyperstimulation syndrome, 6 percent. Patients with polycystic ovary syndrome are prone to hyperstimulation, and facilities for daily ultrasonography and rapid E_2 assays are mandatory for safe monitoring of these patients.

Another method of ovulation induction in patients with polycystic ovary syndrome has been the down-regulation of pituitary secretion of LH using superactive analogues of GnRH, followed by ovarian stimulation with hMG. Overall results of this therapy in 33 cycles (8 women) were: 94 percent of cycles were ovulatory, and there was a 15 percent pregnancy rate per cycle; there were 5 pregnancies, no abortions, and 1 multiple gestation (triplet); hyperstimulation occurred in all 5 pregnancy cycles. Because of the high rate of hyperstimulation, this regimen should be reserved for patients with polycystic ovary syndrome in whom the follicles fail to stimulate with hFSH or who undergo premature luteinization during hFSH therapy. In these patients, during the luteal phase tonic ovarian support by endogenous gonadotropin is impaired; thus, support with progesterone or hCG is indicated. Progesterone in oil in doses of 25 to 50 mg per day is preferred over hCG, again to decrease the possibility of hyperstimulation.

Hypogonadotropic Hypogonadism

Hypoestrogenic women with hypothalamic or pituitary failure respond rapidly to hMG. Although these patients will also respond to hFSH alone, the response to hMG (LH and FSH) is more pronounced and leads to more physiologic follicular maturation. This points to a beneficial effect of LH, in addition to FSH, during ovarian follicular stimulation. Pretreatment with sequential estrogen-progestin combination for 1 or 2 cycles "primes" the endometrium and may result in a better response to hMG. Because tonic ovarian stimulation by pituitary gonadotropin is absent in these patients, luteal phase support with either progesterone or hCG is indicated.

Assisted Reproductive Technology

Assisted reproductive technology (ART) encompasses the various modalities of advanced reproductive therapy available to assist couples achieve a pregnancy. ART includes in vitro fertilization and embryo transfer (IVF-ET), gamete intrafallopian transfer (GIFT), zygote intrafallopian transfer (ZIFT), and other modalities of zygote or gamete transfer.

Success in ART is positively correlated with the number of oocytes retrieved and the number of embryos transferred. This finding has led to the use of multiple regimens of ovarian stimulation, and hMG or hFSH therapy achieves similar numbers of oocytes retrieved per aspiration, fertilization rates, embryos cleaved and transferred, and pregnancies per embryo transfer. However, ovarian stimulation with hFSH results in fewer cancelled cycles and fewer immature oocytes retrieved. The rationale behind the use of hFSH alone in ART is that increased levels of hFSH should result in improved follicular recruitment in those patients with intact endogenous basal LH secretion.

A modification of the stimulation regimens just mentioned involves the combined use of hMG and hFSH early in the cycle, followed by hMG alone until the time of ovulation induction with hCG (hFSH-boost protocol). This manipulation of the LH-FSH ratio in an ovulation-inducing protocol favors the latter, and, theoretically, should result in improved follicular recruitment and development. In practice, this protocol results in a trend toward low cancellation rates, short duration of gonadotropin administration, improved pregnancy per embryo transfer, and increased viable pregnancies per embryo transfer.

A combination of clomiphene citrate and hMG is also frequently used in ovulation induction in ART. Theoretically, this regimen should result in optimal follicular development when compared with a single agent (hMG or hFSH). However, in practice, combined clomiphene citrate–hMG therapy results in similar rates of follicular development, oocyte recovery, embryo transfer, and pregnancy as in the hMG or hFSH protocols. Moreover, the clomiphene citrate–hMG protocol in ART precludes the use of long-acting GnRH analogues for pituitary desensitization in combination with hMG for ovarian stimulation.

The most recent modification of ovarian stimulation for ART involves the use of long-acting analogues of GnRH for pituitary desensitization and endogenous gonadotropin suppression, followed by ovarian stimulation with exogenous hMG. This protocol has the advantage of eliminating endogenous LH surges, and therefore, decreasing the number of cycles cancelled. The GnRH agonist is usually started in the midluteal phase of the menstrual cycle preceding ovarian stimulation. At this time follicle recruitment and selection have not yet taken place. Therefore, the initial agonistic effect of the GnRH analogue is not as prominent. Patients should be warned to use barrier contraception during the cycle preceding ART therapy to avoid the administration of GnRH in a possibly fertile cycle. At the time of menses, when complete pituitary suppression is achieved, as evidenced by low ovarian secretion of E_2 (<20 pg), the GnRH analogue dose is reduced and hMG is added and continued until the time of ovulation induction. The GnRH analogue is stopped along with the hMG on the day of ovulation induction with hCG. The luteal phase must be supported with either progesterone or hCG supplementation, because of the diminished endogenous gonadotropin support of the corpus luteum after the follicular phase pituitary desensitization. Use of this protocol has resulted in increased pregnancy rates without cycle cancellations due to premature ovulation. However, larger doses of hMG for a longer time are necessary to achieve adequate ovarian stimulation. The exact mechanism of this relative resistance of the ovary to stimulation after pituitary desensitization with GnRH agonist is not known. Possible explanations include lack of preantral follicles at the time of the hMG administration because of the downregulation of endogenous gonadotropins or the possible release of pituitary gonadotropin isoforms (nonglycosylated, bio-inactive FSH), which then bind to ovarian LH and FSH receptors and interfere with hMG ovarian stimulation. This, indeed, is the case during use of GnRH antagonists for pituitary desensitization.

Unexplained Infertility

A new and still controversial indication for ovarian gonadotropin stimulation involves patients with long-standing infertility of unknown cause. These patients should first undergo a complete infertility evaluation, including laparoscopy, and specialized tests such as the sperm penetration assay and serum antisperm antibodies. Theoretically, controlled ovarian stimulation with hMG in conjunction with intrauterine inseminations with washed semen should increase the monthly probability of pregnancy. Preliminary reports have established cycle fecundity rates of 19 percent for unexplained infertility, 17 percent for endometriosis, and 29 percent for cervical factor infertility. These results are comparable to those obtained during in vitro fertilization, and, perhaps, this approach can be considered in patients with long-standing infertility and at least one patent tube who are approaching ART as a final therapeutic option.

Timed Initiation of Ovulation

The therapeutic use of hCG relies on the similarity of biologic activity to LH. Controlled ovarian stimulation with hMG and hFSH includes the use of hCG to trigger follicular rupture when the follicle reaches maturity according to ultrasound and E_2 RIA criteria. The minimum dose of hCG to induce ovulation is 5000 U and, more commonly, 10,000 U of hCG is used. During ovarian stimulation with clomiphene citrate, if the patient fails to ovulate on a dose of 100 mg for 5 days, and has good cervical mucus and a mature follicle (≥18–20 mm) as demonstrated by ultrasound, then hCG, 10,000 U, can be given to trigger ovulation. However, if hCG is given too early during folliculogenesis, it may result in luteinization of the theca interna and degeneration of the tertiary follicles leading to inhibition or postponement of ovulation.

Luteal Phase Dysfunction

Inadequate endometrial response to postovulatory progesterone production in the corpus luteum results in recurrent abortions and infertility.

Luteal phase defects in patients unresponsive to progestin or clomiphene citrate therapy can be treated with gonadotropins. Use of gonadotropins is based on the finding of a relative deficiency in FSH, but not LH, during the early follicular phase of cycles, which are later found to have inadequate corpus luteum function. Therefore, hFSH has been used in the follicular phase in patients with luteal phase defects proved by examination of endometrial biopsy specimens. This treatment has resulted in improved endometrial maturation, normalization of the follicular phase length, increased luteal phase length, and cumulative pregnancy rates of 48 percent over 6 cycles.

hCG supports corpus luteum function by its direct steroidogenic effect. hCG therapy thus offers an alternative to exogenous progesterone supplementation in ART cycles, in stimulated cycles during pituitary desensitization with GnRH analogues, or in patients with hypothalamic or pituitary failure. In these cases, corpus luteum function may be adversely affected by altered pituitary gonadotropin tonic stimulation.

hCG therapy during the luteal phase may be given either as a single dose of 5000 U, 1 week after ovulation induction with 10,000 U, or multiple doses of 1000 to 2500 U every 3 days for 3 doses, after an ovulatory dose of 5000 U. These regimens should be closely monitored because of the possibility of triggering the ovarian hyperstimulation syndrome.

CONTRAINDICATIONS, WARNINGS, AND PRECAUTIONS

Gonadotropins should not be used in patients with primary ovarian failure as evidenced by high endogenous gonadotropin levels, because such patients will not respond. Patients with functional ovarian cysts or ovarian enlargement that is not due to polycystic ovarian syndrome should not be started on gonadotropin therapy until such cysts have resolved. Use during pregnancy is also contraindicated. Patients with thyroid, adrenal, or pituitary dysfunction should be thoroughly evaluated and abnormalities treated prior to stimulation with gonadotropins. Women with ovulatory dysfunction resulting from pituitary adenomas will respond to exogenous gonadotropin therapy. However, pituitary adenomas may increase in size during pregnancy with severely deleterious consequences. Thus, a serum prolactin level should be obtained in all women with menstrual irregularities prior to initiating gonadotropin therapy. If the serum prolactin level is elevated, pituitary adenoma should be excluded by appropriate imaging technique and alternative therapies considered (see Chap. 7). Finally, abnormal bleeding of undetermined origin is a contraindication to use of gonadotropins. Facilities for daily monitoring by ultrasonography and E_2 RIA should be readily available 7 days a week to adequately follow patients stimulated with gonadotropins.

METABOLIC EFFECTS, ALTERED LABORATORY VALUES, AND DRUG INTERACTIONS

Gonadotropin administration results in ovarian production of hormones, especially estrogen during the follicular phase and progesterone during the luteal phase. The rise in endogenous estrogens during the follicular phase produces characteristic changes in vaginal smears leading to predominance of superficial cells. In addition, the cervical mucus increases in volume, elasticity, and ferning. After ovulation, with the formation of the corpus luteum, vaginal smears show increased parabasal cells, the cervical mucus becomes more viscous, and beading is present. There are no known drug interactions attributed to the gonadotropins.

ADVERSE REACTIONS

Common side effects seen in patients treated with gonadotropins are: ovarian enlargement, skin irritation at the injection site, gastrointestinal symptoms (nausea, vomiting, diarrhea, and bloating), headaches, and breast tenderness, most likely related to the increased ovarian hormones. More serious side effects include: sensitivity reactions (fever, chills, musculoskeletal pain, and malaise), multiple pregnancies (overall incidence, 2–41%; twins, 2–3%; 3 babies or more, 0–10%), and ovarian hyperstimulation syndrome (0.1–2.0% incidence).

Ovarian hyperstimulation syndrome is characterized by sudden symptomatic ovarian enlargement and increased vacular permeability secondary to abnormally elevated levels of E_2. The resulting third-spacing of fluid causes ascites, pleural effusions (0.4–1.3%), hemoconcentration, decreased renal perfusion, and increased weight. In addition, the ovarian enlargement can lead to rupture and massive hemoperitoneum. Also, increased blood hypercoagulability may lead to thrombotic accidents.

Mild to moderate ovarian hyperstimulation syndrome occurs in as many as 20 percent of patients treated with gonadotropins or hCG and regresses spontaneously within 2 or 3 weeks. These patients usually develop weight gain, abdominal distension, and abdominal pain.

Severe ovarian hyperstimulation syndrome develops rapidly over 3 to 4 days during the 2-week period immediately following gonadotropin or hCG-induced ovulation. Patients should be hospitalized and monitored for increasing ascites, abdominal girth, weight gain, and pleural effusions. Fluid input and output should be closely followed. Pelvic examination should be avoided to prevent ovarian rupture and hemoperitoneum, and, instead, pelvic ultrasonography should be used. Laboratory monitoring should include: serial hematocrits, serum and urinary electrolyte determinations, coagulation profile, serum osmolality, and urine specific gravity. Treatment is primarily geared to relieving symptoms and involves: bed rest, analgesics, and initial fluid and electrolyte replacement followed by fluid restriction to allow for third-space fluid resorption. The ascitic fluid should never be removed because of possible injury to the ovary. If ovarian cyst rupture occurs with hemoperitoneum, conservative surgery with partial resection of the ovary is usually adequate. In order to avoid ovarian hyperstimulation syndrome the ovulatory dose of hCG should be withheld if the E_2 level is greater than 2000 pg/ml and multiple small (diameter <10 mm) follicles are present in addition to the larger, leading follicles.

There are no known teratogenic effects with the use of gonadotropins.

ADMINISTRATION

Patients who are candidates for gonadotropin stimulation should first undergo a thorough infertility evaluation. In addition, facilities for ultrasonography and rapid E_2 RIA monitoring should be readily available to avoid some of the major adverse reactions of gonadotropin therapy.

GONADOTROPIN PREPARATIONS

All available gonadotropin preparations are obtained from the urine of postmenopausal (hMG, hFSH) or pregnant (hCG) women. The manufacturing process for the three gonadotropin products uses several chemical and physical methods that are known to inactivate human immunodeficiency virus (HIV), as well as other viruses. Recombinant DNA technology may soon supply unlimited quantities of the gonadotropins; however, these preparations are still experimental and not commercially available.

Human menopausal gonadotropin (Pergonal [Serono]) is supplied in ampules containing lyophilized LH (75 IU) and FSH (75 IU).

An ampule of sodium chloride diluent is provided. It is also supplied in vials containing 150 IU of LH and 150 IU of FSH per vial. The approximate cost per ampule (75 IU LH/75 IU FSH) is $30 to $40.

hMG is easily dissolved in the sodium chloride solution, and as many as four ampules of powder (300 IU LH, 300 IU FSH) can be dissolved in as little as 2 ml of diluent. hMG is well absorbed after intramuscular injection and the peak effect of activity, reflected by elevated E_2 levels as determined by RIA, occurs 12 to 14 hours after injection. The starting dose of hMG is 1 ampule (75 IU LH, 75 IU FSH) with dosage adjusted during the next 7 to 12 days prior to hCG administration.

Urofollitropin (Metrodin [Serono]) is supplied in lyophilized ampules containing 75 IU of FSH and less than 1 IU of LH per vial. An ampule of sodium chloride diluent is provided. The approximate cost per ampule is $40 to $50.

hFSH is rapidly dissolved and well absorbed after intramuscular injection. The starting dose is 1 ampule (75 IU FSH) to be adjusted over the next 7 to 12 days prior to hCG administration.

Chorionic gonadotropin (APL [Ayerst], chorionic gonadotropin [Quad], Pregnyl [Organon], Profasi [Serono]) is supplied in lyophilized multiple-dose vials with an accompanying 10-ml bacteriostatic water vial for dilution. Vials of 5000 U.S.P. U or 10,000 U.S.P. U per vial are available. The approximate cost per ampule for 10,000 U.S.P. U is $30 to $40 and for 5000 USP U, $15 to $25.

hCG is rapidly dissolved in as little as 2 ml of diluent and rapidly absorbed via intramuscular injection. Usual dose for ovulation induction is 5000 to 10,000 U.S.P. U given 1 day following the last dose of gonadotropins. If corpus luteum support is needed after ovulation, doses of 1250 to 2500 IU are given every 3 or 4 days.

PROTOCOLS

Standard Gonadotropin Protocol—Human Menopausal Gonadotropin or Urofollitropin*

1. Aim: Mature follicle(s) with good estradiol (E_2) production.
2. Definition
   a. Mature follicle is 18–25 mm in diameter as shown by ultrasound.
   b. Good E_2 production is 250–300 pg/ml per mature follicle.
3. Stimulation: Pergonal (hMG) *or* Metrodin (hFSH) is used.
4. Start: Day 2 or 3 of spontaneous cycle or of induced uterine bleeding. Measure E_2 and ultrasound in the morning (baseline studies). Give 2 ampules of hMG or hFSH in the afternoon for 4 days. (Patients with polycystic ovary syndrome should receive 1 ampule of hMG or hFSH in P.M. for 4 days.)
   a. Repeat E_2 determination and ultrasound 5 days later in the morning. If E_2 level is less than 3 times the baseline or less than 200 pg/ml, increase dose by 1 ampule.
   b. Recheck in 2 days if dosage is increased. Increase hMG or hFSH by 1 ampule until E_2 level equals more than 3 times the baseline level or more than 200 pg/ml. Continue at that dosage

* Not for assisted reproductive technology

(*effective dosage*). E_2 determinations and ultrasound should be done daily when E_2 level is 200 pg/ml or higher.
   c. hMG or hFSH dose should be omitted or decreased if the dominant follicle is larger than 10 mm but smaller than 16 mm and E_2 level is 1000 pg/ml or higher.
   d. When the leading follicle is 18 to 25 mm and no more than 3 mature follicles are present, give 10,000 U of hCG.
   e. Hold hCG if:
      (1) E_2 level is 2000 pg or higher
      (2) More than 3 mature follicles are present or 2 or 3 mature follicles and several midsized (14–16 mm) ones are present.
5. *Subsequent Cycle*: If the patient does not conceive, restart therapy at the next cycle at the effective dose level minus 1 ampule, but with at least 2 ampules (1 ampule in patients with polycystic ovary syndrome). Measure E_2 and do an ultrasound. Delay therapy if the E_2 level is higher than twice the baseline of the prior cycle.

Assisted Reproductive Technology Gonadotropin Protocol—Human Menopausal Gonadotropin or Urofollitropin

1. Aim: Multiple mature follicles with good estradiol (E_2) production.
2. End-point: Lead follicle is 18 mm or more in diameter and a secondary follicle is 16 mm or more. Additionally, there must be 4 or more follicles present with a minimum diameter of 10 mm on the day of hCG administration. The minimum E_2 level on day of hCG administration is 750 pg/ml.
3. Start on day 2 of a spontaneous cycle or of induced bleeding.
4. Measure baseline E_2 level and do ultrasound.
5. Dose: Give hMG or hFSH 4 ampules (300 IU) IM at 6:00 P.M. on cycle days 2 and 3. Follow with 2 ampules (150 IU) from day 4 on, until criteria are met.
6. Monitor daily E_2 levels and ultrasound beginning on day 6 and continuing through the day after hCG administration.
7. Reduce the dose if E_2 level is disproportionately high for follicular size and number ($E_2 > 2000$ pg/ml with follicles <14 mm); reduction of hMG or hFSH by 1 ampule (75 IU) must be carried out.
8. The dose is continued until criteria are met. If E_2 level exceeds 2000 pg/ml, give hCG that evening. If E_2 level is less than 2000 pg/ml on the day criteria are met, give hMG or hFSH for one additional day, then give hCG that evening.
9. hCG, 10,000 U IM, is given at 9:00 P.M., approximately 27 hours after the last hMG or hFSH dose.
10. Follicle aspiration: Planned 34 hours after hCG (7:00 A.M.)
11. Cancel cycle if there is:
    a. No follicular development or no estrogen increase after 5 days of hMG or hFSH
    b. A functional cyst (E_2 level is 150–200 pg/ml and "follicle," 20 mm in diameter, is detected on cycle day 6)
    c. A dominant follicle (single follicle reaches 20 mm without at least one other 16 mm)
    d. An unchanged estrogen level for 3 days or a decreasing level for 2 days during hMG or hFSH therapy
    e. Decreasing estrogen level after hCG administration

f. LH elevation (a twofold elevation of baseline LH associated with a decline in E_2 levels)
g. LH surge (plasma LH > 30 mIU/ml).

Note: LH is measured in all blood samples obtained for estrogen monitoring. The last blood sample is obtained immediately prior to hCG injection. All samples are stored frozen at −20°C and analyzed by a rapid radioimmunoassay at the same time, the day after hCG injection.

Assisted Reproductive Technology—GnRH Analogue (Lupron) and Human Menopausal Gonadotropin (Pergonal) Protocol

1. Aim: Endogenous gonadotropin suppression followed by exogenous gonadotropin stimulation to obtain multiple mature follicles.
2. End-point
   a. Complete ovarian suppression by Lupron prior to Pergonal-induced stimulation (i.e., estradiol (E_2) level < 20 pg/ml and no ovarian follicles or cysts as shown by ultrasound
   b. Pergonal stimulation to obtain lead follicle of 18-mm diameter or more and a secondary follicle of 16 mm or more. Additionally, there must be 4 or more follicles present with a minimum diameter of 12 mm on the day of hCG administration. The minimum E_2 level on day of hCG is 750 pg/ml.
3. Start Lupron 1 mg SQ daily, 10 days prior to expected menses of scheduled ART cycle. (*Patients should be instructed to use barrier contraception during the entire cycle preceding ART cycle if fallopian tubes are open.*)
4. Measure E_2 levels during menses or after 12 days, whichever occurs later. The E_2 level must be less than 20 pg/ml before stimulation with Pergonal is initiated. Continue Lupron suppression until E_2 is less than 20 pg/ml and ultrasonography confirms no follicles or cysts.
5. Add Pergonal, 3 ampules (225 IU) IM daily after E_2 is suppressed and resume E_2 and ultrasound monitoring after 5 doses.
6. Continue Lupron at a reduced dose of 0.5 mg SQ daily, along with Pergonal.
7. Monitor daily E_2 levels and ultrasound through the day after hCG administration.
8. If E_2 level is disproportionately high for follicular size and number (E_2 >2000 pg/ml with follicles <14 mm) reduction of Pergonal dose to 1 ampule (75 IU) must be carried out.
9. The dose is continued until criteria are met. Then, if E_2 level exceeds 2000 pg/ml, give hCG on that day. If E_2 level is less than 2000 pg/ml on the day criteria are met, give Pergonal for one additional day, then give hCG.
10. hCG, 10,000 U IM, is given at 9:00 P.M., approximately 27 hours after last Pergonal dose.
11. Follicle aspiration: Planned 34 hours after hCG (7:00 A.M.).
12. Cancel cycle if there is:
    a. No follicular development or no estrogen increase after 5 days of Pergonal
    b. A functional cyst (E_2 is 150–200 pg/ml and "follicle" 18 mm in diameter is detected on day 6 of Pergonal stimulation)
    c. A dominant follicle (single follicle reaches 18 mm without at least one other 14 mm)

d. An unchanged estrogen level for 3 days or a decreasing level for 2 days during Pergonal stimulation

Assisted Reproductive Technology–Clomiphene and Human Menopausal Gonadotropin Protocol

1. Determine baseline estradiol (E_2) level and ultrasound appearance.
2. Administer clomiphene, 100 mg, daily on days 2–6.
3. Give Pergonal (hMG), 2 ampules, IM at 6:00 P.M. daily starting day 2 for 4 days.
4. Daily monitor rapid E_2 levels beginning on day 6; do ultrasound daily beginning day 8 and continuing through day after hCG administration.
5. Reduce hMG dose to 1 ampule (75 IU) if E_2 level is disproportionately high for follicular size and number (E_2 >2000 pg/ml with follicles <14 mm).
6. Hold hMG when 2 follicles reach 18 mm on greatest diameter.
7. Give hCG, 10,000 U, IM at 9:00 P.M. when the above criteria are met (34 hours prior to planned aspiration).
8. There is no modification of this protocol if poor folliculogenesis results.
9. Cycle is cancelled if less than 2 adequate follicles develop by day 12 or if rapid LH at time of hCG administration approximates twice the baseline level or 30 mIU/ml. Also cancel cycle if dominant follicle or functional ovarian cysts are noted.

BIBLIOGRAPHY

Overview

Daughaday, W. H. The Anterior Pituitary. In J. D. Wilson and D. W. Foster (eds.), *Williams Textbook of Endocrinology* (7th ed.). Philadelphia: W. B. Saunders, 1985. Pp. 568–613.

Physiology

Auletta, F. J., and Flint, A. P. F. Mechanisms controlling corpus luteum function in sheep, cows, nonhuman primates, and women especially in relation to the time of luteolysis. *Endocr. Rev.* 9:88, 1988.

Fink, G. Gonadotropin Secretion and Its Control. In E. Knobil and J. Neill (eds.), *The Physiology of Reproduction*. New York: Raven Press, 1988. Pp. 1349–1377.

Goodman, A. L., and Hodgen, G. D. The ovarian triad of the primate menstrual cycle. *Recent Prog. Horm. Res.* 39:1, 1983.

Hodgen, G. D., Goodman, A. L., Stouffer, R. L., et al. Selection and Maturation of the Dominant Follicle and Its Ovum in the Menstrual Cycle. In H. M. Beier and H. R. Lindner (eds.), *Fertilization of the Human Egg In Vitro*. Berlin: Springer-Verlag, 1983. Pp. 57–69.

Karsch, F. J. Central actions of ovarian steroids in the feedback regulation of pulsatile secretion of luteinizing hormone. *Ann. Rev. Physiol.* 49:365, 1987.

Knobil, E., and Hotchkiss, J. The Menstrual Cycle and Its Neuroendocrine Control. In E. Knobil and J. Neill (eds.), *The Physiology of Reproduction*. New York: Raven Press, 1988. Pp. 1971–1994.

Ross, G. T. Disorders of the Ovary and Female Reproductive Tract. In J. D. Wilson and D. W. Foster (eds.), *Williams Textbook of Endocrinology* (7th ed.). Philadelphia: W. B. Saunders, 1985. Pp. 206–258.

Pharmacology

Harlin, J., Khan, S. A., and Diczfalusy, E. Molecular composition of luteinizing hormone and follicle-stimulating hormone in commercial gonadotropin preparations. *Fertil. Steril.* 46:1055, 1986.

Murad, F., and Haynes, Jr., R. C. Adenohypophyseal Hormones and Related Substances. In L. S. Goodman and A. G. Gilman (eds.), *The Pharmacological Basis of Therapeutics* (7th ed.). New York: MacMillan, 1985. Pp. 1362–1388.

Pierce, J. G. Gonadotropins: Chemistry and Biosynthesis. In E. Knobil and J. Neill (eds.), *The Physiology of Reproduction*. New York: Raven Press, 1988. Pp. 1335–1348.

Ryan, R. J., Keutmann, H. T., Charlesworth, M. C., et al. Structure-Function Relationships of Gonadotropins. *Recent Prog. Horm. Res.* 43:383, 1987.

Indications

Anovulation

Pepperell, R. J. A rational approach to ovulation induction. *Fertil. Steril.* 40:1, 1983.

Pergonal (menotropins for injection, USP). Package Insert. Randolph, Mass.: Serono Laboratories, 1986.

Polycystic Ovary Syndrome

Charbonnel, B., Krempf, M., Blanchard, P., et al. Induction of ovulation in polycystic ovary syndrome with a combination of a luteinizing hormone-releasing hormone analog and exogenous gonadotropins. *Fertil. Steril.* 47:920, 1987.

Claman, P., Seibel, M. M., McArdle, C., et al. Comparison of intermediate-dose purified urinary follicle-stimulating hormone with and without human chorionic gonadotropin for ovulation induction in polycystic ovarian disease. *Fertil. Steril.* 46:518, 1986.

McKenna, T. J. Pathogenesis and treatment of polycystic ovary syndrome. *N. Engl. J. Med.* 318:558, 1988.

Metrodin (urofollitropin for injection). Package Insert. Randolph, Mass.: Serono Laboratories, 1987.

Hypogonadotropic Hypogonadism

Couzinet, B., Lestrat, N., Brailly, S., et al. Stimulation of ovarian follicular maturation with pure follicle-stimulating hormone in women with gonadotropin deficiency. *J. Clin. Endocrinol. Metab.* 66:552, 1988.

Assisted Reproductive Technology

Awadalla, S. G., Friedman, C. I., Chin, N. W., et al. Follicular stimulation for *in vitro* fertilization using pituitary suppression and human menopausal gonadotropins. *Fertil. Steril.* 48:811, 1987.

Barnes, R. B., Scommegna, A., and Schreiber, J. R. Decreased ovarian response to human menopausal gonadotropin caused by subcutaneously administered gonadotropin-releasing hormone agonist. *Fertil. Steril.* 47:512, 1987.

Dahl, K. D., Bicsak, T. A., and Hsueh, A. J. W. Naturally occurring antihormones: secretion of FSH antagonists by women treated with a GnRH analog. *Science* 239:72, 1988.

de Ziegler, D., Cedars, M. I., Randle, D., et al. Suppression of the ovary using a gonadotropin releasing-hormone agonist prior to stimulation for oocyte retrieval. *Fertil. Steril.* 48:807, 1987.

Hill, G. A., Diamond, M. P., Maxson, W. S., et al. Combination clomiphene citrate/human menopausal gonadotropin stimulation protocols for *in vitro* fertilization-embryo transfer. *J In Vitro Fertil. Embryo Transfer* 4:34, 1987.

Meldrum, D. R., Wisot, A., Hamilton, F., et al. Timing of initiation and dose schedule of leuprolide influence the time course of ovarian suppression. *Fertil. Steril.* 50:400, 1988.

Navot, D., and Rosenwaks, Z. The use of follicle-stimulating hormone for controlled ovarian hyperstimulation in *in vitro* fertilization. *J In Vitro Fertil. Embryo Transfer* 5:3, 1988.

Scoccia, B., Blumenthal, P., Wagner, C., et al. Comparison of urinary human follicle-stimulating hormone and human menopausal gonadotropins for ovarian stimulation in an *in vitro* fertilization program. *Fertil. Steril.* 48:446, 1987.

Unexplained Infertility

Dodson, W. C., Whitesides, D. B., Hughes, Jr., C. L., et al. Superovulation with intrauterine insemination in the treatment of infertility: a possible alternative to gamete intrafallopian transfer and *in vitro* fertilization. *Fertil. Steril.* 48:441, 1987.

Kemmann, E., Bohrer, M., Shelden, R., et al. Active ovulation management increases the monthly probability of pregnancy occurrence in ovulatory women who receive intrauterine insemination. *Fertil. Steril.* 48:916, 1987.

Melis, G. B., Paoletti, A. M., Strigini, F., et al. Pharmacologic induction of multiple follicular development improves the success rate of artificial insemination with husband's semen in couples with male-related or unexplained infertility. *Fertil. Steril.* 47:441, 1987.

Welner, S., De Cherney, A. H., and Polan, M. L. Human menopausal gonadotropins: a justifiable therapy in ovulatory women with longstanding idiopathic infertility. *Am. J. Obstet. Gynecol.* 158:111, 1988.

Timed Initiation of Ovulation

Abdalla, H. I., Ah-Moye, M., Brinsden, P., et al. The effect of the dose of human chorionic gonadotropin and the type of gonadotropin stimulation on oocyte recovery rates in an *in vitro* fertilization program. *Fertil. Steril.* 48:958, 1987.

Friedrich, F., Kemeter, P., Salzer, H., et al. Ovulation inhibition with human chorionic gonadotrophin. *Acta Endocrinol. Scand.* 78:332, 1975.

Luteal Phase Dysfunction

Blumenfeld, Z., and Nahhas, F. Luteal dysfunction in ovulation induction: the role of repetitive human chorionic gonadotropin supplementation during the luteal phase. *Fertil. Steril.* 50:403, 1988.

Lee, C. S. Luteal phase defects. *Obstet. Gynecol. Surv.* 42:267, 1987.

Minassian, S. S., Wu, C. H., Groll, M., et al. Urinary follicle stimulating hormone treatment for luteal phase defect. *J. Reprod. Med.* 33:11, 1988.

Adverse Effects

Blankstein, J., Shalev, J., Saadon, T., et al. Ovarian hyperstimulation syndrome: prediction by number and size of preovulatory ovarian follicles. *Fertil. Steril.* 47:597, 1987.

Haning, Jr., R. V., Strawn, E. Y., and Nolten, W. E. Pathophysiology of the ovarian hyperstimulation syndrome. *Obstet. Gynecol.* 66:220, 1985.
Scialli, A. R. The reproductive toxicity of ovulation induction. *Fertil. Steril.* 45:315, 1986.

ENHANCED ENDOGENOUS GONADOTROPIN SECRETION BY ANTIESTROGENIC COMPOUNDS AND OPIOID ANTAGONIST

ANTIESTROGENIC COMPOUNDS

An understanding of the regulatory role that ovarian steroid hormones play on gonadotropin release has led to the use of compounds that enhance gonadotropin secretion. One such compound is clomiphene citrate, an antiestrogen with weak estrogenic activity. This drug inhibits or modifies the action of estrogen on the hypothalamo-pituitary-ovarian axis by binding to estrogen receptors, competing for estrogen-binding sites. Thus, it prevents the normal "feedback inhibition," resulting in increased hypothalamic release of GnRH, increased pituitary gonadotropin secretion, and increased ovarian stimulation.

Physiology

The antiestrogens are nonsteroidal compounds with structural similarities to the estrogen diethylstilbestrol. The mechanism of action of antiestrogens involves displacement of estrogen from estrogen receptor–binding proteins in the hypothalamo-pituitary-ovarian axis, leading to decreased negative feedback of endogenous estrogen. This results in enhanced hypothalamic GnRH pulse generator activity, increased pituitary gonadotropin secretion, augmented follicular recruitment, and sustained corpus luteum function. The two antiestrogenic compounds available in the United States for clinical use are clomiphene citrate and tamoxifen. Both are triphenyl-ethylene derivatives. Only clomiphene citrate is approved by the Food and Drug Administration (FDA) for ovulation induction.

Pharmacology

Chemical initiation of ovulation via enhancement of gonadotropin secretion early in the follicular phase of the menstrual cycle can be accomplished with nonsteroidal antiestrogens, such as clomiphene citrate. Structurally, clomiphene citrate is a triphenyl-ethylene derivative. It is supplied as a racemic mixture of stereochemical isomers labeled as enclomiphene (*trans* form), and zuclomiphene (*cis* form), making up 62 percent and 38 percent, respectively. It appears that the cis isomer is responsible for the ovulation-inducing properties of this compound.

Clomiphene citrate is readily absorbed orally, is metabolized via the enterohepatic circulation, and is excreted in the feces. An average of 51 percent of radiolabeled drug is excreted in the feces after 5 days, with small amounts recovered up to 6 weeks after dosing. The estimated half-life of clomiphene citrate is between 5 and 7 days.

Indications

Anovulation

Clomiphene citrate is the agent of choice for induction of ovulation in women with normo- (or inappropriate) gonadotropic, normoprolactinemic anovulation. Patients should first undergo a basic infertility and endocrine evaluation, and they should have adequate endogenous estrogen production, as evidenced by progestin withdrawal. Clomiphene citrate is given in the early follicular phase (beginning day 5 of the menstrual cycle) at a starting dose of 50 mg (1 tablet) and continuing for 5 days. Ovulation occurs 5 to 10 days after the last tablet of clomiphene citrate is taken (average of 7 days). If started earlier than day 5 of the cycle, clomiphene therapy may result in recruitment of additional follicles with possible increase in multiple gestations; if started later than day 5, ovulation may be delayed. If ovulation does not occur, the dose can be further increased by 50 mg each cycle, up to 250 mg daily for 5 days. However, doses higher than 100 mg daily for 5 days are associated with small increments in the conception rate and increased side effects. When the ovulatory dose is reached, no further changes in the dosage are required. Results of clomiphene-induced ovulation are: ovulation, 50 to 94 percent; pregnancies, 22 to 61 percent; abortions, 0.2 to 26.0 percent; multiple pregnancies, 0 to 33 percent (twins, 10%; 3 babies or more, <1%); and congenital abnormalities, 2.5 percent. Approximately two-thirds of all clomiphene-related conceptions occur at doses no higher than 100 mg daily for 5 days, and most pregnancies occur within the first 6 ovulatory cycles.

If a patient fails to ovulate on a dose of clomiphene citrate of 100 mg for 5 days, and has good cervical mucus and a mature follicle (diameter >18–20 mm) as shown by ultrasound, then hCG, 10,000 U, can be given to trigger ovulation. However, if hCG is given too early during folliculogenesis, it may result in luteinization of the theca interna cells and degeneration of the tertiary follicles leading to ovulation inhibition or postponement.

Patients who fail to ovulate using the standard graded clomiphene citrate regimen are candidates for an incremental protocol. Clomiphene citrate is given continuously, starting day 3 to 5 at 50 mg daily for 5 days and increasing the dosage incrementally by 50 mg every 5 days, up to a maximum total dose of 3750 mg (total of 25 days of therapy). The ovarian response is monitored with ultrasound and E_2 RIA every 5 days. With this protocol a small series of 30 patients, who were previously unresponsive to clomiphene citrate in standard dosage, had a 70 percent ovulation rate, a 27 percent conception rate, a 3 percent rate (1 patient) of ovarian hyperstimulation, and minimal side effects. This method is a rapid way to assess whether patients will respond to clomiphene citrate or will require gonadotropin therapy. Occasionally some patients will hyperstimulate even with 50 mg of clomiphene citrate. In such women, the dose may be decreased to 12.5 mg or the duration of therapy limited to 3 days. On occasion, clomiphene responders may be made to ovulate by the administration of small doses of corticoids (i.e., dexamethasone, 0.5 mg, at bedtime or its equivalents) given for a few weeks prior to initiation of clomiphene therapy. Women likely to respond to this regimen usually show signs of increased androgen production with an elevated blood level of dehydroepiandrosterone sulfate (DHEA-S) of higher than 200 mg percent. Corticoid administration results in reduced adrenal androgen production and enhanced pituitary gonadotropin release and ovarian response after clomiphene administration.

Assisted Reproductive Technology

ART encompasses the various modalities of advanced reproductive therapy available to assist couples achieve a pregnancy. Success in

ART is positively correlated with the number of oocytes retrieved and the number of embryos transferred. This finding has led to the use of multiple regimens of ovarian stimulation.

One method of ovulation induction in ART is the use of combination clomiphene citrate and hMG. Theoretically, this regimen should result in optimal follicular development when compared to the use of a single agent (hMG or hFSH). However, in practice, the clomiphene citrate–hMG protocol results in similar rates of follicular development, oocyte recovery, embryo transfer, and pregnancy as in hMG or hFSH protocols. Moreover, the clomiphene-hMG protocol precludes the use of long-acting GnRH analogues for pituitary desensitization in combination with hMG for ovarian stimulation.

Luteal Phase Defects

Infertility and recurrent abortions have been associated with inadequate endometrial response to postovulatory output of progesterone. Adequate corpus luteum function is essential to endometrial receptivity for nidation and maintenance of early pregnancy. The findings of two endometrial biopsy specimens, obtained in consecutive cycles, with endometrial development lagging 2 days behind the expected date according to the onset of menses, confirm the diagnosis of a luteal phase defect. Treatment of patients with luteal phase inadequacy can be in the form of progesterone vaginal suppositories, 25 mg, twice a day or progesterone, 12.5 mg, intramuscular injection daily (50–70% success rates). Clomiphene citrate in the usually prescribed doses has also been effective in the treatment of luteal phase insufficiency with a conception rate of 33 to 41 percent. However, by exercising its antiestrogenic effect on the endometrial receptor, clomiphene citrate can also induce luteal phase defects with a reported incidence of 20 to 50 percent in patients treated. Therefore, when clomiphene therapy does not result in pregnancy in spite of luteal progesterone levels suggestive of ovulation, luteal phase dysfunction should be reassessed with a follow-up endometrial biopsy, and the treatment adjusted accordingly.

Contraindications, Warnings, and Precautions

Clomiphene citrate should only be used in patients with normal liver function because of this drug's enterohepatic circulation. It is not effective in patients with pituitary or gonadal failure. Patients with abnormal uterine bleeding should be evaluated prior to the use of clomiphene to induce ovulation. Clomiphene citrate should not be given to patients with ovarian cysts, as further ovarian enlargement may result. Use of clomiphene during pregnancy is contraindicated. The occurrence of visual symptoms during the course of clomiphene therapy is a contraindication to its continued use.

Metabolic Effects, Altered Laboratory Values, and Drug Interactions

Use of clomiphene citrate during the early follicular phase of the menstrual cycle results in increased production of pituitary LH and FSH. This is accompanied by ovarian follicular recruitment and selection of a dominant follicle with increased levels of plasma E_2. In addition, luteal phase production of progesterone by the corpus luteum is enhanced, with increased levels of circulating plasma progesterone. Clomiphene citrate has not been reported to cause significant abnormalities in hematologic or renal tests, in protein-bound iodine, or in serum cholesterol levels. There are no reported drug interactions attributed to clomiphene citrate.

Adverse Reactions

Side effects of ovulation induction by clomiphene citrate are more common at the higher dosages. The more common side effects during its use are hot flashes (11.0%), abdominal discomfort (7.4%), ovarian enlargement (14.0%), breast tenderness (2.1%), and nausea and vomiting (1.9%). Less common adverse effects are nervousness and insomnia (1.9%), headaches (1.0%), dizziness and light-headedness (1.0%), depression and fatigue (0.8%), urticaria and allergic dermatitis (0.6%), abnormal uterine bleeding (0.5%), weight gain (0.4%), and reversible alopecia (0.3%). All of these side effects are reversible. A serious side effect of clomiphene therapy involves the development of visual symptoms (1.6%): blurred vision, spots, or flashes (scintillating scotomata), and decreased visual acuity. The symptoms tend to disappear within a few days or weeks after discontinuation of therapy. Ovarian enlargement, including severe ovarian hyperstimulation syndrome, is more common in patients with polycystic ovarian syndrome, and these patients should be closely monitored. Because of its antiestrogenic effect on the cervical mucus, administration of clomiphene is at times associated with "hostile" cervical mucus. Thus, if the first ovulatory cycle does not result in pregnancy, a postcoital test should be scheduled in the following cycle approximately 5 days after termination of clomiphene therapy. If deficient cervical mucus is found, small doses of estrogens (0.3 mg of conjugated equine estrogens) should be given from day 10 to 18 of the cycle and the postcoital test repeated. Alternatively, intrauterine inseminations with washed concentrated semen, timed with peak estrogen levels and peak follicular maturation, can be used to bypass the hostile cervical mucus.

The occurrence of multiple gestations in women treated with clomiphene citrate averages 8 percent, of which 7 percent are twins and less than 1 percent are triplets or more.

Use of clomiphene citrate for ovulation induction has also been associated with a severalfold increase in the incidence of ectopic gestations, even after correction for tubal factors related to infertility (relative risk, 4.4).

A theoretical concern of ovulation induction by clomiphene citrate involves its prolonged half-life, and therefore its presence at the time of presumed ovulation, nidation, and steroid-sensitive organogenesis. In patients treated with clomiphene, active metabolites are still present on days 14 to 22 of the menstrual cycle. However, no metabolites are present 60 days after treatment. The incidence of congenital anomalies following clomiphene therapy is 2.5 percent, no different than rates reported in the general population.

Administration

Patients who are being considered for ovulation induction by clomiphene therapy should have a prior basic infertility workup that includes semen analysis, hysterosalpingogram, as well as evaluation for prolactin, thyroid, or adrenal dysfunction (DHEA-S). Also, determination of plasma progesterone levels, postcoital tests, and endometrial biopsy during administration will help assess the effectiveness of the treatment.

Clomiphene Citrate Preparations

Clomiphene citrate (Serophene [Serono], Clomid [Merrell Dow]) is supplied in 50-mg scored white tablets. The approximate cost per tablet is $5 to $10.

Clomiphene citrate is well absorbed orally, and the starting dose is 50 mg daily for 5 days, starting on day 3 to 5 of the menstrual cycle. When higher doses are required, a single daily dosage can be used, because of the drug's long half-life. Tablets of clomiphene citrate should be protected from light, moisture, and excessive heat.

Protocols

Assisted Reproductive Technology–Clomiphene-Pergonal Protocol

1. Measure baseline estradiol (E_2) level and do ultrasound.
2. Administer clomiphene, 100 mg daily, on days 2–6.
3. Give Pergonal (hMG), 2 ampules IM at 6:00 P.M. daily, starting on day 2.
4. Monitor E_2 levels daily, beginning day 6; perform ultrasound daily beginning day 8, and continuing through day after hCG administration.
5. Reduce hMG dose to 1 ampule (75 IU) if E_2 level is disproportionately high for follicular size and number (E_2, >2000 pg/ml with follicles <14 mm).
6. Hold hMG when 2 follicles reach 18 mm on greatest diameter.
7. Give hCG, 10,000 U IM at 9:00 P.M. when above criteria are met (34 hours prior to planned aspiration).
8. There is no modification of this protocol if poor folliculogenesis results.
9. Cycle is cancelled if less than 2 adequate follicles develop by day 12 or if rapid LH level at time of hCG administration approximates twice the baseline level or 30 mIU/ml. Also cancel cycle if dominant follicle or functional ovarian cysts are noted.

Incremental Clomiphene Protocol

1. Baseline estrogen levels are determined.
2. On day 3 to 5 of the menstrual cycle, clomiphene therapy commences at 50 mg a day for 5 days. Estrogen level is measured on day 5 of treatment.
3. Incremental clomiphene therapy is continued, unless baseline estrogen level doubles and reaches a minimum of 200 pg/ml.
4. If clomiphene is continued, dosage is increased in increments of 50 mg a day *every 5 days* up to a maximum of 250 mg a day for 5 days (i.e., 25 days of consecutive treatment with maximum dosage of 3750 mg). If clomiphene is continued, repeat estrogen determinations every 4 or 5 days. Stop clomiphene if estrogen level doubles to about 200 pg/ml as described above.
5. Ultrasound scans should be started 2 days after stopping clomiphene.
6. hCG injection, 10,000 U, is done when largest follicle is 18–20 mm in diameter.
7. Postcoital test is done the next day to assess adequacy of cervical factor.
8. Progesterone assay is performed 8 days after hCG administration.
9. The incremental clomiphene regimen is repeated for 3 more cycles in patients who are initially responsive. If patients are unresponsive, switch to gonadotropin stimulation.

OPIOID ANTAGONIST

Hypothalamic amenorrhea is characterized by low gonadotropin levels and low estrogen levels. The low gonadotropin levels are related to the reduction of hypothalamic GnRH release. Indirect evidence links the decreased GnRH release to increased production of endogenous opioids at the hypothalamic level.

Administration of a long-acting opioid antagonist, naltrexone, in doses of 50 mg per day resulted in the restoration of menses after 4 weeks of administration in 3 patients with hypothalamic amenorrhea. The ensuing luteal phase was characterized by progesterone levels somewhat lower than those found in the normal luteal phase. However, the use of opioid antagonists in the treatment of menstrual disorders is still experimental.

BIBLIOGRAPHY

Overview

Murad, F., and Haynes, R. C., Jr. Estrogens and Progestins. In L. S. Goodman and A. G. Gilman (eds.), *The Pharmacological Basis of Therapeutics* (7th ed.). New York, MacMillan, 1985. Pp. 1412–1439.

Physiology

Adashi, E. Y. Clomiphene citrate: mechanism(s) and site(s) of action—a hypothesis revisited. *Fertil. Steril.* 42:331, 1984.

Pharmacology

Mikkelson, T. J., Kroboth, P. D., Cameron, W. J., et al. Single-dose pharmacokinetics of clomiphene citrate in normal volunteers. *Fertil. Steril.* 46:392, 1986.

Indications

Anovulation

Adashi, E. Y. Clomiphene citrate-initiated ovulation: a clinical update. *Sem. Reprod. Endocrinol.* 4:255, 1986.

Hill, G. A., Diamond, M. P., Maxson, W. S., et al. Combination clomiphene citrate/human menopausal gonadotropin stimulation protocols for *in vitro* fertilization-embryo transfer. *J. In Vitro Fertil. Embryo Transfer* 4:34, 1987.

O'Herlihy, C., Pepperell, R. J., Brown, J. B., et al. Incremental clomiphene therapy: a new method for treating persistent anovulation. *Obstet. Gynecol.* 58:535, 1981.

Pepperell, R. J. A rational approach to ovulation induction. *Fertil. Steril.* 40:1, 1983.

Luteal Phase Defects

Lee, C. S. Luteal phase defects. *Obstet. Gynecol. Surv.* 42:267, 1987.

Adverse Effects

Geier, A., Lunenfeld, B., Pariente, C., et al. Estrogen receptor binding material in blood of patients after clomiphene citrate administration: determination by a radioreceptor assay. *Fertil. Steril.* 47:778, 1987.

Marchbanks, P. A., Annegers, J. F., Coulam, C. B., et al. Risk factors for ectopic pregnancy. A population-based study. *J.A.M.A.* 259:1823, 1988.

Serophene (Clomiphene citrate tablets; U.S.P.). Package insert. Randolph, Mass.: Serono Laboratories, 1987.

Opioid Antagonist

Wildt, L., and Leyendecker, G. Induction of ovulation by the chronic administration of naltrexone in hypothalamic amenorrhea. *J. Clin. Endocrinol. Metab.* 64:1334, 1987.

GONADOTROPIN-RELEASING FACTORS

GnRH is a decapeptide that has been characterized and synthesized, leading to a better understanding of pituitary gonadotropin release, and thereby to clinical application in ovulation induction. Similarly, GnRH agonists have become widely used in the treatment of infertility and endocrine disorders. The use of GnRH antagonists has lagged considerably behind, because of the adverse histamine-releasing property of high doses of potent lipophilic first- and second-generation compounds. With the introduction of third-generation GnRH antagonists it appears that their therapeutic potential may yet be realized.

PHYSIOLOGY

GnRH is secreted in discrete pulses from the arcuate nucleus of the hypothalamus into the hypophyseal-portal circulation. On reaching the pituitary, GnRH binds to specific receptors on specialized cells (gonadotropes), causing the release of pituitary glycoproteins. The interaction of GnRH with cell surface gonadotrope receptors activates intracellular hydrolysis of inositol phospholipids that act as second messengers to initiate exocytosis of secretory granules by a calcium-dependent mechanism. Ovarian steroids have a significant impact on pituitary gonadotropin secretion. Estrogen has a biphasic action first inhibiting, then augmenting hypothalamic pituitary response to GnRH, resulting in the preovulatory surge of gonadotropins. Further amplification of the preovulatory peak of gonadotropin secretion results from increased responsiveness to GnRH itself (self-priming action). The postovulatory rise in ovarian production of progesterone causes a decrease in hypothalamic and pituitary response to GnRH and this action is mediated by endogenous opiate peptides. GnRH is synthesized as part of a larger precursor, with 89 amino acids, which includes a 56 amino acid region, termed gonadotropin-releasing-hormone–associated peptide (GAP), which has prolactin-inhibiting properties. However, most of the peptide released into the hypophysial-portal circulation is in the form of GnRH. The circulatory half-life of GnRH is measured in minutes and the anterior pituitary is rich in peptidases that cause rapid hydrolysis.

In an attempt to prolong the half-life and, therefore, the potency of GnRH, analogues have been synthesized by multiple substitutions of amino acids in the peptide chain, resulting in a 10- to 60-fold prolongation of action. These analogues of GnRH can bind to cell surface gonadotrope receptors resulting in an initial increased production of gonadotropins. Paradoxically, this is followed shortly thereafter by cellular desensitization with loss of occupied GnRH receptors (downregulation), and uncoupling of receptors from the secretory signal (desensitization). This results in a decreased gonadotropin secretion, and a "medical castration" ensues. The hypogonadism that results from long-term use of GnRH analogues has been used therapeutically in gonadal steroid–dependent syndromes.

The use of GnRH antagonists has the theoretical advantage of rapid onset of action without initial stimulatory secretion of gonadotropins. Nevertheless, use of GnRH antagonists in clinical practice has been precluded by their ability to cause mast cell degranulation and thereby anaphylactoid responses in animals. The action of GnRH antagonists is due to competitive binding to GnRH-binding sites on the gonadotropes, without causing a stimulatory signal. However, the clinical results of long-term suppression should not differ between agonists and antagonists.

PHARMACOLOGY

Synthetic GnRH is a decapeptide with the amino acid sequence: pyro Glu-His-Trp-Ser-Tyr-Gly-Leu-Arg-Pro-Gly-NH_2 (Fig. 6-1). This peptide is rapidly hydrolyzed in plasma and excreted in urine with a half-life of about 4 minutes. Intravenous administration of synthetic GnRH results in a bimodal distribution. The first phase is a rapid (half-life of 2–8 minutes) mixing throughout the vascular and extracellular fluid spaces. The second phase has a slower clearance (half-life of 15–60 minutes). The predominant clearance of exogenous GnRH is via the kidneys, with minimal hepatic metabolism. The subcutaneous route of administration of GnRH is characterized by a slower absorption than intravenous administration. This is due to a depot-like property of subcutaneously administered GnRH in tissues, resulting in prolonged absorption. The only synthetic GnRH available in the United States is gonadorelin hydrochloride. It has been approved by the FDA for pituitary function testing.

GnRH agonists are obtained by amino acid substitutions of the synthetic decapeptide. The more potent agonists have modifications at position 6 that result in slower degradation by peptidases. Indeed, the active cleavage sites for proteolysis are the bonds between amino acids 6-7 and 9-10 (see Fig. 6-1). Substitutions that protect from enzymatic degradation (i.e., D-amino acid at position 6 or ethylamide residue in place of amino acid 10 [Gly]) also lead to increased receptor-binding affinity. The only analogue available in the United States for clinical use is leuprolide acetate, which is a nonapeptide with a D-Leu substitution at position 6 and a Pro ethylamide substitution at position 9 of synthetic GnRH. Leuprolide acetate is readily soluble in water and its mean plasma half-life is 2.9 hours. Leuprolide acetate is not active when given orally. Bioavailability, by subcutaneous administration (the preferred route), is comparable to that by intravenous administration. The metabolism, distribution, and excretion of leuprolide acetate in humans have not been determined. The FDA has approved leuprolide acetate for use in prostatic cancer. Since this compound is not FDA approved for use in gynecology, informed consent should be obtained from patients prior to starting therapy. A once-a-month depot form of leuprolide acetate (Lupron Depot) is now available and this promises to make therapy for steroid-dependent conditions easier for patients. Other GnRH analogues under investigation, which should become available in the next few years, are: nafarelin, buserelin, decapeptyl and zoladex, all extensively tested in Europe and Canada (Table 6-1).

The development of GnRH antagonists is based on multiple substitutions of the synthetic decapeptide. Nevertheless, the development of clinically useful GnRH antagonists has been slow and complicated by unwanted side effects (i.e., peptide-induced histamine release). Currently, clinically applicable GnRH antagonists are still under development.

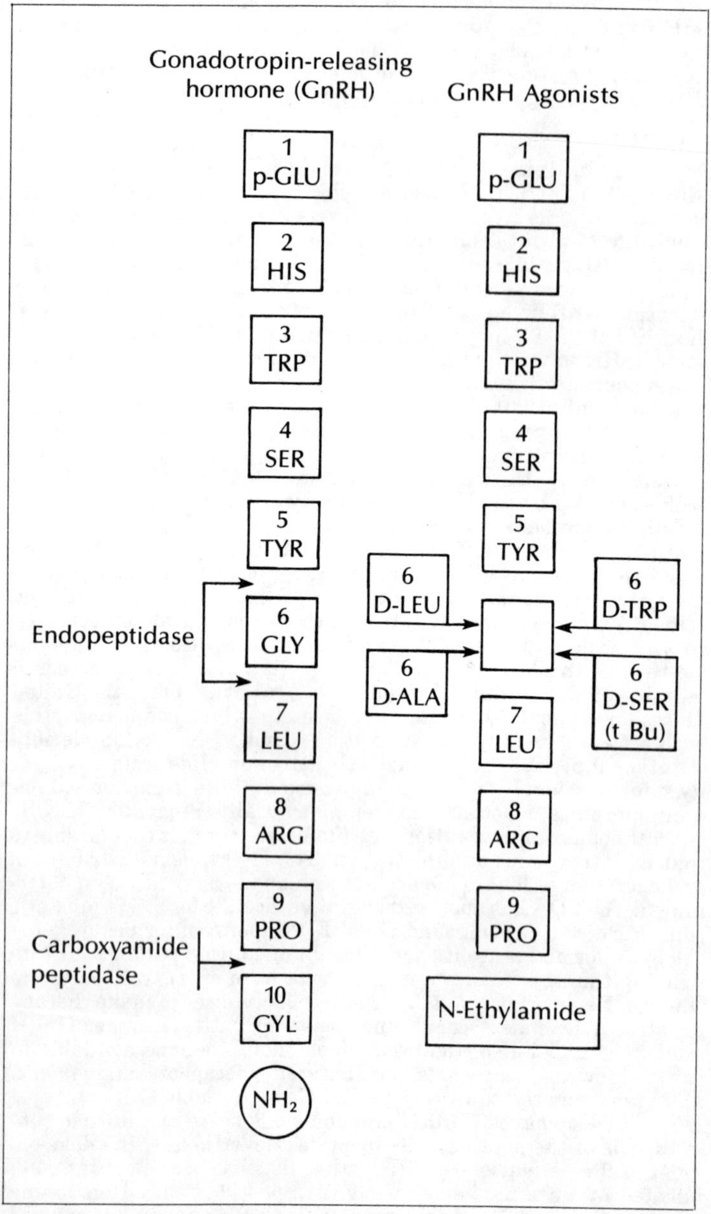

Fig. 6-1. Amino acid sequence of GnRH and GnRH agonist.

Table 6-1. Gonadotropin-releasing hormone agonists under investigation for use in gynecology

Agent	Generic	Substitution	Potency	Half-Life (min)
Factrel	Gonadorelin	—	1	4
Lupron[a]	Leuprolide	D-Leu^6; NHEt^{10}	15	180
Lupron Depot[a]	Leuprolide	D-Leu^6; NHEt^{10}	15	—
Decapeptyl	D-Trp-6-GnRH	D-Trp^6	36	120
Receptal	Buserelin	D-Ser(tBu)^6; NHEt^{10}	50	80
Zoladex	Goserelin	D-Ser(tBu)^6; Az-Gly^{10}	50–100	360
Nafarelin	—	D-Nal(2)^6	100	260
Histrelin	—	D-His (im Bzl)^6; NHEt^{10}	100	—

[a] Approved by the Food and Drug Administration for use in prostate carcinoma.
NHEt^{10} = elimination of 10th amino acid (nonapeptide) and addition of ethylamide.

INDICATIONS

Ovulation Induction

Use of GnRH for induction of ovulation provides a physiologic approach to patients with hypothalamic amenorrhea. These patients have congenital or acquired deficiency of endogenous GnRH, resulting in extremely low circulating gonadotropin levels and clinical features of hypoestrogenism. A thorough assessment of these patients is necessary prior to the start of therapy to exclude conditions that would best be treated otherwise. Women with amenorrhea related to weight loss may have multifollicular ovaries as shown by pelvic ultrasonography. Such ovaries are normal in size or slightly enlarged and filled with cysts measuring 4 to 10 mm on ultrasonography. These women are not hirsute and plasma LH levels and FSH levels are normal and reduced, respectively. The uterus is small, indicating estrogen deficiency. Unlike the typical patients with polycystic ovary syndrome, in whom ovulation induction by GnRH therapy has been disappointing, women with multifollicular ovaries respond very favorably to GnRH therapy both with ovulation and pregnancies.

GnRH for ovulation induction is given by intravenous or subcutaneous routes. The intravenous route is more efficient; however, subcutaneous therapy is much simpler to implement. The rates of ovulation (90–95%) and pregnancy (30–35%) are comparable with both routes. Around-the-clock pulsatile GnRH administration is done with automated minipumps.

In order to mimic the intrinsic pulsatility of endogenous GnRH, the automated minipump is set at pulse frequencies ranging from 60 to 120 minutes. The starting dose for intravenous therapy is 2.5 to 5.0 μg per dose and for subcutaneous therapy, 5 to 20 μg per dose. Patients should be monitored with ultrasound and E_2 RIA. After ovulation occurs, luteal phase support is recommended. This can be accomplished by continuing GnRH pulsatile therapy or, more simply, by daily suppositories or injections of progesterone, or by intermittent doses of hCG injections.

The advantages of GnRH pulsatile administration over gonadotropin therapy (hMG or hCG) are replacement that mimics the normal physiologic secretory pattern; maintenance of intact feedback mechanisms between pituitary and ovary, leading to endogenous ovulation; and decreased instances of ovarian hyperstimulation syndrome and multiple pregnancies. The disadvantages of GnRH therapy are the need for continuous pump infusion with indwelling catheter, the high cost of the autoinfusion minipumps, and the possibility of drug resistance due to GnRH antibody formation.

Use of GnRH analogues for ovulation induction in patients with polycystic ovary or in protocols for ART relies on pituitary gonadotropin downregulation prior to stimulation with hMG. This approach eliminates the aberrant gonadotropin ratio characteristic of polycystic ovary or controls endogenous gonadotropin surges in programs of ART. Leuprolide acetate is usually started during the luteal phase of the menstrual cycle with a daily dose of 1 mg subcutaneously. When GnRH analogues are started during the midluteal phase of the cycle preceding the planned stimulation with hMG, the initial agonist effect occurs at a time when follicle recruitment and selection have not yet taken place. Therefore, the initial agonist effect is not as prominent and results in small increases in corpus luteum function. Subsequently, when menses occurs, pituitary function is usually downregulated and exogenous gonadotropins (hMG) can be added, resulting in direct ovarian stimulation. However, more hMG for a longer period is needed to stimulate the ovaries after the initial pituitary desensitization with the GnRH agonist. Although not clearly understood, this effect may be related to the release of pituitary gonadotropin isoforms (deglycosylated, bio-inactive FSH), which then bind to ovarian FSH receptors and interfere with hMG ovarian stimulation. This, indeed, is the case with use of GnRH antagonists for pituitary desensitization. Alternatively, the downregulation of endogenous gonadotropins results in a lack of preantral follicles at the time of hMG administration.

Precocious Puberty

Puberty involves the maturation of the hypothalamo-pituitary-gonadal axis which leads to sexual maturation and the capacity to reproduce. Precocious puberty is characterized by the appearance of pubertal signs before age 8 in girls and before age 10 in boys. When precocious puberty is due to premature activation of the hypothalamo-pituitary-gonadal axis, it is defined as central precocious puberty. Prior to appropriate management, these children must be thoroughly evaluated. Therapy requires suppression of the elevated gonadotropin and gonadal steroid levels. Long-acting GnRH analogues are the treatment of choice for central precocious puberty. This therapy achieves decreased growth rate and bone maturation, leading to improved predicted adult height. The dosage of injectable preparations ranges from 1 to 40 μg/kg per day. Therapy is continued until epiphyseal fusion occurs, chronological age matches the bone age, or the patient is 12 years old.

Endometriosis

Endometriosis is characterized by the presence of functioning endometrial glands and stroma outside the uterine cavity. It is associated with dysmenorrhea, dyspareunia, pelvic pain, and infertility. Administration of long-acting GnRH analogues in women with endometriosis results in a hypoestrogenic environment that leads to atrophy of endometriotic lesions. However, this "medical ovariectomy" is associated with reversible decreases in bone mineral density. Patients are thus instructed to ingest 1500 mg of calcium daily during therapy.

Treatment is started in the luteal phase of the menstrual cycle, to prevent initial agonist stimulation of ovarian estrogen production, unopposed by progesterone, and therefore to prevent worsening of the endometriosis. Leuprolide is started at a dose of 1 mg subcutaneously daily, 10 days prior to the expected onset of menses, and patients are instructed to use barrier contraception during the entire treatment. Monthly E_2 assays are used to follow the response to agonist therapy, and when E_2 levels fall below 20 pg/ml, dosage can be decreased to alleviate some of the vasomotor symptoms of medical castration. Therapy is continued for 6 to 8 weeks prior to surgery, or 3 months postoperatively. When no surgery is employed, leuprolide is given for up to 6 months. Menses returns 6 to 8 weeks after the discontinuation of treatment.

Uterine Leiomyomata

Uterine leiomyomata are smooth muscle neoplasms found in 20 percent of all women older than 30 years. Growth of these tumors is stimulated by estrogen, and estrogen receptors have been identified in leiomyomata. A hypoestrogenic state is known to prevent further fibroid growth and even reduce fibroid size and gynecologic symptoms. Therefore, GnRH agonists have been used to suppress the hypothalamo-pituitary-gonadal axis in such patients. GnRH agonists are also successful in patients with pulmonary leiomyomatosis. In addition, the recent finding of GnRH-specific–binding sites in uterine leiomyomata suggests a direct effect of GnRH analogues on this tissue.

Treatment with GnRH analogues is started during the luteal phase of the menstrual cycle, to prevent the initial rise of E_2, unopposed by progesterone, and, therefore, to prevent initial growth of the myomas. The percent decrease in uterine volume is related to the degree of hypoestrogenemia achieved by the agonist. Near maximal reduction in uterine volume occurs at 12 weeks of therapy. The bone mineral density shows little change during agonist therapy, and any decreases appear to be reversible. Patients are instructed to ingest 1500 mg of calcium daily during therapy.

The therapy is started at a dose of 1 mg of leuprolide acetate subcutaneously administered daily, beginning 10 days prior to the expected menses. Patients are instructed to use barrier contraception during the entire time of therapy. Monthly E_2 determinations and ultrasonography are used to follow the level of hypoestrogenemia and the degree of myoma volume decrease. Magnetic resonance imaging has also been used to assess myoma's regression. Once the E_2 level is less than 20 pg/ml, the dose may be reduced to decrease vasomotor symptoms. Although administration of medroxyprogesterone acetate (20 mg orally daily) is successful in alleviating vasomotor symptoms, it interferes with the shrinking of the myoma and over one-third of patients have vaginal spotting. Therapy is continued until the myoma volume is markedly decreased or reaches a plateau, or vasomotor symptoms and dyspareunia become incapacitating. Surgery after 3 to 6 months of therapy is easier and less bloody because of the decrease in size and vascularity of the tissues. Menstrual function returns 6 to 8 weeks after discontinuation of therapy. Women whose only complaint is infertility associated with uterine myomas may conceive in the first few cycles after stopping leuprolide therapy without any surgical intervention.

Hirsutism

Hirsutism is related to excessive androgen production by the ovaries or the adrenals, or increased sensitivity of the hair follicle to androgens. A thorough evaluation of possible causes of androgen excess should exclude ovarian or adrenal tumors, Cushing's syndrome, and congenital adrenal hyperplasia. Once it is established that the hirsutism is mainly related to increased ovarian production of androgen, GnRH agonists offer an alternative and effective form of therapy. By suppressing the hypothalamo-pituitary-gonadal axis, GnRH analogue therapy decreases ovarian-produced androgens, hair follicle diameter, and hirsutism score. Leuprolide acetate is administered subcutaneously at a dose of 1 mg and patients are instructed to use barrier contraception throughout the entire time of therapy. Monthly levels of blood E_2, testosterone, androstenedione, and hair growth are measured, and dosage may be decreased when E_2 levels are less than 20 pg/ml to decrease vasomotor symptoms. In order to prevent hot flashes and other effects of hypoestrogenism, concomitant use of estrogen supplementation with monthly progestin withdrawal may be considered. Alternatively, a low-dose oral contraceptive preparation may be used concomitant to leuprolide therapy.

Therapy is continued for 3 months, at which time electrolysis treatments are started. Duration of therapy has not been determined, but reassessment after 6 months of therapy seems prudent in view of the effects of prolonged ovarian suppression on bone mineral density. Menses returns within 6 to 8 weeks. Although little change in bone mineral density has been demonstrated during use of GnRH agonists, any observed change is reversible. Patients are instructed to ingest 1500 mg of calcium daily during therapy. Concomitant estrogen therapy prevents any bone density changes.

Menstrual Cycle-Associated Disorders

Patients with disorders that recur monthly with each menstrual cycle are candidates for GnRH analogue treatment. Indeed, suppression of the hypothalamo-pituitary-ovarian axis should result in resolution of clinical disorders related to hormonal imbalance or sensitivity.

Premenstrual syndrome (PMS) is characterized by recurrent mental and physical changes occurring during the luteal phase of the menstrual cycle. The symptoms usually start during corpus luteum development and disappear when E_2 and progesterone levels reach follicular phase levels at the end of the luteal phase. Inhibition of ovulation and corpus luteum formation with GnRH analogues has been used successfully to treat patients with severe PMS.

Recurrent idiopathic anaphylaxis is characterized by recurring anaphylactic or anaphylactoid attacks of unknown cause. Urticaria, angioedema, upper and lower airway obstruction, vomiting, diarrhea, abdominal bloating, syncope, hypotension, and flushing occur during the attacks. In some of these patients, the attacks are associated with progesterone secretion. Allergy to progesterone or its metabolites has been postulated. Therefore, ovarian suppression with GnRH agonists may benefit women with recurrent idiopathic anaphylaxis who demonstrate sensitivity to progesterone.

Acute intermittent porphyria is an autosomal dominant inherited disorder that presents clinically with recurring abdominal pain and neuropsychiatric symptoms. The disorder is due to a defect of porphyrin and heme synthesis resulting from lack of the enzyme uroporphyrinogen I synthetase. The controlling step in porphyrin biosynthesis precedes the just mentioned reaction and is the inducible enzyme aminolevulinic acid synthetase. This enzyme can be induced by drugs and hormones, including estrogen and progesterone. GnRH agonists have been used successfully to induce suppression of the hypothalamo-pituitary-gonadal axis in women with catamenial acute intermittent porphyria.

All of the just mentioned disorders have been shown to improve in some patients during use of GnRH analogues. Therapy should be started with daily subcutaneous injection of 1 mg of leuprolide acetate and patients should be instructed to use barrier contraception as well as ingest 1500 mg of calcium daily during therapy. Patients with PMS, recurrent idiopathic anaphylaxis, and catamenial acute intermittent porphyria are started on GnRH agonist treatment during the follicular phase of the menstrual cycle. Follow-up consists of monthly monitoring of E_2 level, basal body temperature, and symptoms. Optimum duration of therapy has not been established but reassessment after 6 months seems prudent, in view of the effects of prolonged ovarian suppression on bone mineral density.

Breast Cancer

Gonadal steroids appear to be involved in the development of breast cancer and surgical ovariectomy is often employed in the management of metastatic breast cancer in premenopausal women with positive sex steroid receptors. Thus, "medical ovariectomy" with the administration of long-acting GnRH analogues is an alternative approach in metastatic breast cancer. Moreover, GnRH analogues have been shown to inhibit human breast cancer cells in vitro and specific GnRH-binding sites have been found in some human breast cancer cell lines. Therefore, GnRH therapy may be employed instead of ovariectomy for the palliative treatment of breast cancer in premenopausal women. Disease flare (bone pain) may be experienced in some women during the agonist phase of the GnRH administration concomitant with the temporary rise in estrogen levels. Postmenopausal women with breast cancer are not likely to benefit from GnRH therapy in spite of the suggested direct antitumor effect of the GnRH agonist.

Ovarian Cancer

Ovarian cancer usually presents at advanced stages, and chemotherapy with cis-platinim–based regimens is the norm. Usual response rates to cis-platinum–based therapy are high, but toxicity is considerable and relapses are frequent. GnRH analogues have been tested in patients with advanced ovarian cancers with promising results. The rationale behind GnRH analogue therapy in ovarian cancers is that gonadotropins have been implicated in ovarian carcinogenesis. Indeed, ovarian cancer cell lines grown in vitro were stimulated to grow by administration of LH-hCG preparations. In addition, ovarian cancer tissues have been shown to have LH and hCG receptors, suggesting gonadotropin dependency. A small group of 41 patients with International Federation of Gynecology and Obstetrics (FIGO) stage III or IV ovarian cancers, who had relapsed following conventional chemotherapy, were treated with a long-acting GnRH analogue. Clinical benefits of therapy were seen in 26 percent (11 patients), and overall response rate (partial remission) occurred in 15 percent (6 patients). Therefore, this new approach to the treatment of ovarian cancer may represent a useful adjuvant to current chemotherapeutic regimens.

Contraception

When it became apparent that GnRH agonists were able to disrupt the normal menstrual cycle, their contraceptive effect was soon investigated. At increasing doses, GnRH agonists cause luteal phase defects, anovulation, and amenorrhea. The endometrium will reflect the endocrine milieu, ranging from atrophic to hyperplastic. When given early in the luteal phase, GnRH agonists will cause premature menses, but simultaneous administration of hCG, and by inference early pregnancy, will correct the GnRH-induced decrements of the luteal phase. Furthermore, administration during early human pregnancy does not induce abortion.

In conclusion, the expectation that GnRH agonists would serve as nonsteroidal contraceptives has not been fulfilled. At low doses administration of GnRH agonists results in estrogen production unopposed by progesterone, a condition likely to give rise to endometrial hyperplasia and endometrial cancer. At high doses, GnRH agonists cause marked hypoestrogenism with its deleterious effects on bone metabolism and the cardiovascular system. Additionally, for many young women, prolonged amenorrhea is not socially or psychologically acceptable.

Pituitary Function Testing

The pituitary gonadotropes are under the control of hypothalamic GnRH pulsatile secretion. Gonadotrope function can be assessed by means of a single injection of synthetic GnRH. This test does not measure pituitary gonadotrope reserve, which may require either prolonged or repeated administration of GnRH. This test is useful to evaluate patients with suspected gonadotropin deficiency, whether due to the hypothalamus alone or in combination with anterior pituitary failure.

The GnRH stimulation test can be performed concomitantly with other tests of anterior pituitary function reserve. The test is performed during the early follicular phase of the menstrual cycle (days 1–7) by administering 100 mg of GnRH subcutaneously or intravenously. Venous blood samples for LH and FSH are followed serially for up to 2 hours. Peak LH response in women occurs 70 minutes after subcutaneous injection, or 30 minutes after intravenous injection, with a more pronounced response in the latter. Peak FSH response is delayed approximately 15 minutes with respect to peak LH response.

CONTRAINDICATIONS, WARNINGS, AND PRECAUTIONS

Synthetic GnRH should not be used in patients with pituitary failure, as these patients will fail to respond. Antibody formation has been reported rarely after chronic administration of synthetic

GnRH. An anaphylactic reaction has been reported during intravenous infusion of synthetic GnRH for ovulation induction; therefore, the initial dose of GnRH therapy should be started while the patient is under medical supervision.

Treatment with leuprolide acetate should be started during the luteal phase of the menstrual cycle in patients whose conditions might be worsened by the initial agonist effect. Patients should also be warned of the possibility of pregnancy and barrier contraception should be used in the periovulatory time of the cycle in which leuprolide acetate will be administered, and thereafter. There are no known contraindications to use of GnRH analogues (leuprolide acetate).

METABOLIC EFFECTS, ALTERED LABORATORY VALUES, AND DRUG INTERACTIONS

Synthetic GnRH directly stimulates pituitary gonadotrope secretion of LH and FSH. This is followed by ovarian stimulation, follicular recruitment, and selection, reflected by rising E_2 levels. There are no known drug interactions, and the pituitary stimulation test can be performed concomitantly with other anterior pituitary evaluations.

Leuprolide acetate is a GnRH agonist that directly binds to pituitary GnRH receptors. It causes initial agonist effects resulting in increased gonadotropin (LH and FSH) secretion. This in turn causes elevated levels of E_2 in the ovarian follicle or corpus luteum and progesterone secretion. Subsequently, after about 1 week of use, pituitary desensitization ensues, resulting in hypogonadotropic hypogonadism. There are no known drug interactions with use of leuprolide acetate.

ADVERSE REACTIONS

Nonspecific complaints in taking synthetic GnRH are headaches, nausea, lightheadedness, abdominal discomfort, and flushing. Local reactions, such as swelling, pain, and pruritus at the injection site have been reported after subcutaneous use. Local and generalized skin rashes have been reported after chronic subcutaneous injection.

Intravenous administration of synthetic GnRH can result in hypersensitivity reactions such as bronchospasm, tachycardia, flushing, urticaria, and induration at the injection site. Therefore, initial injection should be performed under medical supervision. Rare cases of antibody formation following chronic administration of synthetic GnRH have been reported.

Use of leuprolide acetate in women has been associated with almost universal occurrence of hot flashes, 3 to 4 weeks after initiation of therapy. These can be ameliorated by decreases in dosage, as long as the patient remains hypoestrogenic, or by addition of progestins (medroxyprogesterone acetate, 20 mg/day orally); however, use of progestins may interfere with the action of GnRH agonists in some situations (e.g., uterine leiomyomata). Other common side effects of GnRH agonists in women are amenorrhea, vaginal spotting, headaches, reduction in breast size, and vaginal dryness. Patients with known allergies to benzyl alcohol, which is a preservative in leuprolide acetate, may develop symptoms of local hypersensitivity, in the form of erythema and induration at the injection site. Mental depression has been reported in some patients taking chronic leuprolide acetate. Reversible decreases in bone mineral density are a side effect of prolonged hypoestrogenemia.

ADMINISTRATION

Patients who are being considered for ovulation induction by synthetic GnRH should have a thorough infertility evaluation to rule out the possible causes of hypogonadotropic hypogonadism. In addition, facilities for monitoring ovulation (i.e., E_2 RIA and ultrasonography) should be readily available.

Clinical therapy with GnRH analogues should be undertaken by personnel with a knowledge of the physiology and pharmacology of these compounds.

DRUG PREPARATIONS

Gonadorelin hydrochloride (Factrel [Ayerst]) is supplied in lyophilized ampules containing 100 μg or 500 μg gonadorelin as the hydrochloride, with 100 mg of lactose. Each ampule is accompanied by a vial of 2-ml of sterile diluent of 2% benzyl alcohol in water for injection. The approximate cost per 100-μg ampule is $50 to $60.

Gonadorelin is rapidly dissolved in as little as 1 to 2 ml of diluent, and is rapidly absorbed after subcutaneous or intravenous injection. Standard dose for pituitary GnRH testing is 100 μg subcutaneously or intravenously. Use of gonadorelin hydrochloride for ovulation induction requires a continuous pulsatile administration via small portable autoinfusion pumps, which cost between $900 and $1500. The starting dose for intravenous therapy is 2.5 to 5.0 μg per dose and for subcutaneous administration, 5 to 20 μg per dose. As an example, 500 μg of gonadorelin hydrochloride dissolved in 5 ml, with 50 microliter of solution to be administered at each pulse, represents a 5 μg dose. Pulse frequencies range from every 60 to 120 minutes, averaging 90 minutes.

Leuprolide acetate (Lupron [TAP Pharmaceuticals]) is supplied as a sterile, aqueous solution for subcutaneous injection. It is available in a 2.8-ml multiple-dose vial containing 5 mg/ml (1 mg/0.2 ml) of leuprolide acetate, sodium chloride for tonicity, 9 mg/ml of benzyl alcohol as a preservative, and water for injection. The approximate cost for 2 weeks (2.8 ml multiple-dose vial) is $150 to $200.

Leuprolide acetate is rapidly absorbed after subcutaneous injection. Standard dose is 1 mg (0.2 ml) subcutaneously daily. Dose may be adjusted down once hypoestrogenemia is established, to decrease vasomotor side effects.

PROTOCOLS

Assisted Reproductive Technology (ART) Lupron-Pergonal Protocol

1. Aim: Endogenous gonadotropin suppression followed by exogenous gonadotropin stimulation to obtain multiple mature follicles.
2. End-point:
   a. Complete ovarian suppression with Lupron prior to Pergonal stimulation (i.e., E_2 <20 pg/ml and no ovarian follicles or cysts by ultrasound)
   b. Pergonal stimulation to obtain lead follicle of 18-mm diameter or more and a secondary follicle of 16 mm or more. Additionally, there must be 4 or more follicles present with a minimum diameter of 12 mm on the day of hCG administra-

tion. The minimum level of E_2 on day of hCG administration is 750 pg/ml.
3. Start Lupron, 1 mg SQ daily 10 days prior to expected menses of scheduled ART cycle. (*Patients should be instructed to use barrier contraception during the entire cycle preceding ART cycle if fallopian tubes are open.*)
4. Measure E_2 levels during menses or after 12 days, whichever occurs later. E_2 must be less than 20 pg/ml before stimulation with Pergonal is initiated. Continue Lupron suppression until E_2 level is less than 20 pg/ml and ultrasonography confirms no follicles or cysts.
5. Add Pergonal 3 ampules (225 IU) IM daily after E_2 levels are suppressed and resume E_2 and ultrasound monitoring after 5 doses.
6. Continue Lupron at a reduced dose of 0.5 mg SQ daily along with Pergonal.
7. Monitor daily E_2 levels and ultrasound through the day after hCG administration.
8. If E_2 level is disproportionately high for follicular size and number (E_2 >2,000 pg/ml with follicles <14 mm) reduction of Pergonal dose to 1 ampule (75 IU) must be carried out.
9. The dose is continued until criteria are met. Then, if E_2 level exceeds 2000 pg/ml, give hCG on that day. If E_2 is less than 2000 pg/ml on the day criteria are met, give Pergonal for one additional day, then give hCG.
10. hCG 10,000 U IM is given at 9:00 P.M., approximately 27 hours after the last Pergonal dose.
11. Follicle aspiration: Planned 34 hours after hCG administration (7:00 A.M.).
12. Cancel Cycle if there is:
    a. No follicular development or no estrogen increase after 5 days of Pergonal
    b. A functional cyst (E_2 level is 150–200 pg/ml and "follicle" is 18 mm in diameter, detected on day 6 of Pergonal stimulation)
    c. A dominant follicle (single follicle reaches 18 mm without at least one other 14 mm)
    d. An unchanged estrogen level for 3 days or a decreasing level for 2 days during Pergonal
    e. A decreasing level of estrogen after hCG administration

GnRH Analogue (Lupron) Protocol for Myomata

1. Measure baseline ultrasound, levels of FSH, LH, and E_2.
2. Start Lupron, 1 mg SQ in midluteal phase. (*Patients should be instructed to use barrier contraception during the periovulatory phase and thereafter if fallopian tubes are open.*)
3. Measure FSH, LH, and E_2 q4 weeks at each dosage.
4. Repeat ultrasound q4 weeks.
5. Reduce Lupron dosage q4 weeks at 0.125–0.25 mg increments if E_2 level is less than 20 pg/ml. Increase if E_2 level is greater than 20 pg/ml.
6. Continue Lupron at the lowest suppressive dose until the size of myomata is unchanged for 8 weeks.
7. Consider surgical versus further medical therapy.

GnRH (Factrel) Pituitary Stimulation Test Protocol

1. Timing: Follicular phase of menstrual cycle (day 1–7).

Table 6-2. Interpretation of the GnRH (Factrel) pituitary stimulation test protocol

Route	Peak LH (mIU/ml)	Maximum LH Increase (mIU/ml)	Time to Peak LH (Min)
SQ	67.9 ± 27.5 100% ≥ 12.5	52.8 ± 26.4 100% ≥ 7.5	71.5 ± 49.6
IV	57.6 ± 36.7 100% ≥ 20.0	44.5 ± 31.8 100% ≥ 7.5	36 ± 24

2. Dose: 100 μg of Factrel administered SQ or IV.
3. Measure LH and FSH levels in venous blood samples
   a. Baseline: average of samples drawn at 15 minutes before and immediately prior to Factrel injection
   b. Postadministration: 15, 30, 60, and 120 minutes after Factrel injection
   c. Peak LH (mIU/ml): highest LH value after GnRH administration
   d. Maximum LH increase (mIU/ml): peak LH value minus baseline LH value
   e. Time to peak: minutes required to reach peak LH value
4. Interpretation: See Table 6-2.
5. Refer to the LH response chart for normal women (i.e., 10th–90th percentile response interval) after subcutaneous or intravenous Factrel injection, in Factrel (Gonadorelin hydrochloride) package insert. Wyeth-Ayerst Laboratories, Philadelphia, Pennsylvania, 1989.

BIBLIOGRAPHY

Overview

Andreyko, J. L., Marshall, L. A. Dumesic, D. A., et al. Therapeutic uses of gonadotropin-releasing hormone analogs. *Obstet. Gynecol. Surv.* 42:1, 1987.

Clayton, R. N. Gonadotrophin releasing hormone: From physiology to pharmacology. *Clin. Endocrinol* 26:361, 1987.

McLachlan, R. I., Healy, D. L., and Burger, H. G. Clinical aspects of LHRH analogues in gynaecology: a review. *Br. J. Obstet. Gynaecol.* 93:431, 1986.

Physiology

Conn, M. P. The molecular basis of gonadotropin-releasing hormone action. *Endocrine Rev.* 7:3, 1986.

Fink, G. Gonadotropin Secretion and Its Control. In E. Knobil and J. Neill (eds.), *The Physiology of Reproduction.* New York: Raven Press, 1988. Pp. 1349–1377.

McCann, S. M. and Rettori, V. Physiology of luteinizing hormone-releasing hormone. *Semin. Reprod. Endocrinol.* 5:333, 1987.

Vickery, B. H., and Nestor, J. J., Jr. Luteinizing hormone-releasing hormone analogs: development and mechanism of action. *Semin. Reprod. Endocrinol.* 5:353, 1987.

Pharmacology

Corbin, A., Bex, F. J., and Jones, R. C. LHRH and analogs: contraceptive and therapeutic considerations. *Int. J. Fertil.* 30:57, 1985.

Handelsman, D. J., and Swerdloff, R. S. Pharmacokinetics of gonadotropin-releasing hormone and its analogs. *Endocr. Rev.* 7:95, 1986.

Karten, M. J., and Rivier, J. E. Gonadotropin-releasing hormone analog design. Structure-function studies toward the development of agonists and antagonists: rationale and perspective. *Endocr. Rev.* 7:44, 1986.

Murad, F., and Haynes, R. C., Jr. Adenohypophyseal Hormones and Related Substances. In L. S. Goodman and A. G. Gilman (eds.), *The Pharmacological Basis of Therapeutics* (7th ed.). New York: MacMillan, 1985. Pp. 1362–1388.

Muse, K., and Wilson, E. A. Endocrine Therapy of Endometriosis: Gonadotropin-Releasing Hormone Agonists. In R. L. Barbieri and I. Schiff (eds.), *Reproductive Endocrine Therapeutics.* New York: Alan R. Liss, 1988. Pp. 187–198.

Indications

Ovulation Induction

Adams, J., Polson, D. W., Abdulwahid, N., et al. Multifollicular ovaries: clinical and endocrine features and response to pulsatile gonadotropin releasing hormone. *Lancet* 2:1375, 1985.

Barnes, R. B., Scommegna, A., and Schreiber, J. R. Decreased ovarian response to human menopausal gonadotropin caused by subcutaneously administered gonadotropin-releasing hormone agonist. *Fertil. Steril.* 47:512, 1987.

Dahl, K. D., Bicsak, T. A., and Hsueh, A. J. W. Naturally occurring antihormones: secretion of FSH antagonists by women treated with a GnRH analog. *Science* 239:72, 1988.

Dodson, W. C., Hughes, C. L., Whitesides, D. B., et al. The effect of leuprolide acetate on ovulation induction with human menopausal gonadotropins in polycystic ovary syndrome. *J. Clin. Endocrinol. Metab.* 65:95, 1987.

Reid, R. L., Fretts, R., and VanVugt, D. A. The theory and practice of ovulation induction with gonadotropin-releasing hormone. *Am. J. Obstet. Gynecol.* 158:176, 1988.

Wong, P. C., and Asch, R. H. Induction of follicular development with luteinizing hormone-releasing hormone. *Semin. Reprod. Endocrinol.* 5:399, 1987.

Precocious Puberty

Laron, Z., Dickerman, Z., and Kauli, R. Treatment of premature and delayed puberty with luteinizing hormone-releasing hormone and its analogs. *Semin. Reprod. Endocrinol.* 5:421, 1987.

Endometriosis

Barbieri, R. L., and Ryan, K. J. Medical therapy for endometriosis: endocrine pharmacology. *Semin. Reprod. Endocrinol.* 3:339, 1985.

Gudmundsson, J. A., Ljunghall, S., Bergquist, C., et al. Increased bone turnover during gonadotropin-releasing hormone superagonist-induced ovulation inhibition. *J. Clin. Endocrinol. Metab.* 65:159, 1987.

Johansen, J. S., Riis, B. J., Hassager, C., et al. The effect of gonadotropin-releasing hormone agonist analog (Nafarelin) on bone metabolism. *J. Clin. Endocrinol. Metab.* 67:701, 1988.

Schriock, E., Monroe, S. E., Henzl, M., et al. Treatment of endometriosis with a potent agonist of gonadotropin-releasing hormone (Nafarelin). *Fertil. Steril.* 44:583, 1985.

Uterine Leiomyomata

Friedman, A. J., Barbieri, R. L., Benacerraf, B. R., et al. Treatment of leiomyomata with intranasal or subcutaneous leuprolide, a gonadotropin-releasing hormone agonist. *Fertil. Steril.* 48:560, 1987.

Friedman, A. J., Barbieri, R. L., Doubilet, P. M., et al. A randomized, double-blind trial of a gonadotropin-releasing hormone agonist (leuprolide) with or without medroxyprogesterone acetate in the treatment of leiomyomata uteri. *Fertil. Steril.* 49:404, 1988.

Healy, D. L., Lawson, S. R., Abbott, M., et al. Toward removing uterine fibroids without surgery: subcutaneous infusion of a luteinizing hormone-releasing hormone agonist commencing in the luteal phase. *J. Clin. Endocrinol. Metab.* 63:619, 1986.

Wiznitzer, A., Marbach, M., Hazum, E., et al. Gonadotropin-releasing hormone specific binding sites in uterine leiomyomata. *Biochem. Biophys. Res. Commun.* 152:1326, 1988.

Hirsutism

Andreyko, J. L., Monroe, S. E., and Jaffe, R. B. Treatment of hirsutism with a gonadotropin-releasing hormone agonist (Nafarelin). *J. Clin. Endocrinol. Metab.* 65:854, 1986.

Steingold, K. A., Judd, H. L., Nieberg, R. K., et al. Treatment of severe androgen excess due to ovarian hyperthecosis with a long-acting gonadotropin-releasing hormone agonist. *Am. J. Obstet. Gynecol.* 154:1241, 1986.

Menstrual Cycle-Associated Disorders

Bancroft, J., Boyle, H., Warner, P., et al. The use of an LHRH agonist, Buserelin, in the long-term management of premenstrual syndromes. *Clin. Endocrinol.* 27:171, 1987.

Hammarback, S., and Backstrom, T. Induced anovulation as treatment of premenstrual tension syndrome. A double-blind cross-over study with GnRH-agonist versus placebo. *Acta Obstet. Gynecol. Scand.* 67:159, 1988.

Norman, R. J., Miller, J., Millar, R. P., et al. Treatment of menstrually induced acute intermittent porphyria by a long-acting gonadotrophin-releasing hormone agonist (D-Trp^6-Pro^9 N ethylamide) LHRH. Case Report. *Br. J. Obstet. Gynecol.* 95:192, 1988.

Slater, J. E., Raphael, G., Cutler, Jr., G. B., et al. Recurrent anaphylaxis in menstruating women: treatment with luteinizing hormone-releasing hormone agonist—a preliminary report. *Obstet. Gynecol.* 70:542, 1987.

Breast Cancer

Blankenstein, M. A., Henkelman, M. S., and Klijn, J. G. M. Direct inhibitory effect of a luteinizing hormone-releasing hormone agonist on MCF-7 human breast cancer cells. *Eur. J. Cancer Clin. Oncol.* 21:1493, 1985.

Manni, A., Santen, R., Harvey, H., et al. Treatment of breast cancer with gonadotropin-releasing hormone. *Endocr. Rev.* 7:89, 1986.

Ovarian Cancer

Parmar, H., Phillips, R. H., Rustin, G., et al. Therapy of advanced ovarian cancer with D-TRP-6-LH-RH (Decapeptyl) microcapsules. *Biomed. Pharmacother.* 42:531, 1988.

Contraception

Corbin, A., Bex, J. F., and Jones, R. C. LHRH and analogs: contraceptive and therapeutic considerations. *Int. J. Fertil.* 30:57, 1985.

Gudmundsson, J. A., Nillius, S. J., and Bergquist, C. Inhibition of ovulation by intranasal nafarelin, a new superactive agonist of GnRH. *Contraception* 30:107, 1984.

Schmidt-Gollwitzer, M., Hardt, M., Schmidt-Gollwitzer, K., et al. Influence of the LHRH analogue buserelin on cyclic ovarian function and on endometrium: a new approach to fertility control? *Contraception* 23:187, 1981.

Pituitary Function Testing

Factrel (gonadorelin hydrochloride). Package insert. Philadelphia: Wyeth-Ayerst Laboratories, 1989.

Contraindications, Warnings, and Precautions

MacLeod, T. L., Eisen, A., and Sussman, G. L. Anaphylactic reaction to synthetic luteinizing hormone-releasing hormone. *Fertil. Steril.* 48:500, 1987.

Serafini, P., Batzofin, J., Kerin, J., et al. Pregnancy: a risk to initiation of leuprolide acetate during the luteal phase before controlled ovarian hyperstimulation. *Fertil. Steril.* 50:371, 1988.

Adverse Reactions and Drug Preparations

Factrel (gonadorelin hydrochloride). Package insert. New York: Ayerst Laboratories, 1988.

Lupron (leuprolide acetate). Package insert. North Chicago: TAP Pharmaceuticals, 1988.

Zacur, H. A. Ovulation induction with gonadotropin-releasing hormone. *Fertil. Steril.* 44:435, 1985.

7

Prolactin Inhibitors

Gary W. De Vane

During the past 20 years prolactin has been identified as a distinct hormone in humans. Elevation of prolactin levels as measured by sensitive radioimmunoassay techniques occurs physiologically during pregnancy and lactation and in pathologic conditions such as prolactin-secreting adenomas of the pituitary gland. Even modest or transient elevations of circulating prolactin levels may result in menstrual irregularity, galactorrhea, and infertility in women and impotence in men.

Historically, ergot preparations were associated with inhibition of lactation indicating a possible role for ergot alkaloids in the suppression of prolactin secretion. The semisynthetic ergot alkaloid, bromocriptine mesylate (Parlodel), was developed in the late 1960s. This ergot derivative with minimal ergotoxic effect functions as a dopamine agonist and is currently the only prolactin inhibitor approved by the Food and Drug Administration (FDA) and available for clinical use in the United States.

The indications for bromocriptine in reproductive endocrinology include the treatment of menstrual dysfunction associated with hyperprolactinemia including amenorrhea with or without galactorrhea, infertility, hypogonadism, prevention of postpartum lactation, and reduction of tumor size in patients with prolactin-secreting adenomas.

NEUROENDOCRINE CONTROL OF PROLACTIN SECRETION

The secretion of prolactin by the pituitary gland is regulated by a neuroendocrine feedback mechanism involving the hypothalamus and pituitary. Prolactin is unique among the hormones of the anterior pituitary in that the primary control mechanism involves one or more prolactin-inhibiting factors (PIF) rather than releasing factors. These PIFs tonically inhibit the secretion of prolactin.

The most important PIF is believed to be dopamine. Dopamine is secreted directly into the hypophyseal portal blood system which transports it to the anterior pituitary. Dopamine binds to dopamine receptors in the pituitary lactotrope cell membrane through which a direct inhibitory effect is exerted on the lactotrope.

Prolactin-releasing factors have also been found in the hypothalamus. The best known of these is thyroid-releasing hormone (TRH). In all probability, other prolactin-releasing factors in the hypothalamus will be identified.

Acting in a short-loop, negative feedback manner, prolactin is the most significant factor in the regulation of its own secretion. Prolactin induces cell bodies in the hypothalamus to secrete dopamine which suppresses secretion of prolactin in the anterior pituitary.

A number of factors are known to raise serum prolactin levels (Table 7-1). These causes of hyperprolactinemia may be physiologic such as sleep-entrained prolactin release or pathologic as associated with prolactin-secreting pituitary tumors. Some drugs can interfere with dopamine action resulting in prolactin release (Table 7-2).

Table 7-1. Causes of hyperprolactinemia

Pituitary lesions
Prolactin-secreting pituitary tumors
Acromegaly
Cushing's disease
Nelson's syndrome
Primary empty sella syndrome
Hypothalamic lesions
Primary hypothyroidism
Chronic renal failure (20%)
Polycystic ovary disease
Irritative chest wall lesions (trauma, herpes zoster, thoracic burns, post-thoracotomy)
Idiopathic hyperprolactinemia
Physiologic
Pregnancy
Breast stimulation
Lactation
Sleep
Food intake

PHARMACOLOGY

Chemical Properties

Bromocriptine is a semisynthetic ergot alkaloid with the formula 2-bromo-alpha-ergocryptine mesylate. The pharmacologic effects of bromocriptine are based on its action as a dopamine receptor agonist. It exerts a direct effect on dopamine receptors in the hypothalamus and pituitary gland. Bromocriptine may also increase the secretion of dopamine in the tuberoinfundibular area of the hypothalamus. In vitro studies have shown that bromocriptine decreases spontaneous and TRH-induced release of prolactin from cultured pituitary tissue by stimulating dopamine receptors on hormone-secreting cells. By acting like dopamine, bromocriptine effectively reduces serum prolactin levels.

Pharmacokinetics

Studies in humans have been performed in part through the use of radiolabeled bromocriptine. The drug is rapidly absorbed from the gastrointestinal tract; 28 percent of an oral dose is absorbed. The maximal plasma levels occur about 1.4 to 3.0 hours following inges-

Table 7-2. Pharmacologic causes of hyperprolactinemia

Reserpine, alpha-methyldopa
Haloperidol, chlorpromazine, metoclopramide
Cimetidine
Tricyclic antidepressants
Opiates (e.g., morphine, methadone)
Estrogens
Verapamil

tion, with a half-life of 3.1 hours. Excretion is primarily (5%) biliary with complete degradation into inactive metabolites. A decline in prolactin levels is evident 2 hours after ingestion, with maximal suppression at 5 hours.

INDICATIONS FOR BROMOCRIPTINE AND THE DISORDERS INVOLVED

Female Reproductive Dysfunction

Bromocriptine is indicated for the treatment of menstrual dysfunctions associated with hyperprolactinemia including amenorrhea with or without galactorrhea, infertility, or hypogonadism. Menstrual irregularity may be classified as either oligomenorrhea (irregular or scanty menses) or amenorrhea (no menstrual cycles).

Ovulatory dysfunction is a frequent manifestation of elevated prolactin levels but in some instances normal menstrual cycles may be present. With careful monitoring, subtle abnormalities of luteal phase progesterone production (luteal phase deficiency) may be present and have been associated with elevated prolactin levels. The actual incidence of hyperprolactinemia-related ovulatory disorders is not known but is estimated to be between 15 and 20 percent of all patients with secondary amenorrhea.

Female Infertility

Almost all women with hyperprolactinemia, regardless of cause, are infertile. While infertility associated with hyperprolactinemia is often associated with menstrual disorders, it has been demonstrated that minimal and transitory increases in serum prolactin levels can induce infertility in women with apparently normal menstrual cycles. Determination of serum prolactin levels is a mandatory part of the evaluation of all reproductive disorders. Even a high-normal prolactin level may not be "normal" because of variation in laboratory testing results.

Prolactinomas

Prolactin-secreting pituitary adenomas are the most common cause of conditions associated with hyperprolactinemia. Tumors are distinguished primarily by size; those less than 10 mm in diameter are microadenomas and those larger than 10 mm are macroadenomas.

Practically all patients with prolactinomas have elevated prolactin levels. In contrast, not all patients with elevated prolactin levels have detectable prolactin-secreting tumor. Generally, the higher the serum prolactin level, the greater the chance that the patient is harboring a prolactinoma.

According to widely accepted criteria, patients with prolactin levels above 100 ng/ml are likely to have pituitary tumors, although there have been reports of patients with prolactinoma who have serum prolactin levels below 50 ng/ml. Thus, examination of the sella is advisable in patients with elevated prolactin levels.

X rays of the sella turcica can reveal alterations in the size and contours of the sella, suggestive of the presence of a tumor, but usually detect large tumors only. In contrast, high-resolution computed tomographic (CT) scanning with direct coronal images can provide evidence of microadenomas as well as anatomic detail that is undetectable on plain film x rays. Magnetic resonance imaging may soon be the preferable diagnostic technique.

Reduction in tumor size has been demonstrated in both male and female patients who have macroadenomas. When neurosurgical excision of adenoma is elected, a course of bromocriptine therapy may be used to reduce the tumor mass prior to surgery.

Prevention of Physiologic Lactation

Bromocriptine tablets are indicated for the prevention of physiologic lactation (secretion, congestion, and engorgement) occurring after parturition when the mother elects not to breast-feed the infant or when breast-feeding is contraindicated and after stillbirth or abortion.

Once bromocriptine is stopped, 18 to 40 percent of patients experience rebound breast engorgement which is usually mild to moderate in severity.

Male Reproductive Dysfunction

While the normal role of prolactin in male reproductive function is not completely understood, clinical studies have clearly shown that elevated prolactin levels can cause male infertility and impotence.

Pseudotumor Cerebri

The possibility exists that prolactin may have a physiologic role in the production of cerebrospinal fluid (CSF) and that excess of CSF prolactin may have a role in the pathogenesis of pseudotumor cerebri. If CSF hyperprolactinemia causes excess CSF production, then bromocriptine mesylate may be a therapeutic agent for pseudotumor cerebri.

Polycystic Ovary Disease

In some women with polycystic ovary disease, as typified by anovulation, hirsutism, and increased body mass but normal prolactin concentration, ovulatory function may be improved by treatment with bromocriptine. Reduction in prolactin levels alone or in combination with ovulation induction (i.e., clomiphene, human menopausal gonadotropin) may provide for normal ovulatory function and fertility. Treatment in women with polycystic ovary disease should be restricted to those patients with high-normal prolactin levels.

Normoprolactinemic Infertility

Certain sensitive, infertile, normoprolactinemic women may benefit from low-dose bromocriptine therapy. These women usually have regular menstrual cycles but may be identified by the presence of expressible galactorrhea or by an exaggerated prolactin release after TRH or metoclopramide dynamic testing. Since these women presumably have intermittent prolactin spikes or nocturnal release, a modified treatment regimen has been shown to have efficacy.

Premenstrual Syndrome

Premenstrual syndrome (PMS) is a poorly understood complex of adverse symptoms affecting women in a cyclic fashion. Certain women with PMS exhibit cyclic fluid retention, edema, and bloating that may respond to prolactin reduction. Those women with elevation of prolactin concentration respond better to this treatment.

Repeated Pregnancy Wastage

The use of bromocriptine empirically in women with repeated pregnancy wastage is not indicated. Both hyperprolactinemia and hypoprolactinemia will induce ovulatory problems. Excessive suppression of circulating prolactin levels has been shown to induce luteolysis. Only documented luteal phase defects with dysfolliculogenesis caused by elevated secretion of prolactin should be considered as an indication for bromocriptine treatment in women with repeated pregnancy loss.

Galactorrhea and Mastalgia

Treatment with bromocriptine will inhibit nonpuerperal breast secretion in women who have elevated as well as normal prolactin concentrations. Patients should be instructed to avoid breast manipulation and to wear a supportive bra. Galactorrhea often recurs following cessation of treatment.

Some women with cyclic breast engorgement and pain may respond to reduction of circulating prolactin levels.

Areas of Controversy

Premenopausal, hypoestrogenic women have been shown to be at risk for development of osteopenia. The possibility that elevated prolactin levels contribute to bone mineral loss is controversial. Some hyperprolactinemic women have been reported to have decreased bone mineral density as compared to both normal and amenorrheic women with normal prolactin levels. Currently, longitudinal studies of hyperprolactinemic individuals compared with control subjects are under way to resolve the influences of prolactin excess and estrogen deprivation on bone mineral content. Estrogen replacement therapy is the therapy of choice to prevent or retard osteopenia. The hyperprolactinemic patient may prove to be at increased risk for osteoporosis. Treatment with bromocriptine to restore normal ovulatory function (endogenous estrogen) may ultimately prove to be more appropriate therapy in premenopausal women than estrogen replacement alone.

CONTRAINDICATIONS, WARNINGS, AND PRECAUTIONS

Sensitivity to Ergot Alkaloids

Warnings

Since hyperprolactinemia with amenorrhea or galactorrhea with infertility has been found in patients with pituitary tumors, a complete evaluation of the pituitary is indicated before treatment with bromocriptine.

Teratogenic Effects

If drug therapy for the restoration of fertility is successful and the patient becomes pregnant, she may have been taking the drug during the period between conception and the confirmation of pregnancy. Thus, the possibility of teratogenic effects of the fertility agent is a prime concern. Another concern is the tendency of some fertility agents to produce multiple births.

Studies assessing the outcome of pregnancies induced by bromocriptine have clearly demonstrated that the incidence of birth defects and multiple births occurring in this group is no greater than in the general population. The report of the drug monitoring center,

Sandoz Limited (Basle, Switzerland), as reported by Turkalj and associates in reviewing 1410 pregnancies, showed 86 percent live births, 11.1 percent spontaneous abortions, 0.9 percent extrauterine pregnancies, 2.5 percent minor malformations, 1.0 percent major malformations, and 1.8 percent twins. Therefore, it appears that patients with both microadenomas and macroadenomas can achieve pregnancy and carry these gestations to term with minimal complications.

Precautions

The safety and efficacy of bromocriptine have not been established in patients with renal or hepatic disease. Care should be exercised when administering bromocriptine therapy concomitantly with other medications known to lower blood pressure.

Hyperprolactinemic States

Since pregnancy is often the therapeutic objective in many hyperprolactinemic patients, a careful assessment of the pituitary is essential to detect the presence of a prolactin-secreting adenoma. Patients who are not seeking pregnancy or those who have large adenomas should be advised to use contraceptive measures, other than oral contraceptives, during treatment with bromocriptine. Since pregnancy may occur prior to reinitiation of menses, a pregnancy test is recommended at least every 4 weeks during the amenorrheic period and, when menses is reinitiated, every time a patient misses a menstrual period. Treatment with bromocriptine should be discontinued as soon as pregnancy has been established. Patients must be monitored closely throughout pregnancy for signs and symptoms that may signal the enlargement of a previously undetected or existing prolactin-secreting tumor. Discontinuation of bromocriptine treatment in patients with known macroadenomas has been associated with rapid regrowth of tumor and increase in serum prolactin levels in most cases.

METABOLIC EFFECTS, ALTERED LABORATORY VALUES, AND DRUG INTERACTIONS

Lack of or decrease in efficacy may occur in patients receiving bromocriptine when they are treated with drugs that have dopamine antagonist activity (e.g., phenothiazines, butyrophenones). This may be a problem, particularly for patients who are treated with bromocriptine for macroadenomas.

Normal individuals who are treated with medications that elevate prolactin secretion often present with menstrual irregularity (see Table 7-2). As a rule, a serum prolactin level must be obtained. Modest elevation of prolactin concentration (40–50 ng/ml) is to be expected. A prolactin level should be obtained every 6 to 12 months in those individuals with menstrual problems who receive such medications. Higher levels of prolactin also are not uncommon. To rule out the possibility of a pituitary tumor contributing to the presumed drug-induced hyperprolactinemia, a baseline CT scan would seem a prudent diagnostic study.

Even birth control pills may cause mild elevations of prolactin release. There is no evidence to indicate residual prolactin secretion or pituitary adenoma formation.

ADVERSE REACTIONS

The incidence of adverse effects is quite high (69%), but the effects are generally mild to moderate in degree. Approximately 5 percent of patients discontinue use because of adverse effects. In decreasing order of frequency these are nausea (49%), headache (19%), dizziness (17%), fatigue (7%), light-headedness (5%), vomiting (5%), abdominal cramps (5%), nasal congestion (3%), and drowsiness (3%).

A slight hypotensive effect may accompany bromocriptine therapy. Adverse reactions may be lessened by temporarily reducing the dosage to a one-half tablet daily, then gradually increasing dosage.

Physiologic Lactation

Twenty-three percent of patients who are treated with bromocriptine within the recommended dosage range for the prevention of physiologic lactation had at least one side effect but it was generally mild to moderate in degree. Approximately 3 percent of patients discontinue use. The most frequently occurring adverse reactions were: headaches (10%), dizziness (8%), nausea (7%), vomiting (3%). fatigue (1%), syncope (0.7%), diarrhea (0.4%), and cramps (0.4%). Transient decreases in blood pressure have occurred in approximately 25 percent of patients at least once during the first 3 postpartum days. Idiosyncratic elevation in blood pressure is a rare but reported complication usually associated with pregnancy-induced hypertensive conditions. The relationship between these adverse hypertensive reactions to bromocriptine is not certain. The use of bromocriptine for lactation suppression is not recommended for patients with uncontrolled hypertension or toxemia of pregnancy. The use of bromocriptine in combination with other ergot alkaloids (ergotamine, methylergonovine maleate, etc.) is also not recommended.

ADMINISTRATION

Bromocriptine should be taken with food. Patients should be evaluated frequently during dose escalation to determine the lowest effective dose.

The initial dose is one-half to one 2.5-mg tablet daily. An additional 2.5-mg tablet may be added to the treatment regimen as tolerated every 3 to 7 days, until an optimal therapeutic response is achieved. The therapeutic dosage usually is 5 to 7.5 mg and ranges from 2.5 to 15 mg per day. On occasion, 1.25 mg (½ tablet) may prove sufficient for treatment.

In those women who experience significant gastrointestinal side effects, vaginal administration of bromocriptine may be a safe and therapeutic mode of therapy. Excellent absorption of bromocriptine in doses of 2.5 to 7.5 mg daily has been demonstrated. Reduction in prolactin concentration occurs approximately 11 hours after vaginal administration with a sustained inhibitory effect demonstrated allowing for single-dose treatment. The incidence of "central" side effects such as headache, dizziness, and hypotension is not different from effects observed with oral therapy.

To reduce the likelihood of prolonged exposure to bromocriptine should an unsuspected pregnancy occur, a mechanical contraceptive should be used until normal ovulatory menstrual cycles have been restored. Contraception may then be discontinued in patients desiring pregnancy. If menstruation does not occur within 3 days of the expected date, bromocriptine therapy should be discontinued and a pregnancy test performed.

BROMOCRIPTINE PREPARATION AND DOSAGE

First synthesized at Sandoz Laboratories, bromocriptine was the first drug developed specifically for suppressing prolactin secretion in humans.

Empirical Formula:	$C_{32}H_{40}BrN_59_5CH_4O_3S = C_{33}H_{44}BrN_59_8S$
Molecular weight:	654.61 + 96.10 = 750.71
Chemical name:	2-Bromoergocryptine mesylate
Name of new drug substance:	Bromocriptine (as the mesylate)
General name:	Bromocriptine mesylate
Trade name:	Parlodel

Parlodel is an ergot derivative with potent dopamine receptor agonist activity. Each tablet for oral administration contains 2.5 mg and each capsule contains 5 mg of bromocriptine (as the mesylate). There is a long-acting injectable preparation (Depo-Parlodel) which is not yet FDA approved.

Other dopamine agonists are not available in the United States.

A second dopamine agonist, pergolide mesylate (Lilly) is effective in the treatment of patients with functional hyperprolactinemia and prolactinoma. Pergolide acts directly at the pituitary to inhibit prolactin secretion and is orally active in a dose range of 25 to 100 μg/day.

A third dopamine agonist, CV 205-502 (Sandoz), is currently under investigation and is similar but slightly more potent than Parlodel.

Lisuride is another class of dopamine agonist with similar characteristics but slightly more side effects.

The therapeutic dose for bromocriptine is usually promoted as 2.5 mg twice daily to 2.5 mg 4 times daily in hyperprolactinemic patients. Much higher doses have been used for nonendocrine related conditions such as in patients with Parkinson's disease. Patients with idiopathic hyperprolactinemia and pituitary adenomas frequently respond to a subtherapeutic dose of bromocriptine. Thus, there is a great deal of variability in the dosage required to elicit the desired therapeutic effect. A logical approach to bromocriptine dosing in patients with various indications for suppression of their hyperprolactinemic condition is to titrate the dose to obtain the desired effect. A gradual increase in dosage should always be used and usually 1.25 mg (½ tablet) is prescribed to be taken at bedtime with food for the first 3 to 7 days. As the dose is increased to the general range indicated below, it is suggested that patients be given 1.25 mg twice daily for 1 week then 1.25 mg orally 3 times daily for 1 week, followed by 2.5 mg twice daily for 1 week, then with increases to 2.5 mg orally 3 to 4 times daily as required. The final maintenance dose is determined by obtaining random prolactin levels while the patient is receiving treatment, with a therapeutic goal of normalizing circulating prolactin concentration. Often, with prolonged therapy, especially in patients with regression of prolactinoma size, patients may be maintained on a reduced dose for extended periods.

PROTOCOLS

For female infertility the dose is usually ½ to 3 tablets (1.25–7.50 mg/day). For infertility associated with borderline and transitory elevations of prolactin, ½ to 1 tablet is taken orally at bedtime or

½ tablet is taken twice a day. For infertility in patients with documented prolactinomas, the dose is 1 tablet taken orally twice a day or 1 tablet taken orally 3 times a day. Menstrual cycle disorders are treated with 1 tablet per day or 1 tablet twice a day.

The protocol for male reproductive dysfunctions varies.

For patients with pituitary macroadenomas the dosage usually given is 5 to 15 mg per day (or higher as required).

The protocol for pseudotumor cerebri is experimental; 1 tablet is taken orally 3 times a day.

A modified regimen for normoprolactinemic infertility is ½ tablet taken orally at bedtime on days 1 to 10 of the menstrual cycle, followed by 1 tablet taken orally on days 11 to 18. This sequence is repeated monthly.

Lactation Suppression

Treatment should be instituted no sooner than 4 hours after a normal delivery. The usual dose is one tablet (2.5 mg) twice daily. The usual dosage range is 2.5 to 7.5 mg daily. Treatment should be continued for 7 to 14 days. Approximately 30 percent of patients experience rebound breast engorgement which usually responds to an additional week of treatment.

The use of bromocriptine for lactation suppression is now the treatment of choice as compared to high-dose estrogen or estrogen-testosterone combinations. Many clinicians continue to use only supportive measures such as breast binding for postpartum suppression of lactation.

INSTRUCTIONS TO THE PATIENT

Bromocriptine acts by inhibiting prolactin secretion at the level of the pituitary. It has also been found to reduce the size of prolactin-secreting pituitary tumors.

The dosage may vary, depending on the cause of prolactin elevation and the degree of elevation. Generally, the dose is started at one-half tablet once daily and is then increased weekly to a specific maintenance dose or as tolerated. You will be given a specific dosage schedule to follow. Periodic prolactin levels will be drawn to evaluate your response to the drug. Most side effects diminish with continued use of Parlodel.

If you are avoiding pregnancy, you should use a reliable form of contraception. Remember that bromocriptine restores ovulation and may increase your chances for pregnancy.

The following are common side effects that are not generally serious: nausea, vomiting, dizziness, and nasal congestion.

If you should experience any of the following symptoms, notify your physician: significant or persistent dizziness, fainting, significant weakness, or persistent vomiting.

BIBLIOGRAPHY

Overview

Goodman, L. S., and Gilman, A. *The Pharmacological Basis of Therapeutics*, ed. 6. New York: Macmillan, 1980. Pp. 1380-1383.

Physiology

Clemens, J. A., and Shaar, C. J. Control of prolactin secretion in mammals. *Fed. Proc.* 39:2588, 1980.

Gibbs, D. M., and Neill, J. D. Dopamine levels in hypophyseal stalk blood in the rat are sufficient to inhibit prolactin secretions in vivo. *Endocrinology* 102:1895, 1978.

Gudelsky, G. A., and Porter, J. C. Release of dopamine from tuberoinfundibular neurons in pituitary stalk blood after prolactin or haloperidol administration. *Endocrinology* 105:526, 1980.

Pharmacokinetics

Herman, T. N., and Molitch, M. E. Bromocriptine: indications and use in patients with endocrine disease. *Hosp. Formul.* 19:784, 1984.

Vermesh, N., Fossum, G. T., and Kletzky, O. A. Vaginal bromocriptine: pharmacology and effect on serum prolactin in normal women. *Obstet. Gynecol.* 72:693, 1988.

Disorders Treated

Menstrual Dysfunction

Del Pozo, E., et al. Prolactin and deficient luteal function. *Obstet. Gynecol.* 53:282, 1979.

Greer, M. E., Moraczewski, T., and Rakoff, J. S. Prevalence of hyperprolactinemia in anovulatory women. *Obstet. Gynecol.* 56:65, 1980.

Infertility

Ben-David, M., and Schenker, J. G. Transient hyperprolactinemia: a correctable cause of idiopathic female infertility. *J. Clin. Endocrinol. Metab.* 57:442, 1983.

Board, J. A., Storlazzi, E., and Schneider, V. Nocturnal prolactin levels in infertility. *Fertil. Steril.* 36:720, 1981.

Coutts, J. R. T., et al. Role of transient hyperprolactinemia in the short luteal phase. *Prog. Reprod. Biol.* 6:187, 1980.

DeVane, G. W., and Guzick, D. S. Bromocriptine therapy in normoprolactinemic women with unexplained infertility and galactorrhea. *Fertil. Steril.* 46:1026, 1986.

Prolactinoma

Vance, M. L., Evans, W. S., and Thorner, M. O. Bromocriptine. *Ann. Intern. Med.* 100:78, 1984.

Impotence

Franks, S., et al. Hyperprolactinemia and impotence. *Clin. Endocrinol.* 8:277, 1978.

Pseudotumor Cerebri

Bates, G. W., et al. Elevated cerebrospinal fluid prolactin in women with pseudotumor cerebri. *South. Med. J.* 75:807, 1982.

Polycystic Ovarian Disease

Seibel, M. M., et al. Treatment of normoprolactinemic polycystic ovary disease with chronic low dose bromocriptine. *Fertil. Steril.* 39:433, 1983.

Osteoporosis

Schlecte, J. A., Sherman, B., and Martin, R. Bone density in amenorrheic women with and without hyperprolactinemia. *J. Clin. Endocrinol. Metab.* 56:1120, 1983.

Therapeutic Usage

Blackwell, R. E., et al. Comparison of dopamine agonists in the treatment of hyperprolactinemic syndromes: a multicenter study. *Fertil. Steril.* 39:744, 1983.

Hesla, J. S., et al. The effects of the ergoline derivative, CU-32085, on prolactin secretion in hyperprolactinemic women. *Fertil. Steril.* 40:555, 1987.

Use in Pregnancy

Turkalj, I., Braun, P., and Krupp, P. Surveillance of bromocriptine in pregnancy. *J.A.M.A.* 247:1589, 1982.

8

Adrenal Hormones

Owen K. Davis and Isaac Schiff

This chapter focuses on the reproductive endocrine applications of drugs that exert their effects, either primarily or in part, on the adrenal gland. An exhaustive survey of adrenal physiology and pharmacology is beyond the scope of this book; accordingly, the ensuing discussion will emphasize those aspects that are most relevant to the practicing gynecologist.

Spironolactone, a potassium-sparing diuretic, appears to be useful in some patients as single-agent or adjunctive therapy for hirsutism. Although displaying prominent target-tissue effects, this agent also affects adrenal and gonadal steroidogenesis, and its net activity likely results from a combination of these factors. Glucocorticoids have also found wide use, both alone and in combination therapy, in the treatment of various reproductive endocrine disorders including congenital adrenal hyperplasia, hirsutism or hyperandrogenism, and anovulation. Glucocorticoids also have diagnostic value, for example, in the performance of suppression tests.

SPIRONOLACTONE

Spironolactone is a 17-spirolactone steroid and is an effective diuretic, useful in the treatment of edematous conditions, essential hypertension, and primary hyperaldosteronism. More recently, it has been shown that spironolactone has significant antiandrogenic properties and is a useful drug in the treatment of hirsutism and possibly hyperandrogenic anovulation. For these latter indications spironolactone can be prescribed either as a single agent or in combination with other therapies, such as oral contraceptives or glucocorticoids.

Pharmacology

Spironolactone is available for oral administration either as the generic drug or as Aldactone (Searle), and is formulated in 25-mg, 50-mg, and 100-mg tablets. It is soluble in alcohol or benzene but is poorly soluble in water. Spironolactone is readily absorbed after oral administration, and its bioavailability exceeds 90 percent. Bioavailability is enhanced 20 to 35 percent in film-coated versus uncoated preparations. Spironolactone is rapidly and extensively metabolized by the liver, and approximately 80 percent of an administered dose is converted to the active metabolite canrenone. Peak serum levels of canrenone are achieved approximately 2 to 4 hours after a dose. In the blood, both spironolactone and canrenone are greater than 90 percent bound to plasma proteins.

The serum half-life of canrenone varies with the frequency of administration. With once or twice daily dosage, its half-life averages 19 hours (range, 13–24 hours) and with administration 4 times a day, the average half-life decreases to 12.5 hours (range, 9–16 hours). The time to peak effect and duration of spironolactone's diuretic action is 2 to 3 days.

The excretion of spironolactone and its metabolites is principally by the renal route, and to a lesser extent by the biliary route. Approximately 70 percent of a single dose of spironolactone is excreted within 5 days. Less than 10 percent of the parent compound is excreted in the urine unchanged.

Mechanism of Action

Spironolactone's diuretic and antihypertensive effects derive from the drug's aldosterone-antagonist properties. As a structural homologue of aldosterone, spironolactone competitively binds aldosterone receptors in the renal distal convoluted tubules, thus affecting sodium and water excretion and potassium retention. This results in an increased urinary sodium-potassium ratio. Further, spironolactone increases calcium excretion through an effect on renal tubular transport.

The antiandrogenic effects of spironolactone appear to be exerted at multiple sites. Spironolactone and its active metabolites bind androgen receptors in target tissues, thus inhibiting the peripheral expression of hyperandrogenism. Additionally, spironolactone may inhibit 5α-reductase activity, thus impeding the peripheral conversion of testosterone to the more potent androgen dihydrotestosterone (DHT). Most investigators believe that these "end-organ" effects are the predominant mode of this drug's antiandrogenic activity.

Several studies have demonstrated that spironolactone has an inhibitory effect on steroidogenesis of sex hormones. Treatment of hirsute women with spironolactone has been shown to result in decreased circulating levels of several androgens, including testosterone, androstenedione, dehydroepiandrosterone sulfate (DHEA-S), and DHT. It should be noted that not all studies have confirmed a significant suppressive effect on all of these androgens, however. Spironolactone impedes the production of androgens primarily through the inhibition of cytochrome P-450. This results in decreased activity of 17-hydroxylase, a key enzyme in the biosynthesis of sex steroids. Further, spironolactone has been shown to inhibit the activities of other gonadal and adrenal enzymes, including the 11β- and 21-hydroxylases, desmolase, and 3β-hydroxysteroid dehydrogenase. Spironolactone may also increase the peripheral aromatization of testosterone to estradiol.

Gynecologic Indications

Hirsutism

Hirsutism is characterized by abnormally increased transformation of vellus to terminal hair, due to either increased circulating levels of androgens or heightened peripheral sensitivity to normal androgen levels (idiopathic hirsutism). In women, this presents clinically as excessive pigmented hair growth in areas such as the face (upper lip, chin, sideburns), chest, and abdomen. Hirsutism may be accompanied by the development of acne or menstrual irregularity, or both. Signs of true virilization, including clitoromegaly, temporal balding, muscle development, and deepening of the voice, are suggestive of marked hyperandrogenism and, along with a history of rapid progression of symptoms, should alert the clinician to the possible presence of an ovarian or adrenal tumor. Once a neoplasm has been ruled out, the differential diagnosis of adult-onset hirsutism in the female consists predominantly of polycystic ovary syndrome and its variants, idiopathic hirsutism and late-onset congenital adrenal hyperplasia. Patients with Cushing's syndrome may also present with hirsutism and acne, but the usual constellation of

Table 8-1. Spironolactone and glucocorticoid therapy in the treatment of hirsutism

Agent	Dose
Spironolactone[a]	100–200 mg PO, qd
Glucocorticoids[b]	
Dexamethasone	0.50–0.75 mg PO, 1hs
Prednisone	2.5–5.0 mg PO, q12h

[a] Check serum electrolyte levels, blood urea nitrogen, and creatinine levels prior to the initiation of therapy. If no improvement of hirsutism is observed within 3–6 months, consider alternative or combination therapy.
[b] Consider glucocorticoids as adjunctive or alternative therapy for hirsutism resistant to standard treatment (e.g., oral contraceptives), particularly when suppressibility of androgens can be demonstrated. Adjust glucocorticoid dosage to maintain morning basal serum levels of cortisol at ≥2.0 μg/dl, to avoid oversuppression.

signs and symptoms should lead to appropriate workup and diagnosis. Late-onset congenital adrenal hyperplasia is most accurately diagnosed by corticotropin-stimulation testing, and first-line therapy consists of glucocorticoids (Table 8-1). Polycystic ovary syndrome and idiopathic hirsutism are amenable to therapy with spironolactone. The mainstay of therapy for polycystic ovary syndrome in patients who do not want to conceive is a combination oral contraceptive. Such therapy results in suppression of luteinizing hormone (LH) levels and increased production of sex hormone—binding globulin (SHBG), with the net effect of decreasing both total and unbound testosterone. Oral contraceptives are also frequently effective in the amelioration of idiopathic hirsutism. Spironolactone is a useful alternative agent for patients in whom a contraindication to oral contraceptives exists or for patients in whom bothersome side effects develop. For example, spironolactone might be a good choice as first-line therapy in a hirsute woman with hypertension, a condition for which oral contraceptives are relatively contraindicated. Spironolactone may also be effective in hirsute patients who show an inadequate response to oral contraceptives or other agents.

When spironolactone is administered as single-agent therapy for hirsutism, a significant clinical response can be expected in 70 to 80 percent of patients. Quantitatively, this improvement is reflected in a 19 to 30 percent decrease in the mean diameter of facial and abdominal anagen hair shafts, in a dose-dependent manner. In hirsute women for whom spironolactone is effective, a positive response is generally seen within the first 3 months of treatment. Suppression of androgens, while measurable within 4 weeks, is maximal after 3 months of spironolactone administration and is maintained thereafter. However, the success of spironolactone therapy should be judged on the basis of degree of clinical improvement of hirsutism, and not on changes in circulating androgen levels per se. Some patients who show a significant symptomatic response to spironolactone will nevertheless have minimal changes in serum androgen concentrations. Of interest, despite strong evidence for a predominantly peripheral effect of spironolactone in many of these women, serum levels of 3α-diol glucuronide (a marker for peripheral androgen metabolism and hirsutism) correlate poorly with improvement of hirsutism.

There is recent evidence that combination therapy consisting of spironolactone coadministered with either oral contraceptives or glucocorticoids may be effective treatment for hirsute women who are unresponsive to single agents. It was found that fully 89 percent of a group of hirsute women failing to respond to single-agent treatment with either spironolactone, oral contraceptives, or dexamethasone had a positive clinical response to combination drug therapy.

Amenorrhea

Although spironolactone is not generally recommended as primary therapy for amenorrhea, it should be noted that cyclic menses will ensue in a majority of amenorrheic patients with polycystic ovary syndrome who are treated with this drug. Spironolactone therapy restored regular although anovulatory menses in all of a group of 34 oligomenorrheic or amenorrheic women with polycystic ovary syndrome. In another study, successful induction of ovulation occurred in 11 (85%) of 13 anovulatory, hyperandrogenic women who were treated with spironolactone in doses of 100 to 150 mg per day.

Method of Use

Preliminary Workup

For patients who are candidates for spironolactone treatment, a medical history should be taken and a physical examination done, with an emphasis on a history of renal disease. The cause of hirsutism should be ascertained, and potentially life-threatening processes such as ovarian or adrenal neoplasia and Cushing's syndrome should be excluded. In the absence of a palpable pelvic or abdominal mass, a serum total testosterone level exceeding 200 ng/dl or a serum DHEA-S level exceeding 700 μg/dl, or both, mandates a thorough workup to rule out an androgen-secreting tumor. Women with signs or symptoms suggestive of Cushing's syndrome should be screened with either an overnight dexamethasone suppression test (discussion to come) or a 24-hour urine collection to determine free cortisol levels. Initial evaluation should also include determinations of serum prolactin concentrations and thyroid function. In patients for whom spironolactone therapy is contemplated, baseline serum electrolyte levels, blood urea nitrogen, and creatinine levels should be assessed because hyperkalemia and impaired renal function are contraindications to the use of this drug. Pregnancy must be excluded, especially in the oligomenorrheic or amenorrheic patient, as the safety of spironolactone use during pregnancy has not been established.

Beginning Spironolactone

Spironolactone is administered in doses ranging from 100 to 200 mg per day in the treatment of hirsutism. Evidence that the frequency of drug-induced side effects correlates with dosage suggests that the spironolactone dosage should be initiated at 100 mg, given either once daily or as two divided doses. Dosage can be increased stepwise to 150 to 200 mg per day in the absence of a satisfactory clinical response. Lack of symptomatic improvement after 3 to 6 months of treatment is indicative of treatment failure, and should lead to consideration of combination or alternative therapy. Although spironolactone is generally prescribed in a continuous fashion, several authors have advocated cyclic therapy from day 4 or 5 through day 21 or 22. Cyclic therapy is predicated on the theories that spironolactone's enzyme-inhibitory effects persist for several days after a single dose and that the incidence of side effects, particularly metrorrhagia, can be reduced by providing a "window" for menstrual bleeding.

Combination Therapy

Hirsute patients refractory to single-agent therapy with spironolactone, oral contraceptives, or glucocorticoids may respond to a regimen combining these agents. In one study, 25 percent of hirsute women who were treated with single agents failed to improve. Combination therapy consisting of spironolactone, 100 to 150 mg, administered daily with either an oral contraceptive or dexamethasone (0.5 mg) resulted in a satisfactory clinical response in 89 percent of these "resistant" patients, based on a doubling of the time interval between adjunctive therapies (e.g., electrolysis) and patient satisfaction.

Use in Pregnancy

Spironolactone and its metabolites may cross the placenta. Although not known to be teratogenic in humans, canrenoate potassium has been shown to exert mutagenic effects in certain in vitro mammalian cell systems. Spironolactone is seldom if ever indicated in pregnant patients. Canrenone, a metabolite of spironolactone, appears in breast milk and the effects of chronic ingestion in infants are not known. Until further data are available, spironolactone should be avoided by nursing mothers.

Side Effects and Toxicity

Initiation of spironolactone therapy often results in a transient diuresis, manifested by polyuria and polydipsia; these symptoms are typically self-limited and confined to the first few weeks of treatment. When spironolactone is given as a single daily dose, administration in the morning can avoid problems with transient urinary frequency at night. Perhaps the most frequent bothersome side effect of spironolactone in hirsute women is menstrual irregularity, specifically metrorrhagia. Most reports describe an incidence of dysfunctional bleeding ranging from 0 to 27 percent. A recent study demonstrated that reducing the initial dosage of spironolactone from 200 to 100 mg per day resulted in a 64 percent reduction in the incidence of metrorrhagia. Other maneuvers that may be attempted include intermittent administration of spironolactone (already mentioned) or addition of cyclic administration of estrogen or progestin. Other less frequently noted adverse reactions include gastrointestinal symptoms, headache, drowsiness, cutaneous eruptions or urticaria, drug fever, and ataxia. Spironolactone may be taken with food, thereby decreasing the likelihood of gastrointestinal upset. Agranulocytosis has been reported in a few patients taking spironolactone. In men, both gynecomastia and impotence have been described. Adverse reactions are usually reversible on discontinuation of therapy.

It should be noted that spironolactone has been shown to be tumorigenic in studies on the effect of chronic toxicity in rats. Although breast carcinoma has been reported in patients taking the drug, a causal relationship has not been established.

One distinct advantage of spironolactone over glucocorticoid therapy is the apparent lack of significant adrenal suppression. Basal levels of serum cortisol and corticotropin are not affected by treatment with spironolactone. There is some evidence that a blunting of the cortisol response to corticotropin-stimulation testing may occur in hirsute women receiving spironolactone, but clinical problems with cortisol insufficiency have not been encountered.

Other Side Effects and Drug Interactions

Coadministration of spironolactone with potassium supplements or other potassium-sparing diuretics may lead to hyperkalemia, and therefore should be avoided. Severe hyperkalemia may also develop if this drug is given to patients with significant renal impairment.

Spironolactone can potentiate the effects of other antihypertensive drugs, and dosages need to be modified accordingly. Spironolactone decreases vascular sensitivity to norepinephrine, and caution must be exercised in patients undergoing general or regional anesthesia.

The serum half-life of digoxin is increased in patients receiving spironolactone, via a reduction in renal clearance, thus increasing the risk of digoxin toxicity. Further, spironolactone may interfere with radioimmunoassays for digoxin.

Contraindications

Contraindications to spironolactone therapy include anuria, acute renal insufficiency, impaired renal function, and hyperkalemia.

GLUCOCORTICOIDS

The glucocorticoids are adrenocortical steroids, both naturally occurring and synthetic, and are used to treat a number of medical problems. As a class, the glucocorticoids display a wide range of actions. Metabolic effects include stimulation of protein catabolism, lipolysis and gluconeogenesis, an increase in blood sugar and hepatic glycogen levels, and inhibition of peripheral glucose utilization. Pharmacologic doses of glucocorticoids inhibit calcium absorption from the gastrointestinal tract, promote bone resorption, and exert anti-inflammatory effects which include stabilization of lysosomes, decreased capillary permeability, suppression of phospholipase A_2 (and hence prostaglandin) activity, and decreased inflammatory cell migration. Immunosuppressive effects impact primarily on the cell-mediated response, but production of humoral antibodies is also impaired. Glucocorticoid activity is important in the physiologic response to stress, as it plays a permissive role in the effect of catecholamines on the cardiovascular system. Further, glucocorticoids augment renal blood flow and increase the glomerular filtration rate.

The therapeutic applications of glucocorticoids are numerous and diverse. Conditions such as allergic diseases, collagen vascular disease, blood dyscrasias, dermatologic disorders, inflammatory gastrointestinal disease, and transplant rejection may be responsive to the anti-inflammatory and immunosuppressive effects of glucocorticoids. Glucocorticoids are indicated as replacement therapy for patients with primary or secondary adrenocortical insufficiency and are the mainstay of treatment for congenital adrenal hyperplasia.

The major reproductive endocrine applications of glucocorticoids include congenital adrenal hyperplasia, hirsutism, ovulation induction, and suppression testing for Cushing's syndrome. The remainder of this discussion will therefore focus on these applications, with an emphasis on the use of dexamethasone and prednisone, the steroids most extensively described in the gynecologic literature.

Pharmacology

Prednisone

Prednisone is available for oral administration both as the generic drug and in a number of brand-name preparations, formulated as 1.0-, 2.5-, 5.0-, 10.0-, 20.0- and 50.0-mg tablets. Prednisone is very slightly soluble in water and slightly soluble in alcohol, chloroform, and dioxane. Prednisone is readily and almost completely (>70%) absorbed after an oral dose. The parent compound has a very low affinity for the glucocorticoid receptor and is essentially inactive. Prednisone is rapidly activated by hepatic reduction to the 11-hydroxyl compound prednisolone, which possesses full glucocorticoid agonist activity. Peak plasma levels of prednisolone are achieved approximately 1 to 2 hours after administration of a dose of prednisone. Plasma proteins bind glucocorticoids to a variable extent, and prednisone and prednisolone are significantly bound by corticosteroid-binding globulin (CBG). Metabolic clearance is therefore affected by CBG concentration.

Prednisone is an intermediate-acting steroid, with a plasma half-life of 3.4 to 3.8 hours and a tissue half-life of 18 to 36 hours. Metabolic inactivation of prednisolone occurs principally in the liver, and to a lesser extent in the kidneys and peripheral tissues. The relative glucocorticoid potency of prednisone is approximately 4 times that of cortisol, whereas its relative mineralocorticoid activity is only 80 percent.

Dexamethasone

Dexamethasone, a synthetic glucocorticoid, is also available in generic and brand-name oral preparations. Tablets are formulated in 0.25-, 0.50-, 0.75-, 1.00-, 1.50-, 4.00- and 6.00-mg doses. Dexamethasone is practically insoluble in water. It is readily absorbed from the gastrointestinal tract and is active without metabolic alteration. Dexamethasone is also bound by CBG in the plasma, although less extensively than prednisone.

Dexamethasone is a long-acting glucocorticoid, with a plasma half-life of 3.0 to 4.5 hours and a tissue half-life of 36 to 54 hours. Metabolic inactivation, as with prednisolone, occurs primarily in the liver. The relative glucocorticoid potency of dexamethasone is approximately 20 to 30 times that of cortisol, whereas mineralocorticoid activity is essentially absent.

Mechanism of Action

The gynecologic endocrine benefits of glucocorticoid therapy derive mainly from suppression of corticotropin release by the adenohypophysis. Corticotropin, a 39 amino acid polypeptide, is derived from the large precursor molecule pro-opiomelanocortin (POMC). Corticotropin secretion is stimulated by the hypothalamic-releasing factor corticotropin-releasing hormone (CRH). Corticotropin binds adrenocortical cell membrane receptors with activation of adenylate cyclase and a resulting rise in intracellular cyclic adenosine monophosphate (cAMP). By this mechanism, corticotropin increases uptake of low-density lipoprotein (LDL) cholesterol and stimulates the conversion of cholesterol to pregnenolone, the rate-limiting step in adrenocortical steroidogenesis. Cortisol secretion peaks within 10 minutes of a corticotropin pulse. Mineralocorticoid production by the zona glomerulosa can also be stimulated by corticotropin, but this is a far less important factor than the renin-angiotensin system.

Inhibitory glucocorticoid feedback is a vital regulatory component of the hypothalamic-pituitary-adrenal axis. This feedback operates at the level of the pituitary and the hypothalamus, and is comprised of both rapid and delayed components. "Fast feedback" is essentially immediate and appears to operate through desensitization of the pituitary corticotrophs to the stimulatory effects of CRH. Delayed, long-term inhibition of corticotropin secretion occurs when there are high levels of glucocorticoid, and entails a suppression of production and release of both CRH and corticotropin.

The antiandrogenic therapeutic effects of the glucocorticoids derive from inhibition of corticotropin release, thereby decreasing the production of adrenal androgens. In patients with congenital adrenal hyperplasia, impaired cortisol synthesis leads to increased release of corticotropin and an overproduction of precursor steroids. Glucocorticoid therapy inhibits corticotropin release and a low, replacement dosage is adequate to suppress androgens in patients with congenital adrenal hyperplasia.

Approximately 50 percent of hirsute or anovulatory patients who have polycystic ovary syndrome have a significant adrenal androgen component to their disease, often manifested by elevated circulating levels of DHEA and DHEA-S. In these women, symptoms may be ameliorated by adrenal suppression with a glucocorticoid, either as a single agent or in conjunction with other drug therapies such as oral contraceptives for hirsutism and clomiphene for anovulatory infertility.

Gynecologic Indications

Congenital Adrenal Hyperplasia

Congenital adrenal hyperplasia results from deficiency of one of several enzymes required to synthesize cortisol from cholesterol. Congenital adrenal hyperplasia therefore refers to a family of disorders, each with a different enzymatic lesion. In all cases, a relative deficiency of cortisol leads to increased release of corticotropins and elevation of corticosteroids proximal to the blocked step. These precursor steroids may then be shunted into androgen synthesis, thus giving rise to hirsutism or ovulatory dysfunction. These defects are generally inherited in an autosomal recessive manner. The 21-hydroxylase deficiency is closely linked to the human leukocyte antigen (HLA) major histocompatibility complex on chromosome 6.

21-Hydroxylase deficiency accounts for 90 to 95 percent of all cases of congenital adrenal hyperplasia. The prevalence of this disorder is increased in certain ethnic populations, notably the Yupik Eskimos and Ashkenazi Jews. The "classic" form of 21-hydroxylase deficiency presents in the neonatal period, and is characterized by virilization and ambiguous genitalia in affected females. Approximately two-thirds of these neonates will suffer from the "salt-wasting" form of the disease, which results from deficient production of aldosterone. These infants may present with vomiting, dehydration, and shock. 21-Hydroxylase deficiency results in impaired conversion of 17-hydroxyprogesterone (17-OHP) to 11-deoxycortisol. Virilization results from the shunting of 17-OHP into androgens such as androstenedione, which can subsequently be reduced to testosterone. The classic form of this disorder is generally diagnosed and managed in the newborn. The "late-onset" form of 21-hydroxylase deficiency is a milder allelic variant. This form of the disease may present either later in childhood or in the peripubertal or postpubertal period with symptoms of hyperandrogenism. Affected women may have hirsutism or menstrual irregularity, and are clinically indistinguishable from patients with polycystic ovary syndrome. The incidence of late-onset 21-hydroxylase deficiency among hirsute women is estimated to be approximately 5 percent, with some investigators reporting rates as high as 20 percent.

Unfortunately, there is considerable overlap of basal androgen and 17-OHP levels between patients with late-onset congenital adrenal hyperplasia and hirsutism due to other causes. Provocative testing with corticotropin, therefore, remains the gold standard for diagnosis. After drawing a baseline blood sample at 8 A.M., 0.25 mg of α 1-24 corticotropin (Cortrosyn [Organon]) is administered as an intravenous bolus, and a repeat blood sample is drawn in 60 minutes. Both samples are then assayed for 17-OHP. An exaggerated rise in the stimulated 17-OHP level is diagnostic of 21-hydroxylase deficiency, and a number of different formulas and nomograms have been devised to standardize the criteria. It has been proposed that a basal serum level of 17-OHP drawn at 8 A.M. during the follicular phase may constitute an adequate screening test. When obtained in this manner, a 17-OHP level of less than 2 ng/ml makes the diagnosis unlikely, whereas a level of greater than 5 ng/ml confirms the diagnosis. During the follicular phase basal levels in the range of 2 to 5 ng/ml are equivocal and should be followed by formal corticotropin stimulation testing.

11β-Hydroxylase deficiency, comprising 5 to 8 percent of cases, is a less frequent cause of congenital adrenal hyperplasia. This disorder may also present either as a classic form, with early diagnosis, or as a milder late-onset version. This enzymatic deficiency results in impeded conversion of 11-deoxycortisol and 11-deoxycorticosterone (DOC) to cortisol and corticosterone, respectively. Shunting of elevated precursors can lead to elevated levels of androstenedione and testosterone, and increased levels of DOC may result in hypertension, a variable finding in these patients. Women with late-onset 11β-hydroxylase deficiency generally present with the postpubertal onset of hirsutism and menstrual disturbance and, again, clinically resemble patients with the polycystic ovary syndrome. Testing for 11β-hydroxylase deficiency is less well standardized than that for 21-hydroxylase deficiency; diagnosis is based on elevated basal or corticotropin-stimulated levels of DOC and 11-deoxycortisol.

Although a relatively rare cause of neonatal congenital adrenal hyperplasia, 3β-hydroxysteroid dehydrogenase (3β-HSD) deficiency may be a less infrequent cause of postpubertal hirsutism, in its late-onset form. Recent evidence suggests that this disorder may have a prevalence among hirsute patients similar to that of late-onset 21-hydroxylase deficiency. 3β-HSD converts Δ^5 steroids to their Δ^4 counterparts. Deficiency of this enzyme results in an accumulation of the Δ^5 compounds 17-hydroxypregnenolone, DHEA, and DHEA-S. A marked elevation in the ratios of 17-hydroxypregnenolone: 17-

OHP and DHEA: androstenedione on corticotropin testing serves to distinguish these individuals from patients with other causes of hirsutism.

Treatment of the various forms of late-onset congenital adrenal hyperplasia consists of replacement with a *physiologic* dose of glucocorticoid. Therapy results in a suppression of corticotropin secretion by the pituitary and normalization of androgen production by the adrenal gland. Dexamethasone appears to be the treatment of choice in so far as mineralocorticoid effects such as fluid retention are minimized. Further, one study demonstrated a greater degree of adrenal suppression with dexamethasone than with equivalent doses of hydrocortisone or cortisone acetate in women with late-onset congenital adrenal hyperplasia. Dexamethasone is administered at a dosage of 0.25 to 0.50 mg nightly. This dose may occasionally need to be increased to 0.75 to 1.00 mg per day. One study suggested that oversuppression of the hypothalamic-pituitary-adrenal axis may be avoided if morning basal serum levels of cortisol are maintained at 2.0 μg/dl or more during treatment. Prednisone has also been shown to be effective in the treatment of late-onset congenital adrenal hyperplasia, and is typically administered twice daily for a total dosage of 5 to 10 mg. A positive clinical response is usually seen within 3 months after initiating glucocorticoid therapy, and is manifested by an improvement of hirsutism and acne and restoration of cyclic menses. Adjunctive therapy with oral contraceptives or spironolactone may be considered in those patients with congenital adrenal hyperplasia who show an incomplete response to glucocorticoid alone, and addition of clomiphene to the therapy can increase the corrected pregnancy rate to as high as 90 percent in those infertile women who fail to conceive during single-agent glucocorticoid suppression.

Hirsutism

There is an increasing body of literature suggesting that many hirsute women with polycystic ovary syndrome have a significant adrenal component to their hyperandrogenism. Approximately 50 percent of patients with polycystic ovary syndrome have elevated levels of androgens such as DHEA-S, 95 percent of which is produced by the adrenals. Nevertheless, the ovaries remain the major source of increased androgen in most of these women.

Patients with polycystic ovary syndrome who fail to show adequate improvement while receiving standard therapy such as oral contraceptives, and who also show evidence for increased adrenal production of androgens, may benefit from the addition of a low-dose glucocorticoid. Such therapy has clearly been shown to be a useful adjunct in ovulation induction with clomiphene, as will be discussed. A number of studies have shown significant decrements in circulating levels of androstenedione, DHEA-S, testosterone, and 3α-diol glucuronide in hirsute women treated with dexamethasone, 0.50 to 0.75 mg per day, or equivalent doses of prednisone. Although elevated baseline levels of DHEA-S suggest that a resistant patient might be a good candidate for glucocorticoid therapy, formal dexamethasone suppression testing has greater predictive value, and should probably be considered given the potential risks of chronic adrenal suppression. Dexamethasone, 0.5 mg, is administered orally every 6 hours for 2 to 7 days. Baseline and posttreatment androgen levels are then assessed for evidence of suppression. This test can aid in the selection of those women who may derive a benefit from glucocorticoid treatment, and avoid the hazards of such therapy in the remainder. Overall, approximately 30 to 50 percent of hirsute patients will show improvement with glucocorticoid therapy.

When glucocorticoid therapy is undertaken, periodic assessment of morning basal serum levels of cortisol, in order to ensure maintenance at levels of 2.0 μg/dl or more, may reduce the risks of oversuppression.

Ovulation Induction

Glucocorticoids have also proved useful as adjunctive therapy for ovulation induction in patients who are unresponsive to clomiphene citrate alone. Most investigators have concluded that such therapy should be predicated on the determination that a patient's serum level of DHEA-S exceeds a threshold level.

In one study, coadministration of oral dexamethasone, 0.5 mg per night, to women who previously failed to ovulate with clomiphene treatment at a dose of 250 mg per day for 5 days resulted in ovulation in 50 percent of patients who received combination therapy. Of note, the women who ovulated after treatment with clomiphene and dexamethasone had significantly higher pretreatment levels of DHEA-S (mean, >300 μg/dl) than those who failed to respond.

Another study compared the efficacy of clomiphene alone with clomiphene and 0.5 mg of dexamethasone in 64 anovulatory women. In the final analysis, 100 percent of those women who received clomiphene with dexamethasone ovulated whereas only 64 percent of those who received clomiphene alone did so. It was observed that the improved ovulatory rate with adjunctive dexamethasone occurred primarily in those patients who had a baseline DHEA-S level that exceeded 200 μg/dl.

It is therefore reasonable to consider adjunctive glucocorticoid therapy in patients who have pretreatment DHEA-S levels of more than 200 μg/dl, if they fail to ovulate after treatment with clomiphene alone.

Dexamethasone Testing for Cushing's Syndrome

Cushing's syndrome results from chronic hypercortisolemia secondary to corticotropin-secreting pituitary adenomas (Cushing's disease), ectopic corticotropin-secreting tumors, adrenal tumors, or iatrogenic glucocorticoid administration. Women with Cushing's syndrome may develop hirsutism (64%), menstrual disorders (60%), or acne (45%). It is therefore important to consider Cushing's syndrome in the differential diagnosis of hyperandrogenism and ovulatory dysfunction. These patients usually display additional signs and symptoms of cortisol excess, including centripetal obesity, hypertension, proximal muscle weakness, easy bruisability, purple striae, and osteoporosis.

A simple screen to rule out Cushing's syndrome is the overnight dexamethasone suppression test (Fig. 8-1). A single oral dose of dexamethasone, 1 mg, is administered at 11 P.M. and a plasma cortisol level is assessed at 8 A.M. the following day. If the cortisol level is suppressed below 5 μg/dl, the diagnosis of Cushing's syndrome is highly unlikely. Typically, afflicted patients will have plasma cortisol levels in excess of 10 μg/dl after the overnight test, and values of more than 5 μg/dl are equivocal. False-positive results are not

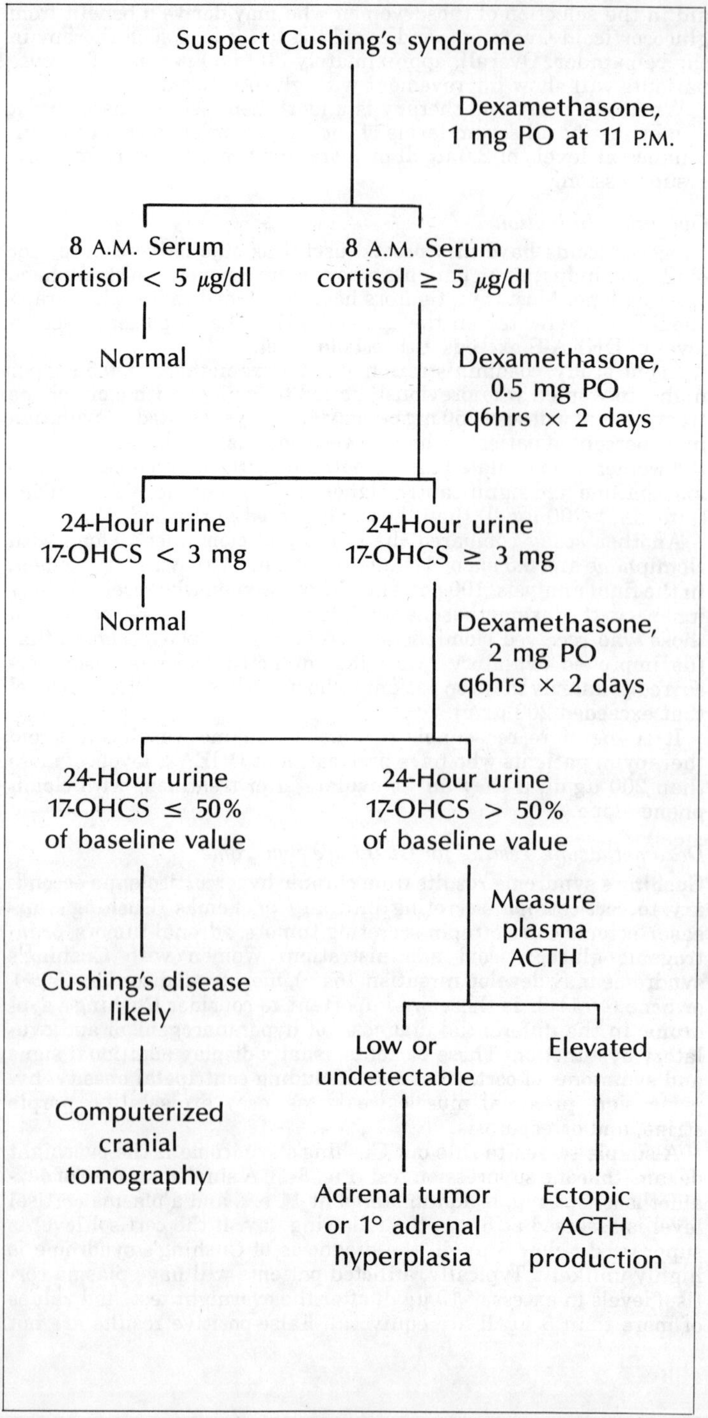
Suspect Cushing's syndrome
Dexamethasone, 1 mg PO at 11 P.M.
8 A.M. Serum cortisol < 5 μg/dl
8 A.M. Serum cortisol ≥ 5 μg/dl
Normal
Dexamethasone, 0.5 mg PO q6hrs × 2 days
24-Hour urine 17-OHCS < 3 mg
24-Hour urine 17-OHCS ≥ 3 mg
Normal
Dexamethasone, 2 mg PO q6hrs × 2 days
24-Hour urine 17-OHCS ≤ 50% of baseline value
24-Hour urine 17-OHCS > 50% of baseline value
Measure plasma ACTH
Cushing's disease likely
Low or undetectable
Elevated
Computerized cranial tomography
Adrenal tumor or 1° adrenal hyperplasia
Ectopic ACTH production

uncommon, and may result from a number of factors including obesity, depression, pregnancy (or exogenous estrogens), and alcoholism.

Patients with a positive or equivocal result on overnight screening test must be evaluated with formal dexamethasone suppression testing. In general, this procedure should be performed and interpreted by an endocrinologist, and is often done on an inpatient basis. The low-dose test is performed after a baseline 24-hour urine collection is done to determine creatinine and 17-hydroxycorticosteroid (17-OHCS) levels. The patient then takes dexamethasone, 0.5 mg, every 6 hours for 2 days, and urine collection is continued. Normal individuals will show a suppression of urinary levels of 17-OHCS to less than 3 mg per 24 hours. A normal result on the low-dose test rules out the diagnosis of Cushing's syndrome.

Patients failing to suppress on the low-dose regimen are then followed with a high-dose test. Dexamethasone is administered at a dose of 2 mg every 6 hours for another 2 days. Suppression of urinary 17-OHCS of 50 percent or more of baseline values suggests a diagnosis of Cushing's disease, and should be followed up with a cranial computed tomography (CT) scan. Failure to suppress by 50 percent generally excludes the diagnosis of Cushing's disease. Plasma corticotropin levels should be measured in these latter individuals; a high plasma level of corticotropin suggests ectopic production (e.g., oat cell carcinoma of the lung), and a low plasma level supports a diagnosis of adrenal adenoma or carcinoma, or primary adrenal hyperplasia. Appropriate imaging techniques are indicated in these instances.

Method of Use

Preliminary Workup

Glucocorticoids are potent agents, and the decision to use them must be based on a careful assessment of potential risks versus benefits. Except in patients with congenital adrenal hyperplasia, these drugs are rarely recommended as first-line therapy for the gynecologic endocrine disorders discussed already, and should therefore be considered only after other therapies have failed.

In patients who are candidates for glucocorticoids, the cause of hyperandrogenism should be determined. A thorough history, physical examination, and assessment of serum testosterone and DHEA-S levels should be performed in an effort to rule out the presence of ovarian or adrenal neoplasia, as previously described. When indicated, suppression testing to rule out Cushing's syndrome and evaluation of serum prolactin levels and thyroid functions should be performed. Diagnosis of congenital adrenal hyperplasia can be made by corticotropin-stimulation testing (Fig. 8-2).

In addition, the presence of other medical conditions that may complicate glucocorticoid therapy should be ascertained. Known hypersensitivity to the medication or systemic fungal infection contraindicates such therapy. A history of latent tuberculosis indicates a risk of reactivation if glucocorticoids are administered, and corneal perforation can occur in corticoid-treated patients who have ocular herpes simplex infection.

Fig. 8-1. Dexamethasone suppression testing. PO = orally, 17-OHCS = creatinine and 17-hydroxycorticosteroids, ACTH = adrenocorticotropic hormone.

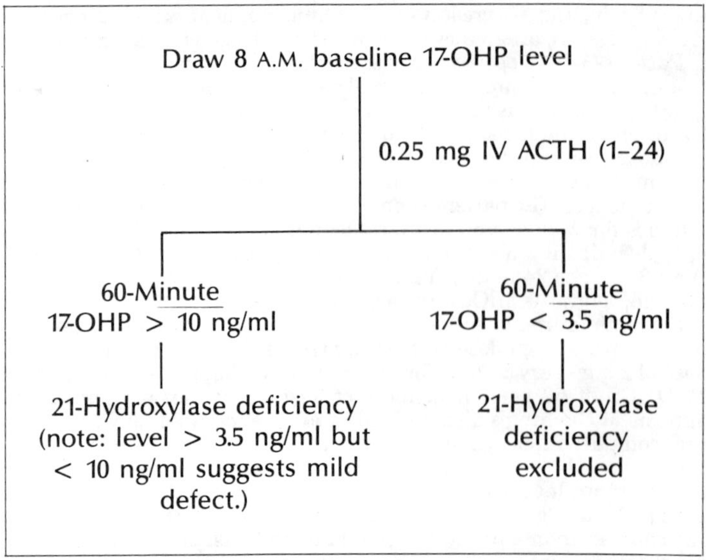

Fig. 8-2. Adrenocorticotropic hormone (ACTH)–stimulation testing for congenital adrenal hyperplasia. 17-OHP = 17-hydroxyprogesterone.

Subclinical or overt diabetes mellitus may worsen during glucocorticoid therapy, and pre-existing psychiatric or emotional disorders may be exacerbated. Caution must also be exercised in administering glucocorticoids to patients with peptic ulcer disease, hypertension, renal insufficiency, osteoporosis, diverticulitis, or recent intestinal anastomosis. Further, individuals with cirrhosis or hypothyroidism show an increased sensitivity to the effects of corticosteroids, and dosage may need to be modified accordingly.

Monitoring Low-Dose Therapy

Most complications of glucocorticoid therapy increase with increasing dosage and duration of treatment. These risks are somewhat reduced in the treatment of congenital adrenal hyperplasia, hirsutism, and anovulation as the recommended doses of glucocorticoid are in the "physiologic" replacement range.

Adrenal oversuppression can be avoided in these patients partly because adrenal androgens are significantly more sensitive than cortisol to glucocorticoid suppression. Work examining the dose-response relationships for suppression of a variety of adrenal steroids by dexamethasone in hirsute women has shown that corticotropin-stimulated DHEA-S and DHEA levels are more sensitive to dexamethasone suppression than stimulated cortisol levels, suggesting that low-dose steroid therapy can improve hyperandrogenism without achieving complete cortisol suppression. A dissociation between cortisol and adrenal androgen secretion in patients taking prednisone on an alternate-day regimen has also been demonstrated. Alternate-day therapy is based on the finding that administration of twice the usual dose of a short- or intermediate-acting glucocorticoid, every other morning, can produce a beneficial clinical response while minimizing adverse effects such as hypothalamic-pituitary-adrenal axis oversuppression or symptoms of glucocorticoid excess. Chronic, low-dose prednisone as alternate-day therapy in patients with systemic lupus resulted in normal baseline corticotropin and cortisol levels despite a decrease in basal androgen levels. Further, CRH-stimulated corticotropin and cortisol levels were blunted only on the day the drug was taken, whereas CRH-stimulated androgen levels were significantly depressed on both days. Alternate-day therapy with prednisone may therefore prove useful in the treatment of adrenal hyperandrogenism.

Nonetheless, women receiving even the low doses of glucocorticoids described in the foregoing discussion must be closely monitored for signs of glucocorticoid excess. It is also clear that therapy with "physiologic" doses of corticoids may place a patient at risk for developing stress-related iatrogenic pituitary-adrenal insufficiency. Dosage should be adjusted so as to maintain morning serum cortisol levels of 2.0 μg/dl or more, in order to minimize this risk. Patients receiving chronic glucocorticoid therapy should be covered with a standard "stress dose" regimen (eg., 100 mg of intravenous hydrocortisone every 6 hours) for surgical procedures or serious acute illness. Such stress coverage should be considered for several months after stopping long-term glucocorticoid therapy. Recovery of normal basal cortisol secretion usually occurs within 1 month after discontinuing prolonged low-dose glucocorticoid treatment, but several months may be required before a normalization of the cortisol response to insulin-induced hypoglycemia is seen.

Use in Pregnancy

Glucocorticoids can cross the placenta. The placenta oxidizes prednisolone to inactive prednisone, thus reducing the placental transfer of active metabolite in prednisone-treated women.

Although glucocorticoids are not known to be teratogenic in humans, animal studies with corticoids have shown an increased incidence of congenital anomalies, including cleft palate. Additionally, glucocorticoid-treated animals have increased rates of placental insufficiency, spontaneous abortions, and intrauterine growth retardation. Since adequate human studies have not been done, the use of glucocorticoids during pregnancy should be undertaken only when clearly indicated. Children of mothers who have received corticoids during gestation should be observed for signs of hypoadrenalism in the neonatal period.

Glucocorticoids are excreted in breast milk, and could theoretically inhibit growth or cause adrenal suppression. Nursing should probably be avoided by mothers taking pharmacologic doses of these agents.

Side Effects and Toxicity

Complications of treatment with glucocorticoids are dependent on the size of the dose and the duration of therapy. Accordingly, the most adverse reactions are seen in patients receiving pharmacologic doses of corticosteroids and are seen only rarely in patients taking physiologic doses such as described in this chapter.

Patients receiving chronic glucocorticoid therapy may have a decreased resistance to infections, and the anti-inflammatory effects may complicate their detection and diagnosis. Individuals may show a decreased antibody response to vaccinations, although this is generally not a problem for patients taking replacement doses. Wound healing may also be impaired.

Adverse effects of glucocorticoid excess are diverse and may impact on fluid balance, the gastrointestinal system, the musculoskeletal system, and the central nervous system. Corticoids may cause water and sodium retention, which can result in hypertension. This is much less common with agents such as dexamethasone, which possess minimal mineralocorticoid activity. Gastrointestinal complications may include peptic ulcer disease and, rarely, pancreatitis. Musculoskeletal effects include steroid myopathy and osteoporosis. Steroid myopathy is manifested by myalgias and weakness, primarily affecting the proximal musculature. Serum enzymes such as creatine phosphokinase and serum glutamic-oxaloacetic transaminase are not elevated in these cases. Osteoporosis is a relatively common complication of prolonged high-dose corticoid therapy, and resembles postmenopausal osteoporosis, often resulting in vertebral compression fractures. Aseptic necrosis of the femoral or humeral head is a serious complication of high-dose glucocorticoid administration, and can occur after short courses of treatment. Ophthalmic side effects such as posterior subcapsular cataracts and glaucoma have also been described. Neurologic effects including psychiatric disorders and pseudotumor cerebri (on steroid withdrawal) may also occur. Metabolic and endocrine effects such as exacerbation of diabetes and adrenal-axis oversuppression were discussed previously.

It must be reemphasized that the appearance of these side effects in patients receiving replacement doses of glucocorticoids is exceedingly uncommon. Most of these manifestations of corticosteroid excess are reversible on discontinuation of the medication.

Drug Interactions

Coadministration of corticosteroids with potassium-depleting diuretics may result in hypokalemia, and patients taking both should be closely monitored. Corticosteroids may inhibit the effects of sodium warfarin (Coumadin). Patients taking oral anticoagulants should therefore be followed with frequent assessment of the prothrombin time.

Other drugs, including ephedrine, rifampin, phenytoin, and phenobarbital, have been reported to increase the metabolic clearance of glucocorticoids, and steroid dosage may need to be modified. This interaction could affect the results of dexamethasone suppression testing, and should be taken into account.

Contraindications

Contraindications to glucocorticoid therapy include systemic fungal infections and hypersensitivity to the drugs.

BIBLIOGRAPHY

Spironolactone

Blum, I., et al. Successful treatment of polycystic ovary syndrome with spironolactone or bromocriptine. *Obstet. Gynecol.* 57:661, 1981.

Evron, S., Shapiro, G., and Diamant, Y.Z. Induction of ovulation with spironolactone (Aldactone) in anovulatory oligomenorrheic and hyperandrogenic women. *Fertil. Steril.* 36:468, 1981.

Helfer, E. L., Miller, J. L., and Rose, L. I. Side-effects of spironolactone therapy in the hirsute woman. *J. Clin. Endocrinol. Metab.* 66:208, 1988.

Lobo, R. A., et al. The effects of two doses of spironolactone on serum androgens and anagen hair in hirsute women. *Fertil. Steril.* 43:200, 1985.

Milewicz, A., Silber, D., and Kirschner, M. A. Therapeutic effects of spironolactone in polycystic ovary syndrome. *Obstet. Gynecol.* 61:429, 1983.

Pittaway, D. E., Maxson, W. S., and Wentz, A. C. Spironolactone in combination drug therapy for unresponsive hirsutism. *Fertil. Steril.* 43:878, 1985.

Serafini, P., and Lobo, R. A. The effects of spironolactone on adrenal steroidogenesis in hirsute women. *Fertil. Steril.* 44:595, 1985.

Shapiro, G., and Evron, S. A novel use of spironolactone: treatment of hirsutism. *J. Clin. Endocrinol. Metab.* 51:429, 1980.

Glucocorticoids

Abraham, G. E., et al. Effect of dexamethasone on serum cortisol and androgen levels in hirsute patients. *Obstet. Gynecol.* 47:395, 1976.

Avgerinos, P. C., et al. Dissociation between cortisol and adrenal androgen secretion in patients receiving alternate day prednisone therapy. *J. Clin. Endocrinol. Metab.* 65:24, 1987.

Birnbaum, M. D., and Rose, L. I. The partial adrenocortical hydroxylase deficiency syndrome in infertile women. *Fertil. Steril.* 32:536, 1979.

Birnbaum, M. D., and Rose, L. I. Late onset adrenocortical hydroxylase deficiencies associated with menstrual dysfunction. *Obstet. Gynecol.* 63:445, 1984.

Boyers, S. P., Buster, J. E., and Marshall, J. R. Hypothalamic-pituitary-adrenocortical function during long-term low-dose dexamethasone therapy in hyperandrogenized women. *Am. J. Obstet. Gynecol.* 142:330, 1982.

Brodie, B. L., and Wentz, A. C. Late onset congenital adrenal hyperplasia: a gynecologist's perspective. *Fertil. Steril.* 48:175, 1987.

Chetkowski, R. J., et al. The incidence of late-onset congenital adrenal hyperplasia due to 21-hydroxylase deficiency among hirsute women. *J. Clin. Endocrinol. Metab.* 58:595, 1984.

Daly, D. C., et al. A randomized study of dexamethasone in ovulation induction with clomiphene citrate. *Fertil. Steril.* 41:844, 1984.

Evans, M. I., et al. Pharmacologic suppression of the fetal adrenal gland in utero. Attempted prevention of abnormal external genital masculinization in suspected congenital adrenal hyperplasia. *J.A.M.A.* 253:1015, 1985.

Hoffman, D., and Lobo, R. A. Serum dehydroepiandrosterone sulfate and the use of clomiphene citrate in anovulatory women. *Fertil. Steril.* 43:196, 1985.

Horrocks, P. M., and London, D. R. A comparison of three glucocorticoid suppressive regimes in adults with congenital adrenal hyperplasia. *Clin. Endocrinol.* 17:547, 1982.

Lobo, R. A., and Goebelsmann, U. Evidence for reduced 3β-ol-hydroxysteroid dehydrogenase activity in some hirsute women thought to have polycystic ovary syndrome. *J. Clin. Endocrinol. Metab.* 53:394, 1981.

Lobo, R. A., et al. Clomiphene and dexamethasone in women unresponsive to clomiphene alone. *Obstet. Gynecol.* 69:497, 1982.

Meikle, A. W., and Odell, W. D. Effect of short and long-term dexamethasone on 3α-androstenediol glucuronide in hirsute women. *Fertil. Steril.* 46:227, 1986.

Pang, S., et al. Late-onset adrenal steroid 3β-hydroxysteroid dehydrogenase deficiency. I. A cause of hirsutism in pubertal and postpubertal women. *J. Clin. Endocrinol. Metab.* 60:428, 1985.

Pugeat, M., et al. Evidence of excessive androgen secretion by both the ovary and the adrenal in patients with idiopathic hirsutism. *Obstet. Gynecol.* 59:46, 1982.

Richards, G. E., et al. The effect of long-acting glucocorticoids on menstrual abnormalities in patients with virilizing congenital adrenal hyperplasia. *J. Clin. Endocrinol. Metab.* 47:1208, 1978.

Rittmaster, R. S., Loriaux, D. L., and Cutler, G. B. Sensitivity of cortisol and adrenal androgens to dexamethasone suppression in hirsute women. *J. Clin. Endocrinol. Metab.* 61:462, 1985.

Steinberger, E., Smith, K. D., and Rodriquez-Rigau, L. J. Testosterone, dehydroepiandrosterone, and dehydroepiandrosterone sulfate in hyperandrogenic women. *J. Clin. Endocrinol. Metab.* 59:471, 1984.

White, P. C., New, M. I., and Dupont, B. Congenital adrenal hyperplasia. *N. Engl. J. Med.* 316:1519, 1987.

Yuen, B. H., and Minsey, E. K. Role of androgens in menstrual disorders of nonhirsute and hirsute women, and the effect of glucocorticoid therapy on androgen levels in hirsute hyperandrogenic women. *Am.* J. Obstet. Gynecol. 145:152, 1983.

9

Thyroid Hormones and Antagonists

Gregory F. Rosen and Sergio C. Stone

The thyroid gland normally functions to produce two active hormones, thyroxine (T_4) and 3, 5, 3′-triiodothyronine (T_3). These protein hormones influence the metabolic rate by making other parts of the body more or less receptive to the effects of other protein hormones including epinephrine, glucagon, insulin, and parathyroid hormone (PTH). Thyroid hormones amplify cyclic adenosine monophosphate (cAMP), the "second messenger," of these hormones. Diseases of the thyroid gland may be manifest by either increased secretion of hormones resulting in a hypermetabolic state, termed hyperthyroidism or thyroid storm, or insufficient hormonal production and a resulting hypometabolic state, termed hypothyroidism or myxedema. Enlargement of the thyroid (goiter) may be associated with either increased, normal, or decreased hormonal production. Thyroid dysfunction should be suspected in patients with galactorrhea and hyperprolactinemia, abnormal sexual development, hirsutism, menstrual irregularity, some forms of infertility, exophthalmos, myxedema, any diffusely or focally enlarged thyroid gland, or a variety of symptoms that will be discussed.

ADULT PHYSIOLOGY

Dietary iodine is absorbed by the gastrointestinal tract and excreted by the kidneys. One of the effects of thyroid-stimulating hormone (TSH) is to cause iodine to be actively transported into the thyroid gland. Once iodine enters the thyroid gland, it is oxidized onto tyrosine in a series of reactions referred to as organification and incorporated onto thyroglobulin. Iodine is first added at the number 3 position on the tyrosine ring and then at the number 5 position. Two of these diiodotyrosine molecules then fuse to yield one T_4 molecule. T_4 is the primary hormone secreted by the thyroid gland. Only 20 percent of the T_3 found in the peripheral circulation is secreted directly by the thyroid gland while the majority of T_3, approximately 80 percent, is derived from peripheral deiodination of T_4. In addition, another thyroid hormone, a nonbiologically active isomer of T_3 called reverse T_3 (rT_3) is also found in small concentration in the circulation of adults. Once T_4 is secreted by the thyroid, as much as 85 percent is metabolized by deiodination to either T_3 or rT_3. Most of this metabolism occurs in the liver. In the circulation, T_4 is bound to the following serum proteins: thyroxine-binding globulin (TBG) (70–75%), thyroxine-binding prealbumin (15–20%), and albumin (5–10%). Most of the T_3 is bound to TBG. Only a very small amount, less than 0.05 percent of T_4 and approximately 0.3 percent of T_3, is found circulating free and these are the biologically active hormones.

Secretion of the thyroid hormones is regulated by a sensitive feedback mechanism between the hypothalamus, pituitary, and thyroid gland. Thyrotropin-releasing hormone (TRH) is a tripeptide, pyroglutamyl-histidyl-proline amide that is manufactured in the hypothalamus. It is released in a pulsatile fashion into the portal circulation, a venous channel that flows from the hypothalamus to the pituitary. TRH binds to its receptor in the pituitary and through the action of cAMP initially causes the release of stored TSH and prolactin and later stimulates their synthesis. TSH is a glycoprotein that is comprised of two subunits, alpha and beta. The oligosaccharides that bind to TSH are essential for its biologic activity. There are at least two forms of TSH, regular TSH and "big" TSH. TSH secretion is also pulsatile but, unlike TRH, it has a circadian rhythm with a nocturnal surge. TSH is responsible for active transport of iodine into the thyroid gland, organification of iodine to tyrosine, the coupling of the iodotyrosine molecules into T_3 and T_4, and the release of thyroid hormones and their rate of synthesis. TSH binds to receptors on the thyroid gland causing an activation of the enzyme adenyl cyclase which increases the concentration of cAMP within the thyroid. This initially causes the release of stored T_4 and T_3 into the circulation but later causes increased hormone synthesis. T_3 and T_4 control their own release in a negative feedback loop that feeds back on the pituitary. Thyroid hormone has two effects on the pituitary: It decreases the number of TRH receptors and thereby decreases the effect TRH has on TSH release and it also directly inhibits the release of TSH. T_3 is the more active hormone moiety in the peripheral circulation and it is also the more active moiety in inhibiting the release of TSH. Normally, a decrease in the level of free hormone in the plasma is followed by an increase in TSH secretion by the pituitary secondary to the increased sensitivity of the pituitary to TRH and the removal of the inhibitory effect of thyroid hormone to its release. There is no evidence that T_3 or T_4 has any effect on the hypothalamic release of TRH.

Other substances that influence the release of thyroid hormone include iodine, somatostatin, levodopa, and glucocorticoids. Iodine deficiency restricts the production of thyroid hormone causing an increase in TSH production. This chronic increase in TSH stimulation causes the gland to hypertrophy in an attempt to maximize the utilization of the iodine available and a goiter may result. Small to moderate physiologic doses of iodine are taken up into the thyroid in a routine fashion; however, with progressively larger doses, the quantity of iodine undergoing organification first increases but then decreases. This is called the Wolff-Chaikoff effect. Pharmacologic doses of iodine block the release of thyroid hormones from the thyroid. Somatostatin decreases the response of pituitary TSH to TRH. Levodopa, which is thought to have the same effect as endogenous dopamine, inhibits the release of TSH and also the response of TSH to a TRH infusion. Glucocorticoids block the conversion of T_4 to T_3 and also decrease the release of TSH.

Palpation of the neck and the thyroid gland is part of any physical examination. The detection of a thyroid nodule is an important finding. Risk factors for malignancy include increased age, the female sex, history of neck irradiation, and a family history of thyroid cancer. The workup of a nodule includes determination of serum T_4 levels (by radioimmunoassay), resin T_3 uptake, thyroid antimicrosomal antibodies and a radionucleotide scan of the thyroid to determine if the nodule is functional. Needle aspiration of the nodule is essential for both diagnostic and therapeutic reasons.

THYROID FUNCTION AND METABOLISM IN OBSTETRICS AND GYNECOLOGY

The serum concentrations and metabolism of thyroid hormones change in states associated with hyperestrogenism. This includes pregnancy and the use of oral contraceptive pills. A rise in estrogen levels stimulates the liver to increase both the synthesis of TBG and the amount of the carbohydrate, sialic acid, bound to this globulin. Sialation is thought to decrease the metabolism of TBG so both processes, augmented synthesis and sialation, cause the concentration of TBG to rise. This leads to an expansion in the number of thyroid hormone–binding sites on TBG and to a parallel increase in total T_3 and T_4 levels. Some studies, however, show no change in T_4 and only an elevation in the T_3 and TBG levels. Another possible cause for increased thyroid function and hormone levels during pregnancy is that human chorionic gonadotropin (hCG) has thyroid-stimulating activity. One unit of hCG contributes about 0.0008 units of TSH-like activity. TSH concentrations are slightly decreased in the first trimester and this is thought to be related to the high levels of hCG. The peak concentration of hCG correlated well with the nadir levels of TSH. TBG, T_4, and T_3 concentrations peak at about 10 to 15 weeks of gestation. Pathologic conditions associated with elevated hCG levels, such as hydatidiform mole and choriocarcinoma, are sometimes associated with increased thyroid function. However, the increased metabolic rate in the second and third trimester of pregnancy is due to increase in body mass and not to an increase in thyroid function. By 6 weeks postpartum, TBG, TSH, T_4, and T_3 are all back to the prepregnancy levels.

HYPERTHYROIDISM

Pathology

The most common cause of hyperthyroidism, about 85 percent of all cases, is Graves' disease and it occurs in women 7 to 8 times more frequently than in men. The clinical history of Graves' disease is not of unremitting hyperthyroidism but is characterized by periods of exacerbations and remissions. Long-standing disease, however, may be associated with progressive thyroid failure probably related to chronic thyroiditis, but about 20 to 30 percent of patients will go into permanent remission without therapy.

Graves' disease may be an immunologic disorder in that patients have an unusual IgG immunoglobulin designated as either "long-acting thyroid stimulators" (LATS) or "thyroid-stimulating immunoglobulins" (TSI). These immunoglobulins bind to TSH receptors causing an increase in release and production of thyroid hormones and, secondarily, a glandular hypertrophy or goiter. This disorder has a triad of manifestations: diffuse goiter, exophthalmos, and characteristic skin changes. The thyroid is diffusely enlarged, soft, and nontender. The eye changes are characterized by inflammatory infiltrates of the orbital content exclusive of the globe. The orbital musculature is enlarged and muscle fibers undergo degeneration and ultimately, fibrosis. There is a thickening of the skin with a lymphocytic infiltrate and a deposition of mucopolysaccharides. The pathogenesis of the ophthalmic and skin components is poorly understood. Other less common causes of hyperthyroidism include thyroiditis, toxic multinodular goiter, toxic adenoma, excess TSH (pituitary tumor), exogenous thyroid production (struma ovarii and metastatic follicular thyroid cancer), states of elevated hCG levels, and iatrogenic hyperthyroidism.

Signs and symptoms of hyperthyroidism can affect every organ system and vary markedly with both age and the degree of hyperthyroidism. Manifestations include nervousness, emotional lability,

Table 9-1. Laboratory indices useful in the diagnosis of thyroid function

Test	Hyperthyroid	Hypothyroid	Pregnancy
T_4 (direct/total)	+/− Increased	+/− Decreased	Increased
T_3 (direct/total)	+/− Increased	+/− Decreased	Decreased
T_4 (free)	+/− Increased	+/− Decreased	Unchanged
T_3 (free)	+/− Increased	+/− Decreased	Unchanged
Resin T_3 uptake	Decreased	Increased	Decreased
Free T_4 index	Increased	Decreased	Unchanged
Thyroid-stimulating hormone	Decreased	Increased	Unchanged
Thyroxine-binding globulin	+/−Increased	+/− Decreased	Increased

T_4 = thyroxine, T_3 = triiodothyronine, +/− (preceding *Increased* or *Decreased*) = respective increase or decrease is uncertain.

insomnia, tremors, palpitations, tachycardia and arrhythmias, heat intolerance, excessive sweating, weight loss, weakness, anorexia, myopathy, myoneuropathy, and osteoporosis. Menstrual irregularities include oligomenorrhea and amenorrhea. Physical examination may demonstrate an anxious, restless, or fidgety patient with warm moist skin. The fingernail sometimes separates from the nail bed (Plummer's nails). The hair is fine and silky. Fine tremors are noticed on the fingers and the toes. Hyperreflexia is characteristic. Ocular signs include the characteristic stare with widened palpebral fissures, infrequent blinking, and lid lag. Cardiovascular findings include a wide pulse pressure, sinus tachycardia, atrial arrhythmias, systolic murmurs, and, at times, cardiac failure. The dermopathy of Graves' disease usually occurs over the dorsum of the legs or feet and is termed pretibial myxedema.

Hyperthyroidism is confirmed by elevated serum levels of T_4 or T_3, or both; a decreased TSH level; and, importantly, an increased resin T_3 uptake, which indicates that either the levels of TBG are low or a greater than normal number of binding sites are filled with thyroid hormone, indicating that there are increased levels of free thyroid hormone (e.g., a hyperthyroid state). The free T_4 index is also elevated (Table 9-1).

Free T_4 index is a laboratory value that is the product of the resin uptake and the serum total T_4 concentration. It correlates extremely well with the free, bioavailable fraction of T_4 and it is easier and less expensive to assay.

Treatment

Since a cure for hyperthyroidism, such as the extirpation of a solitary hyperfunctioning adenoma, can be obtained in only a few patients, there are two major approaches to the control of this syndrome and an optimal method of treatment awaits discovery of the cause of these disorders. The first is to limit the quantity of thyroid hormones that the gland can produce. This is accomplished by using antithyroid agents to block synthesis. The second approach is to destroy or remove the thyroid and give physiologic replacement. This latter modality may be achieved either by surgery or with radioactive iodine.

Table 9-2. Recommended therapeutic agents useful in the treatment of hyperthyroidism[a]

For long-term antithyroid therapy
- Propylthiouracil (approved for use in pregnancy), 100–150 mg, orally, every 6 to 8 hours
- Methimazole (contraindicated in pregnancy), 10–15 mg, orally, every 6 to 8 hours

For ablative therapy
- Iodine 131 (in older patients)
- Subtotal thyroidectomy (in younger patients)

[a] All patients with the diagnosis of hyperthyroidism need to be followed for life for signs and symptoms of hypothyroidism whether during treatment or in remission.

Propylthiouracil is effectively used to manage a majority of patients (Table 9-2). Doses of this medication range from 100 to 150 mg given every 6 to 8 hours except in occasional patients who require larger doses. *Methimazole* is at least as effective as propylthiouracil and is administered at one-tenth the dosage. Both medications inhibit synthesis of thyroid hormone but propylthiouracil has the advantage of inhibiting the peripheral conversion of T_4 to T_3 and thereby brings about a more rapid systemic improvement. Leukopenia that may proceed to agranulocytosis is the principal serious side effect of these medications. Routine blood cell counts are not a good predictor of who will have this side effect so it is recommended that patients have complete blood cell counts immediately with the onset of any infectious-like symptoms (e.g., fever, sore throat, myalgia). Other side effects include a lupus-like syndrome, myalgia, and fever that will remit as soon as the medication is discontinued. Patients should be maintained on therapy for 1 to 2 years before discontinuation and assessment for remission. However, it is very important to follow patients for signs and symptoms of hypothyroidism.

In Obstetrics and Gynecology

Hyperthyroidism has only a theoretical effect on fertility unless the patient is severely hyperthyroid and these patients may be amenorrheic. Hyperthyroidism during pregnancy is associated with a slight increase in fetal wastage but there is a significant increase in prematurity, stillborns, and infants who are small for gestational age. There is also a twofold increase in the risk of preeclampsia.

Thyroid hormone and TSH do not cross the human placenta and although TRH can readily pass through the placenta, the quantities are so small that the fetal thyroid develops autonomously. The signs and symptoms of hyperthyroidism during pregnancy are weight loss or poor weight gain, a resting pulse rate that is greater than 100 beats per minute, and congestive heart failure. Propylthiouracil is the drug of choice for pregnant hyperthyroid women. This medication appears to be less readily transferred across the placenta and into the fetal circulation than is methimazole. However, neonatal hypothyroidism and goiter still occur in about 10 percent of infants of mothers treated with propylthiouracil, though there is no increase in any other congenital anomalies. It is therefore important to use as low a dose as possible in pregnant women and in approximately one-third of patients it is possible to stop their medication prior to delivery. Patients should also have their weight and resting heart rate checked routinely and they should be monitored closely for early signs and symptoms of preeclampsia. The incidence of hyperthyroidism during pregnancy is approximately 0.2 percent and the cause is Graves' disease approximately 85 percent of the time. Neonatal hyperthyroidism secondary to the transplacental passage of the IgG LATS occurs and it is important to follow these infants closely. There is no contraindication to breast-feeding when the mother is taking propylthiouracil since only a minimal amount of the medication crosses into the mother's milk and this has been shown to have no effect on the infant.

Medical ablation of the thyroid, using radioactive iodine 131, is considered by some to be the therapy of choice for the nonpregnant, adult population with Graves' disease. Subtotal thyroidectomy is infrequently used as therapy for all types of hyperthyroidism. It is usually reserved for children and young adults who are unable to take or tolerate propylthiouracil or methimazole. It is important to follow all hyperthyroid patients for life for signs and symptoms of hypothyroidism.

THYROID STORM

Thyroid storm is a very rare life-threatening condition that carries with it approximately a 10 to 50 percent risk of mortality. Most of these patients do not have a previous diagnosis of hyperthyroid disease and an exposure to a new stressful situation, such as trauma, infection, or the onset of labor, leads to the development of thyroid storm. There is no relationship between a prethyroid storm level of hyperthyroidism and the risk of developing this life-threatening disorder.

Thyroid storm is a clinical diagnosis in which treatment must be started without waiting for laboratory confirmation of the diagnosis. The signs and symptoms of thyroid storm include the following: (1) temperature greater than 100°F (38°C); (2) central nervous system changes including stupor, apathy, delirium, coma, psychosis, or disorientation; and (3) signs and symptoms of hyperthyroidism including tremors, nausea, vomiting, diarrhea, abdominal pain, jaundice, pulmonary edema, tachycardia, arrhythmias, congestive heart failure, and shock. All three of these symptom groups *must* occur for the diagnosis of thyroid storm.

Treatment must be very aggressive and it is recommended that all patients with suspected thyroid storm be immediately transferred to an intensive care unit. Initial therapy should include careful monitoring of fluids and electrolyte levels, examination for infections using blood cultures, and treatment of hyperpyrexia with cold packs or a cooling blanket but not with aspirin since aspirin displaces thyroid hormones from TBG. It is recommended that patients be placed on prophylactic, triple antibiotics and then treated with digitalis if signs of cardiac failure or arrhythmias are present. Lastly, patients should be treated with antithyroid medication. There are four approaches to treating hyperthyroidism during hyperthyroid storm. These include:

1. Blocking synthesis of new thyroid hormones. Currently, only oral medications have this ability. Propylthiouracil, 300 to 1000 mg, should be given orally stat. If the patient is comatose, it can be

given through a nasogastric tube. Afterward the dosage should be continued at 150 to 300 mg every 6 hours.

2. Blocking the release of thyroid hormones. Iodine, in pharmacologic doses, blocks the release of thyroid hormones. Sodium iodine should be given approximately 1 hour after propylthiouracil is administered. The dose is 500 to 1000 mg given intravenously every 8 hours.
3. Blocking the conversion of T_4 to T_3 in extrathyroidal tissues. Propylthiouracil acts to block this conversion and so do glucocorticoids. The patient should be given dexamethasone, 2 mg intravenously every 6 hours.
4. Blocking peripheral effects of hyperthyroidism. Beta blockers can be used. Propranolol is given intravenously in doses of 1 mg per minute up to a total of 10 mg every 4 to 6 hours. This also may block the conversion of T_4 to T_3.

HYPOTHYROIDISM

Pathology

Hypothyroidism can result from any of a variety of structural or functional abnormalities that lead to insufficient synthesis and release of thyroid hormone. The classification of hypothyroidism is divided into thyroid or suprathyroid causes. An abnormality within the thyroid, termed primary hypothyroidism, accounts for 95 percent of hypothyroidism while only 5 percent or less is caused by an abnormality of the pituitary or hypothalamus, termed secondary and tertiary hypothyroidism, respectively. In primary hypothyroidism, the inability to synthesize sufficient quantities of thyroid hormones leads to an increased secretion of TSH and potentially a goiter. The commonest cause of hypothyroidism in North America is Hashimoto's disease.

The clinical picture of patients with hypothyroidism varies greatly and depends on the patient's age when the deficiency begins and the severity of the disorder. If severe hypothyroidism occurs and is untreated in the neonatal period, profound developmental abnormalities occur and this condition is termed cretinism. It is present in approximately 1 of every 5000 neonates. It usually manifests itself with abnormally long periods of physiologic jaundice, hoarse cry, constipation, somnolence, and feeding problems in the neonatal period. Current medical practice dictates that all newborns be screened for hypothyroidism. Cretinism leads to short stature, coarse features with protruding tongue, broad flat nose, widely spaced eyes, sparse hair, dry skin, protuberant abdomen, umbilical hernias, and impaired mental development. Radiologic examination reveals delayed bone age and dentition. Juvenile hypothyroidism is found in older children. They have normal somatic and intellectual development initially. The clinical manifestations of hypothyroidism are intermediate between those of neonatal and adult hypothyroidism. However, juvenile hypothyroidism may lead to the development of abnormal pubertal development. In the adult, symptoms may include lethargy, constipation, cold intolerance, stiffness and cramping of muscles, carpal tunnel syndrome, abnormal uterine bleeding, decreased intellectual capacity, decreased motor activity, decreased appetite with or without weight gain, obesity, a thinning of the hair, and a characteristic, nonpitting edema called myxedema. In more advanced stages, it presents as an expressionless face, sparse hair, exophthalmos, ptosis of the upper lids, periorbital puffiness, large tongue, and pale colored skin that feels rough and doughy. A chest x ray may reveal an enlarged heart secondary to both dilation and a pericardial effusion. Adynamic ileus may occur with a resulting intestinal obstruction. Physical examination reveals a prolongation of deep tendon reflexes and there may be respiratory depression leading to changes in the arterial blood gases. Hypothyroidism may be fatal. These patients become hypothermic and progress into a stuporous state called myxedema coma.

The most important screening test for the diagnosis of hypothyroidism is TSH. In more advanced stages, it can be diagnosed by a decrease in thyroid hormone accompanied by an increased resin T_3 uptake and a decreased free T_4 index.

In Obstetrics and Gynecology

Hypothyroidism in reproductive aged women leads to decreased fertility due to ovulatory disturbances. It is important to screen for hypothyroidism in patients who present with dysfunctional uterine bleeding, amenorrhea, and with elevated prolactin levels. The routine screening of infertile patients with a TSH is not warranted or cost-effective. Maternal hypothyroidism does not pose a problem for the fetus since neither TSH, T_4, or T_3 can cross the placenta. It is important to note that thyroid function in utero is not important for fetal well-being. Children born with congenital absence of the thyroid gland are normal at birth. Patients receiving thyroid replacement therapy are at no increased risk for obstetric complications or congenital malformations. It is necessary, however, to monitor their status during pregnancy to assure a euthyroid condition due to the already mentioned changes in TBG. The best screening test in pregnancy is the free T_4 index, a test that takes into account both the total T_4 and the binding capacity of TBG.

It has been taught that pregnancy is goitrogenic. This may be true in countries where iodine consumption in the diet is markedly restricted or deficient. However, there is no evidence that there is any enlargement in the thyroid gland during pregnancy in women who are not iodine deficient.

Treatment

Treatment of hypothyroidism requires hormone replacement. Synthetic hormones include levothyroxine, levotriiodothyronine (liothyronine), or a combination of the two (liotrix). Animal thyroid extracts are of nonuniform potency and therefore we prefer the use of synthetic preparations. Levothyroxine is preferred because ingestion does not lead to an abrupt increase in T_3 concentration which could be dangerous, especially to older patients or patients with coexisting heart disease. It is extremely important that replacement therapy proceeds very slowly in elderly patients, especially those with preexisting heart disease in whom a sudden increase in the metabolic rate may tax the cardiac or coronary reserve and could lead to cardiac compromise. The normal maintenance dose of levothyroxine is approximately 150 to 200 μg per day. However, it is recommended that the initial daily dose be 25 μg and that this be increased by similar increments every 2 to 3 weeks until a normal metabolic state is attained. This can be confimed by measuring the serum TSH or T_3 concentrations. Elevation of the former is indicative of insufficient treatment while elevation of the latter is indicative of excessive treatment.

Numerous patients have been placed on thyroid hormone replacement for questionable reasons. To determine if replacement therapy is necessary, baseline measurements of TSH, T_4, and resin T_3 uptake are necessary. If all of these levels are within the normal range, thyroid replacement treatment should be stopped and the TSH level should be checked again in 4 to 6 weeks. This interval is necessary for the recovery of the hypothalamic-pituitary-thyroid axis.

RECOMMENDED THERAPY IN THE TREATMENT OF HYPERTHYROIDISM

Agent	Dose
Propylthiouracil (approved for use in pregnancy)	100–150 mg, orally, every 6–8 hours

Once a patient is started on therapy, check the complete blood cell count with a differential every month for the first 4 months to evaluate for granulocytopenia. It is extremely important that the patients be informed of this potential side effect and be advised to call with any symptoms of infection to check if this has occurred.

All patients with the diagnosis of hyperthyroidism need to be followed for life for signs and symptoms of hypothyroidism, whether during treatment or in remission, with yearly measurements of TSH, resin T_3 uptake, and T_4.

If the patient is pregnant, because of the potential risks to the developing infant, examine her for signs and symptoms of hyperthyroidism and check the free T_4 index every 2 to 4 weeks and adjust the dosage accordingly. We prefer to have patients slightly hyperthyroid during pregnancy in an attempt to limit the amount of drug exposure to the infant.

RECOMMENDED THERAPY IN THE TREATMENT OF THYROID STORM

All patients with suspected thyroid storm should be immediately admitted to an intensive care unit with appropriate consultations to endocrinology, cardiology, and infectious disease specialists.

Agent	Dose
Propylthiouracil	300–1000 mg stat orally (per nasogastric tube, if necessary), then 150–300 mg orally every 6 hours
Sodium iodine	Give 1 hour after administration of propylthiouracil; 500–1000 mg intravenously every 8 hours
Dexamethasone	2 mg intravenously every 6 hours
Propranolol	1 mg/minute, intravenously, to a total of 5 mg every 4–6 hours as needed to control symptoms
Triple antiobiotics	
Ampicillin	1 gm intravenously every 6 hours
Gentamicin	1.5 mg/kg every 8 hours
Clindamycin	300 mg every 6 hours
Cooling blanket or cold packs	

RECOMMENDED THERAPY IN THE TREATMENT OF HYPOTHYROIDISM

Agent	Dose
Levothyroxine	Start at 25 μg orally every day and increase by 25 μg every 2–3 weeks; 150 μg represents the dose necessary to sustain a normal metabolic rate

Assessment of the proper dosage of levothyroxine requires periodic checking of TSH and T_3 levels. An elevated TSH level indicates that more thyroid replacement is necessary while an elevated T_3 level indicates overtreatment. This should be performed after the patient has been taking 100 μg per day for a month to assess if there is a need to increase the medication. If the patient is still hypothyroid, these tests should be repeated 1 month after increasing the dosage as recommended above. Once the optimum dose is obtained, repeat these tests every 6 to 12 months.

PREPARATIONS

Thyroid Agonists—Treatment of Hypothyroidism

Levothyroxine Sodium (Levothyroid [USV], Synthroid [Flint], Generic)

Synthetic levothyroxine is absorbed by the gastrointestinal tract or via intravenous administration. Oral absorption, however, may be adversely affected by other food stuffs and by malabsorption syndromes. This hormone is indistinguishable from endogenous T_4 and is metabolized identically. Blood levels only vary slightly from dose to dose. Plasma concentrations and ratios of T_4 to T_3 are normal when the patient is euthyroid during levothyroxine therapy. Symptoms of overdosage are identical to those for hyperthyroidism. Usage in pregnancy is not associated with any increase in congenital malformations.

Levothyroxine sodium is supplied as 0.025-, 0.050-, 0.075-, 0.100-, 0.125-, 0.150-, 0.200-, and 0.300-mg tablets.

For oral dosage the average adult will require 0.10 to 0.20 mg per day. Dosage should commence with 0.050 mg per day in healthy adults and be increased by 0.025 mg every 3 weeks, as tolerated, until the patient is taking 0.015 mg per day or is clinically euthyroid. After 1 month of this therapy, a TSH measurement should be obtained. If this is elevated, continue to increase the medication up to a maximum of 0.020 mg per day. Repeat the TSH measurement at each increment. If the TSH level is normal, follow the patient with a free T_4 index every 6 months to ensure proper dosage. If the patient is older or has a history of heart disease, start thyroid replacement at 0.025 mg per day and increase it every month, if tolerated, by 0.025 mg and follow the same protocol as above.

Intravenous dosage should be used only in emergency situations when the patient is unable to take the oral preparation, as in myxedematous coma.

Liothyronine Sodium (Cytomel [Smith Kline & French])

Liothyronine is considered to be approximately 3 times more potent, on a weight by weight basis, than levothyroxine. Due to this medication's shorter half-life, blood levels tend to fluctuate from dose to dose. Liothyronine is also more difficult to monitor than levothyroxine. For these reasons, liothyronine's use in the management of hypothyroidism is uncommon. Plasma T_4 concentrations remain low in patients receiving this form of therapy.

Liothyronine is supplied as 0.005-, 0.025-, and 0.050-mg tablets.

For oral dosage this medication should be given in divided doses, 2 or 3 times a day. The average replacement dose in an adult is 0.050 to 0.075 mg per day. In an otherwise healthy adult, liothyronine, 0.010 mg, may be given twice a day and the dose may be increased by 0.010 mg per day every 3 weeks until the patient is euthyroid. Older adults, cardiac patients, or patients with severe hypothyroidism should be started on 0.0025 mg twice a day and increased by 0.0025 mg per day every month to avoid toxicity and cardiac complications. Follow-up should be identical as with levothyroxine.

Liotrix (Euthroid [Parke-Davis], Thyrolar [Rorer])

Each liotrix tablet contains a ratio, by weight, of 4:1 of levothyroxine: liothyronine. Liothyronine is more readily absorbed through the gastrointestinal tract than is levothyroxine. This fact combined with the increased potency of liothyronine makes this medication less desirable for elderly patients or patients with any cardiac history.

Liotrix is supplied as ¼, ½, 1, 2, and 3 containing the following quantities of levothyroxine/liothyronine: 0.0125/0.0031, 0.025/0.00625, 0.050/0.0125, 0.10/0.025, 0.150/0.0375, 0.20/0.050, and 0.30/0.075 mg.

The oral dosage is identical to that for levothyroxine, starting with a dose of 0.050 of levothyroxine and 0.0125 of liothyronine and increasing by 0.025 mg of levothyroxine (with 0.00625 mg of T_3).

An intravenous dosage is not available.

Thyroid Extract (Armour Thyroid [Rorer], Proloid [Parke-Davis], S-P-T [Fleming], Generic)

This porcine thyroid extract contains a combination of levothyroxine and liothyronine in a ratio of approximately 4:1 (Armour Thyroid, Proloid) or 2.5:1.0 (S-P-T) plus other iodotyrosines and organic compounds. Historically there have been problems with variable potencies from lot to lot.

How thyroid extract is supplied varies with each product.

Oral dosage is not recommended.

Thyroid Antagonists

Propylthiouracil (Generic)

Propylthiouracil has two actions. It inhibits the iodination of tyrosine and thereby inhibits the formation of thyroid hormone and it inhibits the conversion of T_4 to T_3. In pregnant women, propylthiouracil is the preferred medication because it crosses the placenta less readily than methimazole but is still associated with neonatal goiter. The most serious and life-threatening side effects are granulocytopenia and agranulocytosis. This usually occurs in the first few months of therapy and monthly complete blood counts with differentials for the first 3 to 4 months are advised. However, the rapidity of onset of this problem makes it imperative that patients be advised to report all symptoms of malaise, sore throat, etc., and they should be immediately evaluated for this problem at that time. Rash is also a common side effect.

Propylthiouracil is supplied as 50-mg tablets.

In adults, although initial oral doses may be as high as 400 mg 3 times a day, most patients are controlled with 100 to 150 mg 3 times a day. Maintenance doses range from 50 mg 2 times a day to 100 mg 3 times a day.

Methimazole (Tapazole [Lilly])

Methimazole has the same effect on thyroid metabolism as propylthiouracil but it is approximately 10 times more potent and its half-life is longer. This allows for single daily dose administration. Its use, however, is contraindicated in pregnant women due to its ability to readily cross the placenta.

Methimazole is supplied as 5- and 10-mg tablets.

In adults initial oral doses for the control of hyperthyroid crisis range from 5 to 20 mg 3 times a day. A dose of 30 mg, given as one daily dose or divided to 10 mg given 3 times a day, is the usual maintenance dose.

Potassium or Sodium Iodine (Generic But May Be Marketed Under The Name "Lugol's Solution")

Large oral doses of iodine have an antithyroid effect by inhibiting the uptake of iodine by the thyroid gland (Wolff-Chaikoff effect). Potassium or sodium iodine is useful only in treatment of thyroid storm and in an attempt to inhibit the uptake of radioactive iodine in a nuclear accident.

Potassium iodine is supplied as 300-mg tablets or 1 gm/ml solution. Sodium iodine is available in 5 percent and 10 percent solutions, and also in bulk.

For protection of adults and children older than 1 year after nuclear accident the oral dosage is 130 mg per day. For children younger than 1 year the dosage is 65 mg per day. For thyroid storm 250 to 500 mg per day of sodium iodine is administered intravenously 1 hour after the initial dose of propylthiouracil and propranolol.

Propranolol (Inderal [Ayerst], Generic)

Propranolol is a beta-adrenergic blocking agent that will mask the clinical symptom of hyperthyroidism and inhibit the conversion of T_4 to T_3. It is useful in the treatment of thyroid storm to alleviate the symptomatology but is contraindicated in patients with congestive heart failure and should be avoided in patients with asthma or chronic bronchitis and in pregnant women.

Propranolol is supplied as 1 mg/ml solution.

Propranolol should only be intravenously administered in an intensive care unit at a dose of 1 mg per minute to a maximum 5 mg every 4 to 6 hours.

BIBLIOGRAPHY

Thyroid Disease and Physiology

Ingbar, S. H. The Thyroid Gland. In J. D. Wilson and D. W. Foster (eds.), *Williams Textbook of Endocrinology*. Philadelphia: W. B. Saunders, 1985. Pp. 682–815.

Thyroid in Pregnancy

Cooper, D. S. Antithyroid drugs: to breast-feed or not to breast-feed. *Am. J. Obstet. Gynecol.* 157:234, 1987.

Fisher, D. A. Maternal-fetal thyroid function in pregnancy. *Clin. Perinatol.* 10:615, 1983.

Mestman, J. H. Thyroid disease in pregnancy. *Clin. Perinatol.* 12:651, 1985.

Thyroid and Reproductive Physiology

Burrow, G. N. The Thyroid Gland and Reproduction. In S. S. C. Yen and R. B. Jaffe (eds.), *Reproductive Endocrinology*. Philadelphia: W. B. Saunders, 1986. Pp. 424–440.

Thomas, R., and Reid, R. L. Thyroid disease and reproductive dysfunction: a review. *Obstet. Gynecol.* 70:789, 1987.

II
Selected Reviews

10

Endocrine Therapy of Cyclic Hormonal Disorders

Michel E. Rivlin

The three common disorders all related to cyclic ovarian function to be considered in this chapter differ in that diagnosis and therapy of one, primary dysmenorrhea, are generally satisfactory while in the remaining two, premenstrual syndrome (PMS) and cyclic mastalgia, are often frustrating to both patient and doctor. Since all three disorders have in common the presence of cyclic hormonal function, it is clear that there will be some similarities in their treatment. The wide variations of response to such therapy in the individual are probably related to diagnostic difficulties rather than to problems with therapy per se.

PRIMARY DYSMENORRHEA

Primary dysmenorrhea is painful menstruation with no discernible organic basis. It is estimated that more than 50 percent of menstruating women experience the condition and in about 10 percent, the symptoms may be incapacitating. The pain is spasmodic, is situated over the lower abdomen, and may involve the back and thighs. The onset is usually with menses, but may occur some hours earlier. Systemic symptoms such as nausea, vomiting, and diarrhea may accompany the menstrual cramps. The condition usually begins at the menarche or soon thereafter. Generally, the cramps subside within 48 to 72 hours.

The cause of primary dysmenorrhea appears to be the increased production and release of endometrial prostaglandins during menses. Prostaglandin-induced myometrial contractions result in uterine hypoxia and pain. The systemic symptoms, in particular, gastrointestinal hypermotility, are likely prostaglandin related. Prostaglandins are C20 hydrocarbons produced from arachidonic acid in the form of prostaglandins E_2 and $F_{2\alpha}$ by enzyme systems including cyclo-oxygenase, isomerase, and reductase. Uterine contractions are induced by prostaglandin through the action of inducing free calcium within the myometrial cell. Ovulation is central to the mechanism of primary dysmenorrhea. A decreasing progesterone level results in the release of phospholipase from the lysosomes that hydrolyze phospholipids to arachidonic acid. The availability of arachidonic acid together with the endometrial cellular breakdown at the onset of menses stimulates the arachidonic acid cascade leading to prostaglandin production.

In a woman requesting *oral contraception* in whom the diagnosis of primary dysmenorrhea is made, in the absence of the usual contraindications, standard birth control pills can be expected to substantially improve the symptom in up to 90 percent of patients. Oral contraceptives inhibit endometrial development and as a result reduce the amount of prostaglandins in the menstrual fluid. If, however, there is no requirement for oral contraception, then initial management should be with a nonsteroidal anti-inflammatory drug (NSAID). The exception would be in those women with a history of gastric ulceration who should not be given NSAID therapy but should be managed with oral contraceptives. In those women managed with oral contraceptives, if relief is not obtained after 3 to 4 months, NSAID therapy should be given in addition. If the symptom persists after 4 to 6 months of combined therapy, laparoscopy is indicated to exclude the usual causes of secondary dysmenorrhea including endometriosis and chronic pelvic inflammatory disease.

As distinct from oral contraceptives, *NSAIDs* do not affect endometrial development but suppress menstrual fluid prostaglandins through enzymatic inhibition of prostaglandin production. However, like oral contraceptives, the amount of menstrual bleeding is decreased with prolonged use of NSAIDs. Patients who do not have gastroduodenal ulceration or a history of hypersensitivity to NSAIDs can be treated for 3 to 6 months with adjustment in the dose as well as the type of NSAID. Should there be no relief, a trial of oral contraception in addition may be attempted for a further 3 to 6 months. Thereafter, a laparoscopy may be indicated. The majority of patients (80–85%) do obtain relief. In general, if a patient does not respond to an adequate dose of a suitable NSAID, switching to another NSAID is preferable to increasing the dose since the side effects are dose related and there is a plateau analgesic effect for these medications. Patients may respond better to another drug of the same class and this can only be gauged by trial and error. Although there is no proven therapeutic value in starting medication before the onset of symptoms, it is recommended that medication be taken at the first indication of discomfort rather than after increased severity of symptoms. Patients with dysmenorrhea related to the use of an intrauterine device (IUD) respond well to therapy with NSAIDs. This is related to a marked increase in prostaglandins in the endometrium in the vicinity of the IUD. Furthermore, the menorrhagia associated with IUD use is also ameliorated by NSAID administration.

Prostaglandin synthetase inhibitors (NSAIDs) may be grouped according to their structural derivative and their site of pharmacologic inhibition of prostaglandin synthesis. Type I drugs are cyclooxygenase inhibitors and are the most useful for treating dysmenorrhea. Some members of the group are less useful than others; for example, aspirin (a benzoic acid derivative) is inadequate in low doses and has unpleasant side effects at high dosage, and indomethacin, an indole acetic acid, is probably too risky for long-term monthly therapy. Most appropriate choices are probably alkanoic (Arylpropionic) acid derivatives such as ibuprofen (Motrin, Rufen, Advil, Nuprin, Medipren, Haltran), 400 mg given 4 times a day; naproxen sodium (Anaprox) 275 mg given 4 times a day; and fenoprofen (Nalfon), 200 mg given 4 times a day. Other effective type I inhibitors are fenamate derivatives such as mefenamic acid (Ponstel), 250 to 500 mg given 4 times a day; however fenamate derivatives are not recommended for monthly therapy because of a high incidence of marrow toxicity. Piroxicam (Feldene) is representative of the oxicam group of NSAIDs and because of its long serum half-life is effective in single daily doses of 20 to 40 mg. Type II drugs inhibit isomerase and reductase enzymes and therefore do not reduce the formation of cyclic endoperoxides, prostacyclins, and thromboxanes, which are also uterotonic. These drugs are buterophanes and include phenylbutazone and oxyphenbutazone. For the reasons already mentioned, they are therefore little used in the therapy of dysmenorrhea.

It is not clear why 15 to 20 percent of patients do not have an adequate response to NSAIDs. One possible explanation is that arachidonic acid is metabolized by a second important enzyme system, a 5-lipoxygenase enzyme leading to leukotrienes. These substances also increase uterine contractility. The development of lipoxygenase inhibitor therapy may therefore be useful in patients who do not respond to cyclo-oxygenase inhibitors. Also, calcium antagonists such as nifedipine (Procardia, Adalat) have been used with success in a limited number of resistant patients. However, nifedipine may produce facial flushing, headaches, and, if conception should occur, may be embryotoxic. In general, patients with secondary dysmenorrhea do not respond well to NSAIDs and a trial of drug therapy may help select out the patients who need to undergo laparoscopy. The fear that arises is that pain relief given by these medications may mask a progressive, damaging process such as endometriosis. As endometriosis is now being found in younger patients, this may become a growing concern.

All NSAIDs are absorbed rapidly after oral administration. The onset of analgesic effects generally occurs within 1 hour. The drugs are tightly bound to plasma proteins, especially albumin. The liver is the major site for metabolism and the major pathway for excretion is the kidney, although significant amounts are excreted in the feces. Adverse effects of NSAIDs include a variety of gastrointestinal, dermatologic, and central nervous system symptoms as well as renal, hepatic, hematopoietic, and allergic reactions. Although all NSAIDs have been associated with such reactions, there are differences that often provide the basis for drug selection. The prolonged administration of large doses of these drugs, as in rheumatic disease, enhances the probability and potential severity of reactions. Nevertheless, considering the widespread use of these drugs, they are relatively safe. Ingestion with food can reduce gastrointestinal disturbance while intestinal ulceration is a contraindication. Because NSAIDs impair platelet aggregation and prolong bleeding time, they should be discontinued 24 to 48 hours before surgery (several days for aspirin). The occurrence of a hypersensitivity reaction is a contraindication to subsequent use and sensitivity is usually shared with other NSAIDs. Patients with a history of asthma, urticaria, hay fever, or nasal polyps are at increased risk and should be given these drugs only if necessary and with great care. Drug interactions of importance occur with anticoagulants and hypoglycemic agents, the action of which is enhanced. Combining two NSAIDs confers no additional benefit. These drugs should not be used in pregnant women or in nursing mothers.

PREMENSTRUAL SYNDROME

Like primary dysmenorrhea, PMS is characterized by its cyclicity related to ovarian function and in that the severity of symptoms may vary greatly from month to month in the same woman. The symptoms themselves are less important than the timing of their appearance. Diagnosis depends on the use of a menstrual calendar prospectively following at least two cycles to verify the cyclic nature of the symptoms. An estimated 20 to 40 percent of all women experience some difficulty, but only approximately 5 percent report a significant impact on work or life-style. Most symptoms fall into one of four subgroups related to either anxiety, depression, fluid retention, or carbohydrate intolerance.

Since the pathophysiology of PMS has not been adequately delineated and in the absence of a definitive diagnostic test, the definition of rational therapy must await further investigation. Presently, pharmacologic intervention is very much an issue of trial and error. All patients with mild PMS can be adequately treated with education, diet, and exercise. Some patients with moderate symptoms also respond readily to these types of conservative therapy. Some patients with moderate symptoms and most of those with severe PMS require medication to alleviate some of their symptoms.

Because PMS does not appear prior to puberty, is eliminated by natural (menopause) or surgical cessation of ovarian function, and is absent during pregnancy, but is unaffected by hysterectomy, pharmacologic suppression of the cyclic production of ovarian hormones would appear to be a logical approach. For this reason, *oral contraception*, especially when contraception is requested, or menorrhagia and dysmenorrhea coexist, is a commonly employed therapy. However, some women first experience PMS while taking these preparations and a constant state of symptoms may be precipitated. It is stated that oral contraceptives improve, do not affect, or worsen PMS in one-third of women so treated. Other estrogen and progesterone treatments employing subcutaneous estradiol implants with cyclic oral progestins claim better results. *Danazol* in daily doses of 100 to 400 mg may be helpful for certain PMS symptoms, but the significant side effects suggest that it is not suitable as a long-term, first-line drug in the treatment of PMS. "Medical ovariectomy" with *gonadotropin-releasing hormone* (*GnRH*) *agonist* therapy creates an acyclic anovulatory state without use of synthetic sex steroids that have been known to precipitate PMS-like symptoms. Early results of this modality are encouraging but long-term use is not recommended because of the estrogen deficiency related to these medications. Possibly, low doses, enough to block the surge of luteinizing hormone (LH) but not completely suppress ovarian steroidogenesis, combined with intermittent progestin therapy may prove useful.

Progestational treatment of PMS is common although there is no evidence to justify this expensive and cumbersome treatment since there are no double-blind, placebo-controlled studies of progesterone therapy in PMS that have shown progestational therapy to be of benefit. The dosage of natural progesterone is 50 to 100 mg daily by intramuscular injection or 200 to 400 mg twice daily by vaginal or rectal suppositories. Treatment should be started 5 days before symptoms are expected and continued until menses or the symptoms abate. The advent of oral micronized progesterone provides a simpler alternative. Patients may be given a 100-mg capsule in the morning and two 100-mg capsules at bedtime, started some 3 days after ovulation. Synthetic progestins such as medroxyprogesterone acetate (Provera) have not generally relieved PMS and may exacerbate some symptoms, especially depression.

Nutritional measures include a reduction in dietary salt and refined sugars, avoidance of methylxanthine-containing substances such as coffee, tea, and chocolate, together with a regular exercise routine. *Vitamin* B_6 supplementation in doses of 300 to 500 mg daily may be helpful. Peripheral neurotoxicity can occur at higher dosage levels so that patients should not increase the amount of medication taken. *Alpha tocopherol* (vitamin E) supplementation in doses of 400 IU daily may also be helpful in some women. *Gamma-linolenic acid* (evening primrose oil) may be helpful for breast discomfort. Alcohol consumption frequently increases in the premenstruum and this should be discouraged.

Symptomatic therapy is commonly used for individual symptoms or symptom complexes. Thus, *diuretics* may be used for symptoms of bloating and swelling and these should be used only as needed. Hydrochlorothiazide, 25 to 50 mg every other day for 10 days prior to menses, may be prescribed with a potassium supplement; spironolactone, 25 mg 3 times a day, provides an alternative treatment.

In selected patients, and especially if prolactin levels are elevated, *bromocriptine* may be prescribed for mastalgia. *Prostaglandin inhibitors* can be used for symptoms of dysmenorrhea and menorrhagia if these are present. *Ergotamine tartrate*, an ergot derivative, may be beneficial for those women who complain of migraine headaches. The drug is used sometimes in combination with a mild sedative plus an anticholinergic. In general, however, because of the chronic nature of the disorder, the use of narcotics or long-acting anxiolytic drugs should be strongly discouraged.

In patients with marked anxiety and irritability, but not those who are at high risk of addictive behavior, newer short-acting antianxiety agents such as *alprazolam* (Xanax) are helpful and are as effective as imipramine and superior to diazepam. The initial dose is 0.25 mg 3 times a day. If drowsiness is a problem, the dosage may be decreased. No more than 0.5 mg 3 times a day should be used. The medication should be used only on the symptomatic premenstrual days. Those women with marked depression should be referred to a psychiatrist for antidepressant medication. These medications are taken daily and improvement is generally seen after 2 to 3 weeks. They are generally required for patients who have an underlying affective disorder exacerbated by PMS. Lithium is not advocated. Monoamine oxidase inhibitors are often effective for depression associated with PMS exacerbation, but not for patients who are free of symptoms during the follicular phase.

The physician and the patient should both be aware of the placebo effect. PMS shows a strong response to placebo, often quoted as 50 to 60 percent, but rates as high as 94 percent have been reported. The duration of the placebo response varies but generally is back to pretreatment levels by 6 months. The psychosocial, subjective component of medicine makes the placebo process a legitimate part of every patient-physician interaction. It is very likely that successful therapy of PMS, regardless of the agent or method used, depends to a significant degree on the placebo process.

CYCLICAL MASTOPATHY

Cyclical mastopathy comprises swelling, tenderness, or enlargement of breasts which typically begins during the luteal phase, increases as menses approach, and resolves quickly with menstruation. The condition affects an estimated 30 to 40 percent of premenopausal women and is severe enough to interfere with normal activity in about 8 percent. Breast pain (mastalgia, mastodynia) may also occur in a noncyclical fashion or be secondary to infection, trauma, or tumor and these conditions must be excluded. Cyclical mastopathy is often a part of PMS and these disorders may be separate entities as the varying components of PMS may respond differently to treatment.

The pathophysiology of benign breast changes is not well understood. The breast reacts to ovarian secretion like the endometrium.

Thus, estradiol induces cell proliferation into mammary ducts while progesterone slows down cell multiplication, acting as an antiestrogen. Steroid hormones are therefore implicated in the evolution of breast lesions and it is possible that the differences observed in the respective degree of cellular hyperplasia and even atypia in the lesions may be related to the duration of the disease. Continuation of an abnormal hormonal milieu in the breast may therefore lead to the clinical findings of nodularity and lumpiness in the breasts often referred to as "fibrocystic disease" and "chronic cystic mastitis." There is no proof that the same hormonal environment plays a major role in the development of breast cancer but it is possible that the lack of progesterone secretion is a common risk for development of both benign breast disease and cancer. The relationship of both benign and malignant breast disease to diet has also implicated a role for serum lipids in the pathophysiology of breast disease. It is hypothesized that the cyclical nature of the symptoms may be attributable to superimposition of the normal cyclical variations in lipid metabolism that have been reported to occur during the menstrual cycle on the underlying lipid disorder.

Theoretically, excellent management of benign breast disorders would alleviate mastodynia, resorb lumps and nodularity, and avoid the mitogenic effects of estrogens. Unfortunately, the wide range of advocated treatments bears testimony to the lack of complete understanding and therefore management of these disorders. Most women do not require medical treatment and wish only to be reassured that no damaging pathologic process is involved. Firm support by a good brassiere together with mild analgesics usually proves adequate for the symptomatology. Caffeine in large doses can cause breast pain in susceptible women; therefore, reduction in methylxanthine intake may be recommended. Dietary fat reduction from 40 to 20 percent of caloric intake has been shown to significantly reduce cyclic breast symptoms. *Evening primrose oil* (Efamol), an essential fatty acid supplement that contains cis-linoleic acid and gamma-linolenic acids, is believed to act as a precursor of prostaglandin synthesis resulting in an increase in the levels of some prostaglandins which in turn may decrease prolactin activity locally. Improvement has been reported in a dosage of 6 capsules per day. Vitamin E has not proved helpful in this condition.

Several approaches have been attempted for the hormonal therapy of cyclic mastopathy. *Bromocriptine* (Parlodel), a dopaminergic agonist that inhibits release of prolactin from the pituitary gland, may be given in a luteal phase dose of 2.5 mg twice daily. The side effects of nausea, vomiting, dizziness, and hallucinations may make its long-term use uncomfortable. The drug is therefore used more often for galactorrhea due to a pituitary prolactinoma. *Bellergal*, which contains ergotamine tartrate, a compound that acts in a manner similar to bromocriptine, also contains belladonna alkaloids and a barbiturate and has been used for PMS. *Danazol* (Danocrine), an androgen derivative (17α-norethindrone), has improved mastodynia, nodularity, and thermographic abnormalities. It may be given in a luteal dose regimen of 100 to 400 mg per day for 2 to 6 consecutive months. Danazol suppresses ovarian function resulting in amenorrhea at higher doses. It is expensive and side effects including acne, hirsutism, hot flushes, and weight gain are major disadvantages. Further, its effects on fetal development are not known and a decrease of up to 50 percent in high-density lipoprotein cholesterol accompanies its use. More recently, *GnRH agonists* at dosages sufficient to inhibit ovarian secretion have been proposed as an alternative; however, this approach entails marked estrogen deprivation and therefore cannot be given for a long period of time.

Tamoxifen, an antiestrogen, reduces estrogenic activity by blocking estrogen receptors. Although tamoxifen is effective in relieving mastalgia, the underlying undefined endocrine abnormality is only suppressed by the treatment. Thus, about half of the patients relapse after discontinuation of therapy. In addition, some patients complain of menstrual irregularity, nausea, hot flushes, depression, and bloating. The dosage is 10 mg daily for a 3-month course. At this time its use must still be regarded as experimental in this context.

Progestational agents have been widely used for the treatment of benign breast disease. The most effective are estrane derivatives. Progestins in this series are derived from 19-nortestosterone. Their androgenic activity is relatively high and this is probably responsible for their antigonadotropin potency which is much greater than that of pregnane derivatives. The two readily available are norethindrone and norgestrel. The antiestrogen activity of estrane derivatives is strong. *Lynestrenol* has proved to be effective in the relief of breast abnormalities measured clinically and thermographically, but is not available in the United States. An alternative approach is to use medroxyprogesterone acetate, 10 mg per day, from day 4 to 25 of the cycle, or a progestin-dominant oral contraceptive containing, for instance, 1 mg of norethindrone acetate and 0.02 mg of ethinyl estradiol (Loestrin 1/20). However, it must be pointed out that although a beneficial effect of oral contraceptives on benign breast disease has been described, mastodynia may first appear during oral contraceptive therapy and be relieved by cessation of the medication. Side effects of progestin therapy also include weight gain and acne.

BIBLIOGRAPHY

Primary Dysmenorrhea

American Medical Association. *Drug Evaluations* (6th ed.). Philadelphia: W. B. Saunders, 1986.

Dawood, M. Y. Current concepts in the etiology and treatment of primary dysmenorrhea. *Acta Obstet. Gynecol. Scand.* [*Suppl.*] 138:7, 1986.

Dawood, M. Y. Nonsteroidal anti-inflammatory drugs and changing attitudes toward dysmenorrhea. *Am. J. Med.* 84:23, 1988.

Fraser, I. S., and McCarron, G. Ibuprofen is a useful treatment of primary dysmenorrhoea. *Aust. N.Z. J. Obstet. Gynaecol.* 27:244, 1987.

Pasquale, S. A., Rathauser, R., and Dolese, H. M. A double-blind, placebo-controlled study comparing three single-dose regimens of piroxicam with ibuprofen in patients with primary dysmenorrhea. *Am. J. Med.* 84:30, 1988.

Rees, M. C. P., et al. Leukotriene release by endometrium and myometrium throughout the menstrual cycle in dysmenorrhoea and menorrhagia. *J. Endocr.* 113:291, 1987.

Smith, R. P., and Powell, J. R. Simultaneous objective and subjective evaluation of meclofenamate sodium in the treatment of primary dysmenorrhea. *Am. J. Obstet. Gynecol.* 157:611, 1987.

Premenstrual Syndrome

Chakmakjian, Z. H., and Zachariah, N. Y. Bioavailability of progesterone with different modes of administration. *J. Reprod. Med.* 32:443, 1987.

Chihal, H. J. Indications for drug therapy in premenstrual syndrome patients. *J. Reprod. Med.* 32:449, 1987.
Johnson, S. R. Premenstrual syndrome. *Clin. Obstet. Gynecol.* 30:365, 1987.
Muse, K. N., Cetel, N. S., and Futterman, L. A. The premenstrual syndrome effects of "medical ovariectomy." *N. Engl. J. Med.* 311:345, 1984.
Reid, R. L. Premenstrual syndrome. *Curr. Prob. Obstet. Gynecol. Infertil.* (February) 8:1, 1985.
Smith, S., et al. Treatment of premenstrual syndrome with alprazolam: results of a double-blind, placebo-controlled, randomized crossover clinical trial. *Obstet. Gynecol.* 70:37, 1987.
Vellacott, I. D., and O'Brien, P. M. S. Effect of spironolactone on premenstrual syndrome symptoms. *J. Reprod. Med.* 32:429, 1987.
Wood, C., and Jakubowicz, D. The treatment of premenstrual syndrome symptoms with mefenamic acid. *Br. J. Obstet. Gynaecol.* 87:627, 1980.

Cyclic Mastopathy

Colin, C., Gaspard, U., and Lambotte, R. Relationship of mastodynia with its endocrine environment and treatment in a double blind trial with lynestrenol. *Arch. Gynaekol.* 225:7, 1978.
Doberl, A., Tobiassen, T., and Rasussen, T. Treatment of recurrent cyclical mastodynia in patients with fibrocystic breast disease. *Acta Obstet. Gynecol. Scand.* 123:177, 1984.
Durning, P., and Sellwood, R. A. Bromocriptine in severe cyclical breast pain. *Br. J. Surg.* 69:248, 1982.
Fentiman, I. S., and Powles, T. J. Tamoxifen and benign breast conditions: the end or just the beginning? *Lancet* 2:1070, 1987.
Goodwin, P. J., Neelam, M., and Boyd, N. F. Cyclical mastopathy: a critical review of therapy. *Br. J. Surg.* 75:837, 1988.
Love, S. M., et al. Benign Breast Disorders. In J. R. Harris, S. Hellman, I. C. Henderson, and D. W. Kinne (eds.), *Breast Diseases*. Philadelphia: J. P. Lippincott, 1987.
Mansel, R. E., Wisbey, J. R., and Hughes, L. E. Controlled trial of the antigonadotrophin danazol in painful nodular benign breast disease. *Lancet* 1:928, 1982.
Preece, P. E., Mansel, R. E., and Hughes, L. E. Mastalgia: psychoneurosis or organic disease? *Br. Med. J.* 1:29, 1978.
Preece, P. E., et al. Evening Primrose Oil (Efamol) for Mastalgia. In D. F. Horrobin (ed.), *Clinical Uses of Essential Fatty Acids*. Montreal: Eden Press, 1982. Pp. 147–154.

11

Hormone Therapy in the Pediatric and Adolescent Female Patient

Michel E. Rivlin

The development of the capacity for reproduction commences in utero and continues through puberty. During the fetal stage, gonadotropin secretion increases progressively with patterns and levels comparable with the onset and first half of puberty. Gonadal steroidogenesis increases and episodic release of gonadotropins indicates that negative feedback mechanisms and differentiation of the hypothalamic-pituitary-gonadal (HPG) axis are functional. During the neonatal phase, hormonal secretion is greater than during childhood. For a few weeks, secretion persists at pubertal levels but without overt physical changes. In the childhood phase, downregulation results in hormone levels equivalent to those in hypogonadotropic hypogonadal adults. The low levels of secretion are a function of decreased hypothalamic stimulation which is under control by the central nervous system (CNS). The final phase of development is puberty which is marked by a resurgence of gonadotropin and sex steroid secretion. This begins with pulsatile, sleep coincident, pituitary gonadotropin release. With further maturation, the pattern becomes regularly episodic over the entire 24-hour period. Many of the problems in pediatric and adolescent patients are related to disturbances in maturation of the HPG axis presenting as disorders of puberty and menstruation.

PRECOCIOUS PUBERTY

In girls, normal puberty is accompanied by an acceleration of growth and by breast development (thelarche). Pubic and axillary hair then develop (adrenarche), followed by menses (menarche). The appearance of signs of sexual maturation such as breast development before the age of 8 years or menarche before the age of 10 years constitutes a working definition of sexual precocity. True or central precocious puberty indicates gonadotropin-dependent changes following premature development of the HPG axis, leading to pulsatile production of gonadotropins with sex hormone elaboration. The normal clinical sequence of pubertal changes is preserved. In peripheral or gonadotropin-independent precocious puberty (precocious pseudopuberty), primary disease of the gonads or adrenals is implicated. Alterations in the normal sequence of pubertal changes may occur. Change consistent with the sex of the individual is called isosexual precocity, while heterosexual precocity indicates the presence of virilization in the female. Those disorders in which development is mild or not progressive, including the entities of precocious thelarche and adrenarche, are sometimes termed incomplete sexual precocity.

Although the appearance of secondary sex characteristics is the presenting manifestation, these conditions are also characterized by an accelerated rate of growth and bone maturation. Deranged statural growth may lead to premature fusion of the epiphyses and a shorter final height. The majority of children presenting to the primary care physician will have the benign disorders of precocious thelarche or adrenarche which are typically nonprogressive. A thorough history, careful abdominal and rectal examination, and determination of bone age by x ray may suffice for initial evaluation. When there is evidence of progressive changes or when more sustained hormonal effects are noted, further studies including determinations of gonadotropin levels, (follicle-stimulating hormone [FSH], luteinizing hormone [LH]), are indicated. Further assessment including pelvic ultrasound and neurologic evaluation (computed tomography [CT] or magnetic resonance imaging [MRI] scan, etc.) may be necessary. The presence of pubic hair requires an assessment of androgen levels of both ovarian and adrenal origin to exclude tumors or enzymatic defects of these organs. Measurements of dehydroepiandrosterone-sulfate (DHEA-S), testosterone, and 17-hydroxyprogesterone levels are helpful in this regard. Dexamethasone suppression and corticotropin stimulation testing may be indicated.

Central Precocious Puberty

Central precocious puberty is usually idiopathic but may be caused by CNS disorders including congenital anomalies, tumors, trauma, or infection. An example is provided by hypothalamic hamartomas, congenital tumors containing gonadotropin-releasing hormone (GnRH) neurosecretory cells. They are slow growing and seldom cause other neurologic symptoms. The diagnosis of central precocious puberty is based on the demonstration of a pubertal response to GnRH administration where there is a marked increase in gonadotropins following intravenously administered GnRH. Neurologic examination with CT or MRI scan is necessary to evaluate the presence of a tumor or anomaly. On occasion, primary removal of the pathologic tissue is possible but in most patients management is medical consisting of either progestin or GnRH analogue therapy.

Progestins

Medroxyprogesterone acetate (MPA), a 6-methyl derivative of 17-hydroxyprogesterone, may act directly on the gonads to reduce steroid biosynthesis and may also suppress gonadotropin secretion. The dose utilized is 10 mg (Provera) given orally daily or 150 mg (Depo-Provera) administered intramuscularly every 2 weeks. If gonadotropins, gonadal steroids, or both, are not suppressed toward the prepubertal range, up to twice the starting dose may be used but doses must be individualized for each patient. If secretion cannot be suppressed, treatment can be discontinued. Although MPA often eliminates menses, regression of secondary sexual characteristics is variable and there is little effect on skeletal growth or final adult height. Since the side effects are often considerable—excessive weight gain, rounded plethoric facies, hirsutism, adrenal suppression, and hypertension (all suggestive of glucocorticoid excess)—it may be better to avoid treating the child whose menarche is between the ages of 6 and 8 years. An alternative medication that also acts via central (feedback) and peripheral actions of sex steroids is *cyproterone acetate*, an antiandrogen derived from hydroxyprogesterone. This drug is not available in the United States but is available in Europe; it is used in a daily dose of 80 to 100 mg/sq m orally. The effect on secondary sex characteristics is satisfactory but the action on bone age and height is no better than that with progestins. Side effects are similar to those for MPA and include the development of gynecomastia. Another medication used for this condition, danazol, is no longer thought to be suitable for use in this context.

Agonists of Gonadotropin-Releasing Hormone

Potent synthetic agonists of GnRH given intermittently in long-acting form suppress pituitary gonadotropin secretion after a transient stimulatory phase. The agonists have been administered subcutaneously, intranasally, and intramuscularly (in depot form). Dosages vary depending on the potency of the specific analogue used and the route of administration. The initial stimulation may present as menses during the first month of therapy in some patients. Thereafter, there is a reduction in sex hormone levels, a decrease in growth velocity, and regression in secondary sexual characteristics. There is an increase in predicted adult height and improved psychosocial adaptation at home and in school. Monthly examination for clinical changes and growth are accompanied by random determinations of gonadotropin and sex hormone levels to assess the degree of suppression. Stimulation tests with 100 μg of the native decapeptide GnRH followed by measurement of serum FSH and LH levels at 3- to 6-month intervals are performed to ensure gonadotropin suppression. Bone age is determined every 6 months. Leuprolide acetate is given in doses in the range of 20 to 50 μg/kg/day (mean dose, 40 μg/kg/day) by subcutaneous injection. A long-acting form given as monthly intramuscular injections is preferred and appears to act equally well. Nafarelin acetate is given by intranasal aerosol in doses of 800 to 1600 μg per day usually as a single bedtime dose. However, nasal absorption tends to be poor and nonpredictable. Side effects of therapy have not presented a problem, other than occasional hot flashes and a significant incidence of withdrawal bleeding during the first 3 months, as a result of estrogen suppression. At the time of writing, no agonists have been approved by the Food and Drug Administration (FDA) for therapy of precocious puberty; however, in practice, leuprolide acetate, which is approved for use in prostatic cancer, can be administered provided informed consent is obtained. As long-term results of this therapy are not in, further experience will clarify the range of responses that can be expected and at this time these drugs appear to represent the treatment of choice. Therapy is continued until the child reaches the average age for her pubertal stage. Hormonal levels generally return to pretreatment values within 8 weeks after cessation of therapy. Results are related to early diagnosis and therapy, although even patients with advanced bone age can still benefit from regression in secondary sex characteristics.

Gonadotropin-Independent Precocious Puberty

Gonadotropin-independent precocious puberty, or precocious pseudopuberty, may be the result of many conditions. *Isosexual* pseudopuberty in girls may be due to estrogens formulated by ovarian follicular cysts, granulosa-theca cell tumors, or thecomas. Tumors that secrete both LH-like substances (e.g., human chorionic gonadotropin) and estrogen (primary ovarian choriocarcinoma) can cause precocious development. Hypothyroidism is a rare cause and on occasion the use of estrogen-containing creams and medications may be implicated. The McCune-Albright syndrome (polyostotic fibrous dysplasia, precocious puberty, and cafe-au-lait pigmentation) is another rare cause.

Heterosexual precocity arises from excess androgen production from an adrenal or ovarian source which results in acne, hirsutism, and virilization. Causes include some milder forms of congenital adrenal hyperplasia, adrenal tumors, Cushing's syndrome, and masculinizing ovarian tumors (Sertoli-Leydig cell, lipoid cell). Conditions causing peripheral precocity may secondarily evoke true, early onset of CNS maturity. Particularly, this can occur in patients with congenital adrenal hyperplasia and with the McCune-Albright syndrome.

Surgical removal of a hormone-secreting tumor should be promptly undertaken in patients with ovarian or adrenal neoplasms. Medical therapy for patients with precocious pseudopuberty varies with the cause. Children with McCune-Albright syndrome may be treated with *testolactone*, an inhibitor of aromatase, thus inhibiting the biosynthesis of gonadal hormones. The drug is administered in doses of 20 to 40 μg/kg/day in four divided doses with minimal side effects. Results have been promising with regard to regression of secondary sex characteristics, cessation of menses, and reduction in skeletal maturation. Patients with congenital adrenal hyperplasia should receive *glucocorticoid replacement* therapy (e.g., hydrocortisone, 13 to 25 mg/sq m/day divided into three daily doses). However, although adequate glucocorticoid replacement therapy is usually effective, when treatment begins after the ages of 4 to 8 years, premature activation of the hypothalamic-pituitary axis may occur and is recognized when pubertal development continues despite adequate replacement and when diagnostic criteria for central precocious puberty are met. In these circumstances, addition of GnRH agonists to the glucocorticoid therapy is indicated to suppress further pubertal development.

DELAYED PUBERTY—PRIMARY AMENORRHEA

Pubertal delay in girls is defined as the lack of breast budding or pubic hair by the age of 14 years or the absence of menarche by 16 years. The average age at the onset of breast bud is 10.5 years, plus or minus 2.5 years. Adrenarche begins at an average age of 11, plus or minus 2 years. The average age at menarche is 12.8 years, plus or minus 2.5 to 3.0 years. Delayed puberty is much more common than precocious puberty. The clinical workup of these girls begins with a good history and a thorough physical including a pelvic examination. The initial clinical findings determine further investigations, which generally include a thyroid function screen, determination of prolactin and gonadotropin levels, and a karyotype. The etiologic factors may be considered firstly at anatomic levels, with *hypothalamic* causes including anorexia nervosa, obesity, drugs (e.g., phenothiazines), stress, competitive athletics, and familial factors. *Pituitary*-related causes include tumors (prolactinoma, craniopharyngioma) and idiopathic hypopituitarism. At the *ovarian* level, gonadal dysgenesis, ovarian failure, polycystic ovary syndrome, and tumors must be considered. *Adrenal* causes via androgen excess include congenital adrenal hyperplasia and tumors. *Uterine* causes include agenesis of the müllerian duct and testicular feminization and at the *cervical* and *vaginal* level, agenesis, transverse vaginal septum, and imperforate hymen.

If there is no uterus, the problem is either uterine aplasia or male pseudohermaphroditism and these are differentiated by karyotype. If some pubertal development has occurred (breast development is a good biologic assay for endogenous estrogen production), a *pro-*

gestin challenge is given to see if the uterus will respond with withdrawal bleeding. Progesterone-in-oil, 100 mg given intramuscularly, or MPA (Provera), 10 mg given twice daily for 5 days, is used as the challenge. If bleeding occurs, the implication is that estrogen is adequate and anatomy is normal; the problem is then that of anovulation. If bleeding does not occur, it is assumed that estrogen was produced previously but not at the present time. Gonadotropin levels help to differentiate between an ovarian cause and a CNS cause. In the absence of breast development, either primary ovarian failure or failure of gonadotropin stimulation is possible and the distinction is made by finding high or low gonadotropin levels. The thyroid profile and prolactin level may indicate a diagnosis of hypothyroidism. If bleeding does not occur with a progestin challenge, conjugated estrogen (Premarin), 1.25 mg administered on days 1 to 21, and MPA (Provera), 10 mg given on days 15 to 21, are given and if no bleeding occurs, uterine abnormality is the likely diagnosis.

Management

Girls with delayed puberty are often small for their age. Because of the importance of body image in adolescence, if reassurance does not restore self-esteem, initiation of estrogen replacement should be considered even though this may lead to a smaller final adult height. Girls with nutritional problems who are either underweight as in the chronically ill or dancers, athletes, and so on, or overweight should be managed at nutritional and counseling levels. Many may consciously choose to continue their training and nutritional course at the expense of their endocrine status. In girls with no prospects of future fertility (e.g., gonadal dysgenesis, uterine aplasia), this should be discussed and counseling provided. Their capability of a normal sex life should be emphasized. In girls whose problems can be managed successfully with medications (e.g., gonadotropin therapy for hypopituitarism), these options should be explained. Those short, healthy girls with a normal karyotype, retarded bone age, and a prepubertal response to GnRH are likely to have constitutional delay of puberty. Most will eventually experience normal development and should not be given estrogen unless there are major psychologic difficulties as a result of the pubertal delay. They should be followed at 6-month intervals.

Gonadal Dysgenesis

Short stature is invariably present in girls with Turner's syndrome. Estrogen deficiency clearly plays a role in the lack of the pubertal growth spurt in these girls. However, gonadal failure is unlikely to be the sole cause of the short stature as these children grow poorly throughout childhood. It is likely that growth hormone, estrogen, and androgen, used alone or in combination, may be potentially useful agents for accelerating growth rate in these girls. Long-term outcome of these therapies is uncertain at this time.

Therapy is begun between the ages of 10 and 12 years with low doses of *ethinyl estradiol* (100 ng/kg/day). In those girls who do not respond with an adequate increase in growth rate (2–3 cm/year over pretreatment growth velocity), therapy with *oxandrolone* is substituted. This is a weak androgenic anabolic steroid and is given in dosages ranging from 0.07 to 0.25 mg/kg/day and results in a significant increase in growth velocity, especially in the first year of treatment. Whether adult height is increased is unclear. Potential androgenic side effects include voice changes, hirsutism, acne, and clitoral enlargement. *Growth hormone* given in conjunction may further augment the growth spurt, but this medication costs about $25,000 per year; it is generally not used at this time because the effect on adult height is not known. Once linear growth appears to be leveling off, hormonal therapy for sexual development is begun using the same regimen as for other girls with sexual infantilism. It must be emphasized that in those patients whose karyotype includes a Y chromosome, the dysgenetic gonads may develop a gonadoblastoma and should be removed before the age of onset of puberty because the risk of malignancy increases with age.

Hypogonadotropism

The age at which estrogen therapy is begun must be individualized and is usually in the range of from 11 to 15 years. These girls may have isolated hypogonadotropism or panhypopituitarism. In the latter, treatment with growth hormone may have resulted in a relatively normal stature and estrogen may be started earlier than in the girl whose growth is severely compromised. Estrogen therapy can be started with 0.3 mg of conjugated estrogens (Premarin) given daily. If no breast development occurs after 3 months, the dose is increased to 0.625 mg per day. Conjugated estrogen alone is continued for 12 to 18 months or until vaginal bleeding occurs. Cyclic menses are then induced with conjugated estrogen for days 1 to 21 of each month and MPA (Provera), 5 to 10 mg for days 7 to 21 of each month. After 1 to 2 years, the dosage of conjugated estrogen is increased to 1.25 mg per day by some, while others prefer a 0.625-mg dosage. Oral contraceptives are not advised for replacement therapy since the dose of estrogen is at pharmacologic rather than physiologic levels in these preparations.

SECONDARY AMENORRHEA

Many of the causes of delayed menarche are also responsible for secondary amenorrhea. The most common causes of missed periods in the adolescent are pregnancy and stress. While many teenagers have irregular menses in the first 2 to 3 years after menarche, since the initial workup comprises a clinical examination, pregnancy test, and progesterone challenge, there is usually no need to postpone these basic investigations. Most patients who have withdrawal bleeding on progesterone challenge are normal, although disorders such as the polycystic ovary syndrome, ovarian tumors, and thyroid disease should be excluded. Polycystic ovary syndrome is diagnosed by demonstrating increased LH levels with slightly suppressed FSH levels. Androgen levels including testosterone are elevated. Teenagers with hypothalamic amenorrhea with response to progesterone are well estrogenized and may be treated with MPA, 10 mg given orally for 5 to 10 days every 3 months to prevent endometrial hyperplasia. Behavioral and weight counseling are important in many instances when exercise, eating habits, or both, are contributing factors. Patients with polycystic ovary syndrome may be treated similarly, but if progressive hirsutism is present, oral contraceptive preparations containing 30 to 35 μg of ethinyl estradiol should be prescribed to suppress androgen production. In these patients, levels of DHEA-S should be measured and if they are elevated, this adrenal androgen should be suppressed with dexamethasone. Dexamethasone is given at bedtime, 0.5 mg for 30 days, then the dose is lowered to 0.25 mg, and after 6 to 12 months it is discontinued and DHEA-S levels rechecked 1 month later.

In patients who fail to respond to the progesterone challenge, the estradiol value is usually below 40 pg/ml. Gonadotropin levels in these patients may be low or normal suggesting the diagnosis of chronic disease, CNS tumor, or hypothalamic amenorrhea. The first step is to exclude a prolactinoma with a determination of serum prolactin level remembering that such tumors may be present in the absence of galactorrhea. If the prolactin level is elevated, such causes as hypothyroidism and drugs must be excluded and CT or MRI studies of the sella turcica may be necessary. If the diagnosis of microadenoma is made, therapy is indicated because of estrogen deficiency. *Bromocriptine* is usually prescribed starting with 1.25 mg taken at bedtime. The prolactin level is rechecked in 2 to 3 weeks. Dosage thereafter is titrated based on the response, with the aim of suppressing prolactin to below 20 mg/ml. Good results with lesser side effects (nausea, headache, dizziness, nasal congestion, fatigue, postural hypotension) and lower dosage have been noted with vaginal bromocriptine. Careful follow-up is essential and may include visual field studies. In young adolescents with anorexia nervosa, hormone replacement is not indicated; however, older girls may need estrogen replacement to prevent osteopenia. Periods may not return for months or years after normal weight is reestablished. Replacement therapy is given with conjugated estrogen, 0.625 mg/day given from days 1 to 25 of the month together with MPA, 5 mg given daily from days 14 through 25. Generally this is given to girls aged 17 and older who have serum estrogen levels below 30 pg/ml.

Patients with high gonadotropin levels may have gonadal dysgenesis or ovarian failure. Premature ovarian failure may follow radiotherapy or chemotherapy, or may be related to autoimmune disease. Estrogen replacement as for Turner's syndrome is usually necessary. If secondary amenorrhea is associated with evidence of androgen excess then the diagnosis must be made between polycystic ovary syndrome, late-onset adrenocortical hyperplasia, Cushing's syndrome, and ovarian and adrenal tumors.

DYSFUNCTIONAL UTERINE BLEEDING

When an adolescent presents with dysfunctional uterine bleeding the first priority is to stop the bleeding. Clinical evaluation with some basic laboratory studies is usually enough to rule out pregnancy, pelvic infection, bleeding dyscrasias, and thyroid disease, leaving the usual problem which is anovulation secondary to immaturity of the hypothalamic-pituitary-ovarian (HPO) axis. Generally, in mild to moderate cases, the use of a progestin is sufficient to arrest hemorrhage; norethindrone, 10 to 15 mg per day administered for 3 weeks, is usually adequate. Thereafter, a low-dose oral contraceptive or MPA, 10 mg per day for 10 to 14 days each month for a few months, is indicated. Some clinicians avoid prescribing oral contraceptives in the sexually inactive in an attempt to not interfere with maturation of the HPO axis. Others believe that there is no proof that the halt in HPO axis maturation caused by their use is irreversible and are willing to use these agents if cyclic progestins do not provide good cycle control. Oral iron supplements should be provided as indicated.

In severe cases, volume and blood replacement may be necessary and the use of high-dose estrogens to provide rapid hemostasis is indicated in order to provide temporary relief and allow time for intensive progestin therapy thereafter. A preparation of intravenous conjugated estrogens (Premarin), 20 to 25 mg given every 4 hours, should stop the bleeding. Thereafter, therapy with MPA, 10 mg given once or twice daily for 10 days, is followed by a withdrawal bleed and the patient is then placed on a low-dose oral contraceptive or on cyclic progestins.

An alternative therapy is to use oral contraceptives and several effective regimens exist. One such is the use of norethindrone and mestranol (Ortho-Novum 1/50) given every 4 hours until bleeding stops (usually 4–8 tablets), and thereafter twice daily or daily for the remainder of the cycle as per the response and in the event nausea is a problem. The long-term prognosis is not always favorable and persistent problems are evident in half the patients after 4 years and in 30 percent after 10 years. These girls are at increased risk of infertility and endometrial carcinoma later on. Careful follow-up is indicated.

ANDROGEN OVERPRODUCTION

The major circulating endogenous androgens are dehydroepiandrosterone (DHEA), its sulfate conjugate, DHEA-S, androstenedione, and testosterone. The androgens are derived from the adrenals and ovaries and from peripheral conversion of steroid precursors. The primary steroids produced by the fetal adrenal are pregnenolone and DHEA, which are converted by the placenta to estrogens. Androgen levels are high in newborns and are primarily of adrenal origin. These levels fall rapidly during the newborn period and remain low until girls approach puberty. DHEA and DHEA-S levels increase between ages 6 and 8 years and continue in parallel with age and pubertal stage. Significant increases in androstenedione and testosterone occur at ages 8 to 10 and 12 to 14 years, respectively. DHEA secretion is probably controlled, at least in part, by corticotropin secretion. The changes of pubarche are probably secondary to the androgen increase. The ovarian contribution to androgen levels during childhood is unknown. The primary ovarian androgen in the ovulating female is androstenedione, although testosterone and DHEA are also synthesized. Approximately one-half of testosterone production in ovulating females is due to peripheral conversion of androstenedione or DHEA to testosterone.

Congenital Adrenal Hyperplasia

Congenital adrenal hyperplasia is a family of inherited inborn errors of steroidogenesis characterized by specific enzyme deficiencies that impair adrenal cortisol production. Those usually affected are 21-hydroxylase, 11-β-hydroxylase, and 3-β-hydroxysteroid dehydrogenase. Decreased cortisol levels result in increased corticotropin levels which in turn increase C19 androgens and lead to the accumulation of precursor steroids in the impeded pathways. A reduced aldosterone synthetic capacity may occur in the 21 and 3-β defects and these variants are termed "salt wasting." By contrast, the 11-β form results in an increased mineralocorticoid action because of overproduction of 11-desoxycorticosterone resulting in a form of low-renin hypertension. Salt-wasting 21-hydroxylase deficiency and its simple virilizing counterpart, both characterized by androgen excess, are the most commonly found forms of congenital adrenal hyperplasia. In the *classic form* of congenital adrenal hyperplasia, adrenal androgens before the ninth week of gestation cause virilization of the external genitalia in genetic females who present with genital ambiguity at delivery. Therefore, it is essential to evaluate the adrenal function of any neonate presenting with ambiguous genitalia. The appropriate diagnostic procedures and hormonal therapy with glucocorticoids must be initiated immediately.

Treatment with glucocorticoids is lifelong. For infants and children, hydrocortisone is given 2 or 3 times daily in a dose of 15 to 20 mg/sq m/day. Clinical progress based on height velocity, bone age, and Tanner stage is assessed together with hormone levels. The best indices of hormonal control are serum 17-hydroxyprogesterone and androstenedione for 21-hydroxylase deficiency, DHEA and 17-hydroxy-delta 5 pregnenolone for 3-β deficiency, and 11-deoxycortisol or 11-desoxycorticosterone for 11-β deficiency. If control is not adequate, dosage may be increased to 20 to 25 mg/sq m/day. However, overtreatment may suppress growth and delay puberty so that long-acting drugs including prednisone and dexamethasone should be avoided in children. Furthermore, excessive weight gain, hypertension, and cushingoid features may develop. Adults, however, may be treated with dexamethasone, 0.25 to 0.50 mg, taken at bedtime. For conditions of stress as in surgery or severe infection, the daily dose should be increased threefold to fourfold given in three or four doses intramuscularly or intravenously and should be maintained 3 to 5 days after surgery or illness.

The *salt-wasting forms* require the addition of mineralocorticoids to the replacement regimen. Infants generally require 0.1 to 0.2 mg of fludrocortisone acetate (Florinef) per day. In children, the average dose is 0.05 to 0.10 mg per day. Sodium chloride supplementation is also necessary via addition to the infant's formula. Adequacy of replacement is determined by plasma renin activity. Infants with salt-wasting 21-hydroxylase deficiency are at risk of adrenal crisis (acute adrenal insufficiency) within 1 to 2 weeks after birth and require urgent treatment. Stress, particularly associated with trauma, infection, or surgery, may also predispose to adrenal crisis in steroid-dependent patients. Management of crisis is beyond the scope of this chapter and may be found in standard medical texts.

Mild steroidogenic enzyme deficiencies, termed *nonclassic adrenal hyperplasia*, may appear in later life as premature pubarche, hirsutism, acne, and irregular menses or infertility. These signs of hyperandrogenism may be treated with glucocorticoids in similar or lesser dosages than in the classic forms. Prenatal diagnosis and treatment of congenital adrenal hyperplasia are possible and pregnant women at risk who have an affected child should be managed accordingly. Male pseudohermaphroditism may occur with 3-β deficiency as a result of low testosterone secretion leading to incomplete virilization. In some instances, female assignment may be appropriate and replacement therapy at the time of puberty should conform to the sex of assignment.

Hyperandrogenism in the Adolescent

Girls usually have adult levels of free testosterone by the time they achieve Tanner stage 3 of breast development and within the year before menarche. Measurements of serum total testosterone and DHEA-S levels are useful screening tests in those with clinical evidence of androgen excess, to rule out tumors of the ovary or adrenal gland. Total testosterone levels of greater than 200 ng/dl or DHEA-S levels of greater than 700 μg/dl require more complete evaluation to rule out an ovarian or adrenal tumor, respectively. Dexamethasone suppression tests, corticotropin stimulation studies, or both, may be helpful as an adjunct in selected patients.

The majority of patients who have progressive hirsutism and menstrual irregularities will be found to have polycystic ovary syndrome. Obese patients should be encouraged to lose weight since weight loss may decrease elevated androgen and estrone levels. If severe acne is the main problem, *isotretinoin*, a synthetic vitamin A analogue, may be used in its treatment. If birth control is required, low-dose *oral contraceptives* increase sex hormone–binding globulin, diminish free testosterone, and suppress LH-dependent hyperandrogenism. Both ovarian and adrenal androgens are suppressed. *Spironolactone* given (100–200 mg daily) from day 4 to 22 of the cycle has been used with moderately good response. The drug displaces androgens from their cellular binding sites. Side effects include polydipsia, polyuria, headache, and increased appetite and weight, but are usually transient. Metrorrhagia may occur but responds to decreased dosage. *Cyproterone acetate* with ethinyl estradiol has been used with success in Europe but is unlikely to be approved for use in the United States because of concern about progestin-associated teratogenicity and carcinogenesis. For those girls with a significant adrenal component to their androgen excess, *glucocorticoid* suppression (dexamethasone, 0.5 mg daily) may be helpful, alone or in combination with oral contraceptives. If cortisol levels are maintained at greater than 2 μg/dl on alternate morning assays, significant long-term problems with prolonged adrenal suppression are unlikely.

Elevated serum testosterone and androstenedione levels can be reduced to castrate levels by a GnRH agonist, with resultant decreased facial hair growth and pigmentation. Typical doses are *leuprolide acetate*, 0.5 mg or 1.0 mg per day. The higher dose is reserved for those women who do not show ovarian suppression at the lower dose. The major limitation with this therapy is associated with the risk of osteoporosis secondary to the profound estrogen suppression. This problem might be avoided by combining the therapy with oral contraception but this approach has not yet been studied.

LABIAL ADHESIONS

Mild degrees of labial adherence are commonly seen in prepubertal children and more than half are detected before the age of 2 years. If the child is asymptomatic, no therapy is required. Dysuria and recurrent vulvar vaginitis are the cardinal symptoms and treatment is necessary. A 2- to 4-week course of topical estrogen cream (Premarin) applied twice daily usually results in separation of the labia. Recurrences of labial fusion are quite common due to the fact that the estrogen-deficient state exists until puberty. Improved perineal hygiene, removal of irritants from the vulva, and the application of petroleum jelly or cortisone cream for 2 weeks after estrogen therapy may help to prevent recurrences.

LICHEN SCLEROSUS

Genital lichen sclerosus is a relatively uncommon condition in prepubertal girls. The vulva characteristically has white atrophic skin and evidence of chronic inflammation and ulceration. Involvement of the perianal area as well as the labia frequently gives the affected area an hourglass configuration. The age of onset, severity of symptoms, and the presence or absence of extragenital lesions are not related to persistence of the condition. The advent of puberty is frequently not associated with improvement of the condition, which may appear and disappear unrelated to pubertal changes. Long-term sequelae with persistent lesions or relapses are relatively common, leading to moderate or severe atrophy in adult life. The diagnosis is made clinically and with confirmatory findings in a biopsy specimen.

Current therapies in premenarchal girls include a combination of good hygiene, elimination of local irritants and vaginitis, and loose-fitting cotton garments. A short course of topical corticosteroids (e.g., fluocinolone acetonide [Synalar] 0.025%), followed by a course of 1% hydrocortisone ointment for an additional few months, provides symptomatic relief but does not affect the disease process. Local application of 100 mg of progesterone-in-oil per 1 oz of Aquaphor applied twice daily has been reported as beneficial. Topical testosterone propionate 2 percent ointment is used in adults and has resulted in reversal of symptoms, lesions, and histologic changes; however, it must be used indefinitely. Systemic side effects of this therapy are unusual. However, because of the possibility of mild clitoral hypertrophy and because of the fear of systemic absorption and its effect on bone growth, use in children has been avoided. Nevertheless, in those premenarchal children who have disabling symptoms or who are developing atrophic sequelae, the benefits of topical testosterone may outweigh the theoretic risks. A tissue diagnosis would be needed prior to long-term testosterone therapy in children. Menarchal children may be treated as adults.

BIBLIOGRAPHY

Resources

Bardin, C. W. (ed.). *Current Therapy in Endocrinology and Metabolism-3*. Toronto: Dekker, 1988.

Emans, S. J. H., and Goldstein, D. P. *Pediatric and Adolescent Gynecology* (2nd ed.). Boston: Little, Brown, 1982.

Lavery, J. P., and Sanfilippo, J. S. *Pediatric and Adolescent Obstetrics and Gynecology*. New York: Springer, 1985.

McDonough, P. G. (ed.). Pediatric gynecology. *Clin. Obstet. Gynecol.* 30:1987.

Precocious Puberty

Kulin, H. E. Precocious puberty. *Clin. Obstet. Gynecol.* 30:714, 1987.

Lee, P. A. Medroxyprogesterone therapy for sexual precocity in girls. *Am. J. Dis. Child.* 135:443, 1981.

Lee, P. A. Pubertal neuroendocrine maturation: early differentiation and stages of development. *Adoles. Pediatr. Gynecol.* 1:3, 1988.

Pescovitz, O. H., et al. The NIH experience with precocious puberty: diagnostic subgroups and response to short-term luteinizing hormone-releasing hormone analogue therapy. *J. Pediatr.* 108:47, 1986.

Rudd, B. T. Precocious and delayed sexual development in children. *Acta Endocrinol. (Copenh.)* 288:66, 1988.

Sonis, W. A., et al. Behavior problems and social competence in girls with true precocious puberty. *J. Pediatr.* 106:156, 1985.

Styne, D. M., et al. Treatment of true precocious puberty with a potent luteinizing hormone–releasing factor agonist: effect on growth, sexual maturation, pelvic sonography, and the hypothalamic-pituitary-gonadal axis. *J. Clin. Endocrinol. Metab.* 61:142, 1985.

Delayed Puberty

Charest, N. J., and French, F. S. Primary amenorrhea: delayed puberty. In C. W. Bardin (ed.), *Current Therapy in Endocrinology and Metabolism-3.* Toronto: Dekker, 1988.

Linder, B., and Cassoria, F. Short stature: etiology, diagnosis, and treatment. *J.A.M.A.* 260:3171, 1988.

Mashchak, C. A., et al. Clinical and laboratory evaluation of patients with primary amenorrhea. *Obstet. Gynecol.* 57:715, 1981.

Rosenfeld, R. G., et al. Methionyl human growth hormone and oxandrolone in Turner syndrome: preliminary results of a prospective randomized trial. *J. Pediatr.* 109:936, 1984.

Ross, J. L., et al. Effect of low doses of estradiol on six-month growth rates and predicted heights in patients with Turner syndrome. *J. Pediatr.* 109:950, 1986.

Tho, P. T., and McDonough, P. G. Gonadal dysgenesis and its variants. *Pediatr. Clin. North Am.* 28:309, 1981.

Secondary Amenorrhea

Board, J. A., et al. Identification of differing etiologies of clinically diagnosed premature menopause. *Am. J. Obstet. Gynecol.* 134:936, 1979.

Drossman, D. A., Ontjes, D. A., and Heizer, W. D. Anorexia nervosa. *Gastroenterology* 77:1115, 1979.

Franks, S. Primary and secondary amenorrhoea. *Br. Med. J.* 294:815, 1987.

Kletzky, O. A., et al. Classification of secondary amenorrhea based on distinct hormonal patterns. *J. Clin. Endocrinol. Metab.* 41:660, 1975.

Kletzky, O. A., et al. Clinical categorization of patients with secondary amenorrhea using progesterone-induced uterine bleeding and measurement of serum gonadotropin levels. *Am. J. Obstet. Gynecol.* 121:695, 1975.

Varga, L., Wenner, R., and del Pozo, E. Treatment of galactorrhea-amenorrhea syndrome with Br-ergocriptine (CB154): restoration of ovulatory function and fertility. *Am J. Obstet. Gynecol.* 117:75, 1973.

Dysfunctional Uterine Bleeding

Fayez, J. A. Dysfunctional uterine bleeding. *Am. Fam. Physician* 25:109, 1982.

Frazer, I. S., et al. Pituitary gonadotropins and ovarian function in adolescent dysfunctional uterine bleeding. *J. Clin. Endocrinol. Metab.* 37:407, 1973.

Strickler, R. C. Dysfunctional uterine bleeding in ovulatory women. *Postgrad. Med.* 77:235, 1985.

Androgen Excess

Andreyko, J. L., Monroe, S. E., and Jaffe, R. B. Treatment of hirsutism with a gonadotropin-releasing hormone agonist nafarelin. *J. Clin. Endocrinol. Metab.* 63:854, 1986.

Bates, G. W. Hirsutism and androgen excess in childhood and adolescence. *Pediatr. Clin. North Am.* 28:513, 1981.

Couzinet, B., et al. Comparative effects of cyproterone acetate or a long-acting gonadotropin-releasing hormone agonist in polycystic ovarian disease. *J. Clin. Endocrinol. Metab.* 63:1031, 1986.

Hatch, R., et al. Hirsutism: implications, etiology and management. *Am. J. Obstet. Gynecol.* 140:815, 1981.
New, M. I., et al. An update of congenital adrenal hyperplasia. *Recent Prog. Horm. Res.* 37:105, 1981.
Steingold, K. A., et al. Treatment of severe androgen excess due to ovarian hyperthecosis with a long-acting gonadotropin-releasing hormone agonist. *Am. J. Obstet. Gynecol.* 154:1241, 1986.
Thomas, C. G., et al. Hyperadrenalism in childhood and adolescence. *Ann. Surg.* 199:538, 1984.

Labial Adhesions and Lichen Sclerosus

Aribarg, A. Topical oestrogen therapy for labial adhesions in children. *Br. J. Obstet. Gynaecol.* 82:424, 1975.
Redmon, C. A., Cowell, C. A., and Krafchik, B. R. Genital lichen sclerosus in prepubertal girls. *Adolesc. Pediatr. Gynecol.* 1:177, 1988.

12

Hormone Therapy in the Male Patient

George Rodney Meeks

The testes are similar to the ovaries and adrenal glands in the biosynthesis of hormones and regulatory mechanisms. Testes produce peptide and steroid hormones that regulate male sexual differentiation and sexual function and produce sperm. Testosterone synthesis and secretion and sperm production are controlled by complex hypothalamic-pituitary-gonad (HPG) interaction. Testosterone, unlike ovarian estradiol and the adrenal hormones, has few direct actions, but serves as prehormone for 5α-reduced androgens (dihydrotestosterone) and estrogen (estradiol). Testicular hormones are required for male differentiation during embryogenesis. Sperm are produced continuously unlike the cyclic production of ova.

Testicular failure may occur because of (1) abnormal hypothalamic synthesis and release of gonadotropin-releasing hormone (GnRH); (2) dysfunction of pituitary synthesis and secretion of follicle-stimulating hormone (FSH), luteinizing hormone (LH), or prolactin; and (3) dysfunction of the testes. Clinical consequences are dependent on the phase of life in which abnormal testicular function develops. Testicular dysfunction may be manifest by female phenotype, ambiguous genitalia at birth, failure of puberty, infertility secondary to absent or reduced sperm production, and sexual dysfunction. Female phenotype occurs if the testicle fails to form or if the testicle degenerates before testosterone production. Ambiguous genitalia, microphallus, hypospadias, or cryptorchidism occur with poor testicular function during fetal development. Failure of puberty, delayed puberty, and arrest of sexual differentiation are manifestations when testicular dysfunction occurs during infancy or childhood. Regression of adult sexual features, sexual dysfunction, infertility, and disordered sperm production are features of testicular dysfunction during adulthood. Hypopituitarism may occur at any stage of life and may be secondary to congenital abnormalities, trauma, tumor, surgery, or radiotherapy. Hypopituitarism may be associated with other hormone deficiencies. Therefore, the secretion status of cortisol, adrenal androgens, thyroid, and insulin must be considered as well as the evaluation of the production of GnRH, LH, FSH, prolactin, testosterone, and estradiol. Acute and chronic systemic illnesses such as autoimmune syndromes, cirrhosis, hemochromatosis, and drug abuse involving opiates, alcohol, and marijuana are associated with testicular dysfunction and gonadotropin deficiencies.

Infertility has reached epidemic proportions and 10 to 15 percent of couples are infertile. Approximately 50 percent of the problems identified are related to the male partner. Male reproductive capability requires each of the following complex mechanisms to function flawlessly: spermatogenesis, spermiogenesis, acquisition of dynein arms for cilial motility, epididymal transit, ejaculation-emission, penetration of cervical mucus, capacitation, acrosome reaction, and spermatozoa penetration of ovum. Assessment requires semen analysis, determination of male reproductive duct patency, evaluation of sexual performance, and, at times, examination of testicular biopsy specimen. The recent attention directed toward male factor infertility has engendered a new term, "andrology," to embrace this common interest shared by scientists with diverse training.

The incidence of testicular dysfunction is difficult to assess. Female phenotype with male genotype occurs in 1 per 60,000 births. The appearance of external genitalia leaves the sex assignment of infants in doubt in 1 infant per 1000 births. Genetic abnormalities such as XXY have an incidence of 1 per 1000 births. As many as 8 million males are infertile and subtle abnormalities in the HPG axis may account for 40 percent of infertility. Testicular function declines with aging. In perspective, 4 million men have diabetes.

MALE DIFFERENTIATION AND ANDROGEN METABOLISM

Male phenotype requires a normal Y chromosome, müllerian-inhibiting factor (MIF), testosterone, and dihydrotestosterone (DHT). For the first 7 weeks of embryologic life, the gonad is indifferent. Both wolffian ducts (male) and müllerian ducts (female) are present. The signal for development of the indifferent gonad into testes has been localized on the short arm of the Y chromosome and is termed testis-determining factor (TDF). This is separate from the H-Y antigen that is located on the long arm of the Y chromosome. Primitive germ cells enter the gonadal ridge. Coelomic epithelium cells grow into the gonad, surround the germ cell, and differentiate into Sertoli's cells. Interstitial cells derived from gonadal ridge mesenchyme differentiate into Leydig's cells and primitive seminiferous tubules (SNT) develop. The Sertoli's cell produces MIF which inhibits the fallopian tubes, uterine fundus, cervix, and upper one-third of vagina. It also causes the tissue surrounding the testis, which would otherwise anchor it in the retroperitoneal space, to degenerate. Testosterone from the Leydig's cell provokes the wolffian duct system to form the epididymis, vas deferens, and seminal vesicles. Testosterone is converted to DHT by intracellular 5α reductase. DHT is necessary for the normal development of the external genitalia and prostate and for contracture of the gubernaculum, which pulls the testis through the inguinal canal and into the scrotum.

SNTs, Sertoli's cells, and Leydig's cells must function in harmony to ensure normal sperm production. Leydig's cells are found in the stroma of the testes and are in highest concentration around the SNT. The SNT are composed of spermatogonia, Sertoli's cells, which have special nurturing roles for the spermatogonia, and a central lumen. The outer one-third consists of tightly bound Sertoli's cells and spermatogonia. The intraluminal two-thirds is composed of spermatocytes in advancing stages of spermatogenesis.

The major function of androgens include: (1) regulation of HPG system, (2) formation of male phenotype, (3) promotion of sexual maturity and adult sexual function, and (4) initiation and maintenance of spermatogenesis. Androgen synthesis and secretion are under control of the HPG axis. The hypothalamus produces GnRH, a decapeptide, in a pulsatile fashion beginning early in embryogenesis and continuing until birth. Following delivery, GnRH production is quiescent until puberty.

GnRH is secreted in pulsatile fashion and stimulates production of FSH and LH by the basophilic cells of the pituitary. A pulse frequency of 90 to 120 minutes is necessary for normal LH and FSH concentration. More frequent pulses cause downregulation (i.e., reduced gonadotropin output). If pulse frequency is reduced to 4 hours or longer, LH concentration is lowered and FSH concentration is elevated. Testosterone decreases LH while estradiol increases LH concentration. Both are mediated by GnRH. Norepinephrine and other alpha adrenergic compounds increase GnRH pulse frequency, and endorphins and enkephalins limit pulse frequency. Steroid-induced feedback on GnRH is mediated by endogenous opioids. Exogenous opiates interfere with normal feedback and produce changes associated with impotence and infertility.

LH stimulates testosterone production by Leydig's cells. Leydig's cells are most efficient when approximately 10 percent of LH receptors are bound. Downregulation occurs following exposure to LH. LH is regulated by a classic monotropic negative feedback with testosterone. One goes down, the other goes up, and vice versa. The regulatory role of FSH is less clearly defined. FSH does not have this trophic-target modulation. Testosterone, estradiol, and inhibin regulate FSH. Inhibin is present in semen but has not been identified in serum. It seems to be produced by the germ cells. As germ cell mass declines (as with aging) inhibin production by the germ cells is reduced and FSH concentration increases. It decreases as FSH rises and vice versa. Testosterone reduces GnRH pulse frequency, and estradiol reduces GnRH pulse amplitude, thus modulating FSH.

Testosterone is derived from cholesterol which may be synthesized de novo from acetylcoenzyme A or come from the plasma pool of low-density lipoprotein (LDL) particles. Both mechanisms seem important in the human male. LH enhances testosterone by stimulating the enzymes responsible for cleaving the side chains from cholesterol. Testosterone is 95 percent bound to testosterone-binding globulin (TeBG) and 2 percent is unbound. The unbound or free testosterone is available to target tissue. Testosterone is a prohormone and is metabolized to active compounds. Approximately 6 to 8 percent of testosterone is metabolized to DHT, the key active metabolite. DHT is not metabolized further. Approximately 0.5 percent of testosterone is metabolized to estradiol. The other metabolites are 17-ketosteroids (40%) and polar metabolites (50%). Urinary excretion accounts for 90 percent of the elimination of metabolites—mainly in the form of 17-ketosteroids.

Male adolescence follows an orderly sequence of adrenarche, spermarche, and gonadarche. Adrenarche is the development of pubic and axillary hair, which is produced by adrenal androgens especially dehydroepiandosterone (DHEA). Gonadarche, which is triggered by increased testosterone production, is manifest by penile enlargement, scrotal development, beard growth, heightened libido, deepening voice, and acne. Spermarche is sandwiched between adrenarche and gonadarche but does not mature until after gonadarche when intratesticular testosterone concentration increases. The pattern of androgen production is vulnerable to a myriad of noxious influences. Disruption of androgen production may adversely affect male sexual and reproductive function at any locus from gametogenesis to maturation of HPG axis (Table 12-1).

SPERMATOGENESIS AND SPERMIOGENESIS

The spermatogenic cycle consists of three processes that occur in an orderly fashion: (1) multiplication of germ cells; (2) reduction of the

Table 12-1. Abnormalities affecting male fertility

I. Gametogenesis
  a. Klinefelter's syndrome
  b. Noonan's syndrome

II. In utero
  a. Androgen resistance
    1. Testicular feminization
    2. Reifenstein's syndrome
    3. Phenotypically normal men
  b. 5α-reductase deficiency
  c. Undescended testes

III. Infancy and childhood
  a. Premature adrenarche
  b. Delayed adrenarche
  c. Adrenogenital syndrome
  d. Precocious puberty
  e. Delayed puberty

number of chromosomes to the haploid state; and (3) metamorphosis of cellular structure that allows motility, generation of energy, and protection of the chromosomal package. Spermatogenesis occurs within the SNT and spermiogenesis occurs in the epididymis and vas deferens. Spermatogenesis in the SNT process requires approximately 70 days and spermiogenesis in the epididymis, an additional 12 to 21 days.

Somewhat unfortunate terminology creates confusion when trying to separate the processes into its components. All terms begin with "spermat" as the first two syllables. The cells nearest the connective tissue barrier of SNT are the sperma*togonia*. These are the earliest stages of germ cells. Sperma*tocytes* have completed the mitotic phase of duplication and are closer to the lumen. Sperma*tids* are cells that have entered meiosis, have completed chromosomal reduction, and are haploid. Sperma*tozoa* are mature male gametes containing the X or Y chromosome. Each primary spermatogonium ultimately gives rise to 16 spermatocytes. Each spermatocyte through meiosis gives rise to 4 spermatids and ultimately 4 spermatozoa. Therefore, each spermatogonium is capable of producing 64 sperm.

The commitment of spermatogonia to this process does not occur randomly. Contiguous groups of cells develop in teams and mature toward the SNT lumen. The Sertoli's cell orchestrates spermatogenesis and Sertoli's cell function is regulated by FSH. High intratesticular testosterone concentration is also necessary to maintain normal spermatogenesis in the SNT and Sertoli's cell complex. This process is poorly understood but cyclic adenosine monophosphate (cAMP) and androgen-binding protein (ABP) have important roles. Sertoli's cells produce ABP under the synergistic action of FSH, testosterone, and insulin. It has many properties of other carrier proteins such as TeBG. ABP is secreted into the SNT lumen and passes to the epididymis. Increased cAMP increases synthesis of protein. High-affinity androgen receptors in cytoplasm and nucleus are also present in SNT. How each of these steps works is not known for certain. Testosterone is necessary for mitosis. FSH is necessary for meiosis and spermatid development.

During epididymal transit, spermatids mature into spermatozoa. Spermatids undergo ultrastructural changes and are transformed into motile spermatozoa with fertilizing potential. A high concentration of ABP is necessary for this process. Aromatase activity in the Sertoli's cell and estradiol production may also be important. Nuclear chromatin condenses and moves to an eccentric position in the cell and cytoplasm is reduced. This portion of the sperm is known as the head. Condensed Golgi apparatus form an acrosome that contains hyaluronidase and other enzymes necessary for the acrosome reaction—a prelude to penetrating the zona pellucida. The mitochondria migrate caudally to form the midpiece and flagellum. Androgens, especially DHT, are necessary for motility and they seem to enhance compounds that allow mobility. Glycerol phosphorylcholine (GPC), carnitine, Ca^{2+}, and cAMP are necessary to establish normal motility. Aged sperm lose motility.

MEDICAL HISTORY

Age, especially for women, is critical. Peak fecundity is at the age of 24 years and declines rapidly after the age of 30. This would also seem to be true for men, although it is less well documented. One must inquire as to any developmental abnormalities at birth such as cryptorchidism. The timing and extent of sexual maturation, rate of beard growth, and current libido will give information regarding the adequacy of androgen production. Sperm production is best evaluated by previous fertility history. Specific injuries to the testicles such as mumps orchitis and testicular torsion may lead to damaged germ cells. Specific medications may interfere with sexual potency and these include alpha-methyl dopa, reserpine, guanethidine, propranolol, and spironolactone. Histamine (H_2) receptor agonists display potent antiandrogenic properties. Recurrent respiratory infections may herald cystic fibrosis which is an abnormality where bronchial tree and male genital tract secretions form obstructive plugs. Sperm are unable to reach the ejaculate. Kartagener's syndrome is caused by a defect in cilia function secondary to absent dynein arms. Sperm motility is completely lacking and thus the patient is infertile. Frequency of emission seems to be a concern only if the initial quality of semen is poor.

Autonomic nervous system (ANS) dysfunction, which leads to impaired emission and ejaculation disorders, is common in men with diabetes mellitus. Symptoms of ANS dysfunction include orthostatic hypotension, dyshidrosis, and incomplete bladder emptying in the absence of prostatic enlargement.

Recreational drugs may lead to reproductive failure. Tobacco smoking seems to reduce sperm count and is associated with increased abnormal sperm forms. In men with otherwise normal findings on semen analysis, smoking is probably not significant but in oligozoospermic men, counts may be reduced to significantly low values. Alcohol is directly toxic to the Leydig's cell and therefore reduces testosterone levels. Likewise, it increases conversion of testosterone to estradiol. If liver dysfunction occurs, especially alcoholic cirrhosis, estradiol metabolism is impaired and gynecomastia is common. Once gynecomastia is present, men suffer decline in libido and potency, and spermatogenesis is impaired. Marijuana (tetrahydrocannabinol [THC]) interferes with gonadotropin release and testosterone production and spermatogenesis. Exogenous opiates (i.e., morphine and heroin) disrupt GnRH pulsatile response by competing with the endogenous opiate system that regulates GnRH release. Use of opiate derivatives strikingly impairs sexual function.

PHYSICAL EXAMINATION

While focusing on specific points relative to sexual maturation and fertility, one should examine all organ systems and not just the genitalia. Body habitus is important. When arm span exceeds total height by 5 inches (12.5 cm) or when lower body-upper body ratio is increased, gonadal dysfunction should be suspected. Klinefelter's syndrome is often associated with such eunuchoid proportions. Elevated blood pressure may be associated with adrenal gland hyperfunction. Low blood pressure, especially orthostatic change, is associated with ANS dysfunction. Beard pattern and density indicate androgenic status. Visual field changes and fundoscopic changes may indicate craniopharyngioma or pituitary tumor. Gynecomastia, except during puberty, often indicates elevated estrogen and occasionally elevated prolactin levels. Penile length and breadth vary greatly in normal men. If the penis fails to protrude beyond the scrotal folds, length is deficient. The urethra should be centrally located and at the distal glans. Examination of the erect penis will confirm Peyronie's disease—a fibrous plaque resulting in deviation of the penis to one side. Sometimes this disease is so severe as to limit intercourse. It is often best to allow the patient to photograph the erect penis with a Polaroid-like camera. A testis should be present in each side of the scrotum and should be symmetric. The testes are characteristically firm, range from 3.5 to 5.5 cm in length and have a volume of 12 to 25 ml. Volume may be estimated with the Prader orchidometer. Since SNT account for 95 percent of testicular volume, reduced germ cell mass may lead to reduced testicular volume and soft consistency. Varicoceles are often apparent only when the male is standing. Valsalva may make the varicocele more prominent or demonstrate an occult one. Prostate palpation allows one to determine evidence of infection and enlargement.

LABORATORY EVALUATION

Following a thorough history and physical examination, one must decide which laboratory tests to perform. In an otherwise normal male, semen analysis is the appropriate first choice. Normal findings on semen analysis all but ensure that the remainder of the laboratory findings will be normal. If the results of semen analysis are abnormal, additional tests are warranted. Low semen volume may indicate ejaculatory duct obstruction, congenital absence of the seminal vesicles or vas deferens, or retrograde ejaculation. Fructose is produced by the seminal vesicles. If fructose is present in the ejaculate, the genital ducts are most likely patent. Azoospermia and extreme oligozoospermia (<5 million/ml) seem to be related and may be from a central nervous system (CNS) cause, genetic cause, testicular cause, aplasia or obstruction of the ductal system, or retrograde ejaculation. Microscopic examination of postejaculation urine helps determine retrograde ejaculation. Vasograms can help pinpoint the site of vas obstruction. Varicoceles have been associated with poor semen parameters, which sometimes improve following ligation of the varicocele. The abnormalities include oligozoospermia, necrospermia, and athenospermia. Men with varicoceles associated with abnormal findings on semen analysis do, however, father pregnancies and indeed, men awaiting surgery have impregnated their wives. Sperm antibodies are associated with infertility. Antibodies, however, are present in 2 percent of fertile men, but 13 percent of subfertile men. Sperm antibodies may impair spermatogenesis, spermatozoal motility, cervical mucus penetration, and acrosomal reaction and zona pellucida binding.

If the results of semen analysis are abnormal or if male sexual maturation is not normal, one must evaluate all aspects of androgen metabolism. Oligozoospermia may be associated with dysfunction of the hypothalamus, Leydig's cell, or germ cell. Hypothalamic secretion of GnRH controls FSH and LH and thus testosterone and sperm production; it is subservient to the central nervous system neurotransmitters, norepinephrine and dopamine, and to the endogenous opioids, the endorphins. Central defects can be diagnosed by determining FSH, LH, prolactin, and testosterone concentrations. Provocative testing utilizing the antiestrogen clomiphene citrate, GnRH and its analogues, menopausal gonadotropins, purified FSH, and human chorionic gonadotropin is sometimes employed to ensure appropriate responsiveness. Leydig's cell and germ cell response may be evaluated by measurement of testosterone and semen analysis. Primary testicular abnormalities may require examination of a biopsy specimen. For the most part, evaluation of biopsy specimen is required in azoospermic men with normal size testes. This most likely occurs in men with obstructed ducts and normal spermatogenesis. Normal germ cell function is associated with normal FSH concentration, while it is rare to see spermatogenesis progress beyond the primary spermatocyte stage with elevated FSH concentration. Chromosome analysis may document genetic abnormalities such as Klinefelter's syndrome. Table 12-2 summarizes the significant elements of medical history, physical examination, and laboratory evaluation.

Table 12-2. Clinical evaluation of male infertility

History
- Age at onset of puberty
- Mumps
- Frequency of erections
- Frequency of shaving
- Medications

Examination
- Body habitus, height, arm span, upper body-lower body ratio
- Hair thickness and distribution on scalp, pubis, axillae, body, and limbs
- Presence of gynecomastia
- Voice
- Breadth of penis
- Consistency, location, and size of testes
- Blood pressure while standing and lying

Laboratory investigations
- Semen analysis
- Measurement of testosterone, gonadotropins, and prolactin levels
- Testicular biopsy
- Chromosome analysis
- Skull x-ray film; radiologic bone age
- Vasography

Semen Analysis

Semen analysis is one of the main tools for determining fertility potential. Because the quality of the ejaculate will vary, two or three semen analyses must be done for accurate evaluation. Four practical factors may affect semen evaluation. These are frequency of emission, days to previous emission, age of specimen, and method of collection. Some laboratory personnel suggest a 48-hour period of abstinence prior to collection of semen for analysis. Others suggest no special period of abstinence, but obtain a specimen at one of the predicted intervals of the couple's usual sexual frequency. The specimen should be collected by masturbation to ensure that no semen is lost and that contamination is kept to a minimum. Occasionally, a patient will have religious or moral proscriptions against masturbation. In this situation, a sample may be obtained by use of a Silastic condom during intercourse. Samples must be evaluated within 2 hours because sperm motility declines rapidly thereafter as a function of time.

The term "spermia" is a suffix and denotes relating to seminal fluid. Aspermia is often used to denote absence of sperm but wrongly so. It means absence of semen, a very rare phenomenon. Oligospermia likewise is incorrectly used to denote decreased sperm but means a semen volume of less than 2 ml. Low volume is also known as hypospermia. Hyperspermia is a volume in excess of 10 ml. Normal volume is 2 to 6 ml. Reduced volume is often associated with abnormalities in the male genital tract or low testosterone concentration. Congenital absence of the vas deferens is often associated with absence of seminal vesicles. This results in low volume and absent sperm. Retrograde ejaculation results in semen being expelled into the urinary bladder and is associated with neurologic disorders such as those associated with diabetes mellitus, multiple sclerosis, and spinal cord injury. Bladder neck dysfunction also leads to retrograde ejaculation.

Semen is produced at ejaculation and is composed of seminal fluid in which spermatozoa are suspended. Normal semen is a grey-yellow opalescent fluid. The normal color may be altered by urine, blood, and jaundice. The seminal plasma is made up of fluid from the testes and all the accessory glands of the male genital tract including the seminal vesicles, prostate, bulbourethral glands, and urethral glands. The testes provide the sperm and approximately 5 percent of semen volume. This fluid is rich in androgens. The epididymis and efferent ductules add carnitine, the main energy source for sperm and epididymal motility protein that coats sperm and appears to induce motility. The seminal vesicles may produce up to 80 percent of a given ejaculate and quantitatively are most important in terms of volume. Fructose, an important energy source for sperm, is added to semen by the semen vesicles. Exclusion of the seminal vesicle component will result in almost completely immotile sperm. The enzyme vesiculase induces the clotting that occurs in semen. The prostate gland provides up to 33 percent of the ejaculate. This portion of semen is rich in biochemically active compounds. Vesiculase is present as are proteolytic enzymes that liquify the semen. The ejaculate forms a gel-like clot but will normally liquify in 5 to 20 minutes. Absence of normal liquification may indicate absence of the prostatic secretions. Viscosity of semen must also be assessed and must not be confused with absence of liquification. Viscosity is the property of a liquid to flow. It is standardized by dropping semen from a standardized pipette. A relationship between viscosity and fertility has not been established. Spermine is a bacteriostatic amine that gives a characteristic odor. Large quantities of acid phosphatase, citrate, calcium, and zinc are also present. The bulbourethral and urethral glands contribute approximately 5 percent of the total ejaculate but they secrete mucoprotein and IgA immunoglobulin. These secretions may contain sperm antibodies. The ejaculate is a very complex fluid. Malfunction of any of the components may severely restrict sperm function and thus fertility.

Sperm concentration and total sperm per ejaculate are critical values in assessing fertility potential. The majority of laboratories use the Neubauer counting chamber (hemocytometer), but the Markler counting chamber is easy to use and both provide accurate counts. Azoospermia is total absence of sperm. Oligozoospermia refers to reduced concentration or total count and is used to describe less than 20 million/ml and less than 50 million/ejaculate, respectively. Polyzoospermia denotes increased counts usually in excess of 350 million/ml. Sperm movement and forward progression are usually assessed visually and subjectively graded on a scale of 0 to 4. Recently, motion has been assessed by computerized strobe light photography or videomicrography which also may be used to determine velocity. Counts of less than 20 million/ml are associated with reduced fertility as is reduced sperm motility.

Sperm morphology may be assessed by light microscopy and various stains including hematoxylin, eosin, Papanicolaou, Giemsa, and nigrosin. Normal head shape is ordinarily tapered with an acrosomal cap. Large, small, ill-shaped, or amorphous heads and cytoplasmic droplets in the head are abnormal. Tail anomalies including coiled tails, eccentric tails, multiple tails, and midpiece (mitochondrial helix) anomalies are associated with infertility. Microscopic assessment of other cellular components is important. A few white cells are normal but increased numbers are associated with infection and reduced fertility. Germinal cells are abnormal and associated with varicocele and increased turnover of germ cells.

Additional tests include measurements of sperm antibodies in both male and female members of the couple, and hamster egg penetration. The technique of these assays is beyond the scope of this discussion.

CLINICAL SITUATIONS

Clinical situations may give insight into the role of peptide and steroid hormones and germ cells. Abnormalities of GnRH may be manifest in childhood or adulthood. *Precocious puberty* is a pure regulatory disorder. GnRH is secreted in an adult pattern, LH secretion is adultlike, and therefore Leydig's cells respond in an adult manner. The abnormality is that the GnRH pulse occurs too early. The pulse frequency can be suppressed by therapy with GnRH analogues which result in downregulation of secretion. Abnormalities can occur in adults. Both frequency and amplitude of GnRH secretion must be normal. *Idiopathic hypogonadotropic hypogonadism* is common and may be secondary to hypothalamic dysfunction. *Kallman's syndrome* is idiopathic hypogonadotropic hypogonadism associated with anosmia. Both can be treated by GnRH administered by intermittent pulse pump.

The role of FSH, LH, and prolactin may also be revealed by unique clinical situations. The *fertile eunuch syndrome* is associated with low LH, normal FSH, and low testosterone concentration. Most individuals are impotent but spermatogenesis proceeds normally. In those capable of emission, semen analysis shows normal seminal plasma, and sperm with normal size, shape, and motility. *Isolated FSH deficiency* occurs very rarely. While LH concentration is in normal range, testosterone concentration is borderline. These individuals are potent but have oligozoospermia or azoospermia. Germinal aplasia, hypospermatogenesis, or spermatogenic arrest may be seen in testicular biopsy specimens. These patients respond to FSH and a few will respond to clomiphene citrate. The *Sertoli-cell–only syndrome* is associated with elevated FSH and normal LH concentrations. Examination of testicular biopsy specimen shows Leydig's cells and Sertoli's cells but no germ cells. More commonly, concentrations of both LH and FSH are low as part of *hypogonadotropic hypogonadism* which is often associated with panhypopituitarism. All peptide and steroid hormone levels are reduced and azoospermia is present. Combined LH-FSH replacement will reverse these findings. It is best to prime testes with LH first and then add FSH. This increases both intratesticular and peripheral testosterone concentrations.

Prolactin is unique in that it is the only pituitary hormone under tonic inhibitory control. Any problem that interferes with the inhibition may result in *hyperprolactinemia*. Elevated prolactin levels impair HPG axis interaction. Hyperprolactinemic men are hyposexual, impotent, and infertile. It seems to interfere with normal GnRH release. Men with elevated prolactin levels should have computerized axial tomography (CAT) scans. Hyperprolactinemic men with normal appearing CAT scans or microadenomas can be treated with bromocriptine. Macroadenomas may require surgery.

Abnormalities of gametogenesis lead to absent gonad development or early gonadal failure. *Noonan's syndrome* (sometimes known as male Turner's syndrome) has normal genetic makeup but the gonads have failed to develop. The body habitus does not mature because of absence of testosterone production. The stereotypical genital abnormality is *Klinefelter's syndrome*. Nondisjunction results in XXY genotype. The patient with Klinefelter's syndrome is a male phenotype with normal external genitalia. Normal Leydig's cells are identified by examination of testicular biopsy specimens at puberty. Müllerian derivatives are absent because MIF is produced. Testosterone is present at puberty and levels are equal to those in normal males. Following puberty one sees progressive loss of testicular function. Leydig's cells atrophy, seminiferous tubules fail to develop normally, testicles are small, and FSH and LH concentrations are elevated indicating loss of Leydig's and Sertoli's cells. Damage to the germ cells is profound and spermatogenesis is not possible. Karyotyping is often necessary to separate the diagnosis of Klinefelter's syndrome and infertile azoospermia in a man who may have other forms of primary hypogonadism.

Androgen resistance may be profound or mild because androgen receptors are absent or defective. The classic androgen resistance is *testicular feminization*. The presentation is a phenotypic female with amenorrhea. Examination reveals a blind vaginal pouch. Testosterone levels are slightly above normal male levels and LH levels are elevated because the feedback mechanism is defective. DHT binding in genital skin is reduced. The testes are intraabdominal and they should be removed because of the risk of malignant degeneration. *Reifenstein's syndrome* is androgen resistance but with variable phenotypic expression. Incomplete testosterone manifestations are seen. Scrotal testes are present. Leydig's cells and Sertoli's cells appear normal. There is germ cell arrest and only primary spermatocytes are seen, possibly because of poor testosterone affect. DHT binding is abnormal but less severe than testicular feminization. Phenotypically normal men who have azoospermia or oligozoospermia may have mild resistance. Occasionally, testosterone and LH concentration will be slightly elevated. The diagnosis is confirmed by showing reduced DHT binding. This very mild abnormality may account for 40 percent of infertile males. Androgen resistance is often manifest at puberty with incomplete or absent sexual maturation. The *5α reductase deficiency syndrome* is manifest at birth by ambiguous genitalia because DHT is responsible for development of external genitalia. A high testosterone-DHT ratio is characteristic. Females have no problems. *Cryptorchidism* occurs in up to 40 percent of males. Failure of descent leads to reduced sperm production. When this is identified in early childhood, orchiopexy is recommended. Unless the procedure is done before the age of 2 years, it does not seem to improve reproductive potential. Even with surgery, abnormal histologic findings and distorted seminiferous tubules are seen. These individuals have reduced reproductive potential.

Sexual function and spermatogenesis cease with *hypophysectomy*. If LH is given, sexual function is restored and FSH replacement stimulates spermatogenesis. High doses of testosterone will suppress LH and FSH, and sperm counts will be reduced. Replacement of FSH and LH will increase counts but not to presuppression levels.

THERAPY

The evaluation and treatment of male infertility can be confusing and algorithms can simplify the approach to evaluation. Swerdloff and Boyers designed an algorithmic approach based on semen analysis and LH, FSH, and testosterone concentrations (Figs. 12-1 to 12-5). The most critical aspect of therapy in the male is accurate and specific diagnosis. Therapy must then be directed to this specific entity. Treatment must consider desired outcome and a cost-benefit analysis of several options must be analyzed. From an infertility standpoint one must not neglect the female member of the couple. One must be sure that the woman has no obvious impediments to fertility since combined male and female factors are identified in as many as 20 percent of couples.

Phenotypic females should be reared in female gender roles. Patients with ambiguous genitalia must be evaluated and managed on an individual basis. Therapy for the phenotypic male with delayed puberty is to mimic normal sexual development and to obtain maximum growth rate.

Fig. 12-1. Diagnostic evaluation of potentially fertile men. LH = luteinizing hormone, FSH = follicle-stimulating hormone, T = testosterone, N = normal. (Reproduced with permission. Adapted from Swerdloff, R. S., and Boyers, S. P. Evaluation of the male partner of an infertile couple: An algorithmic approach. *J.A.M.A.* 247(17):2419. Copyright 1982, American Medical Association.)

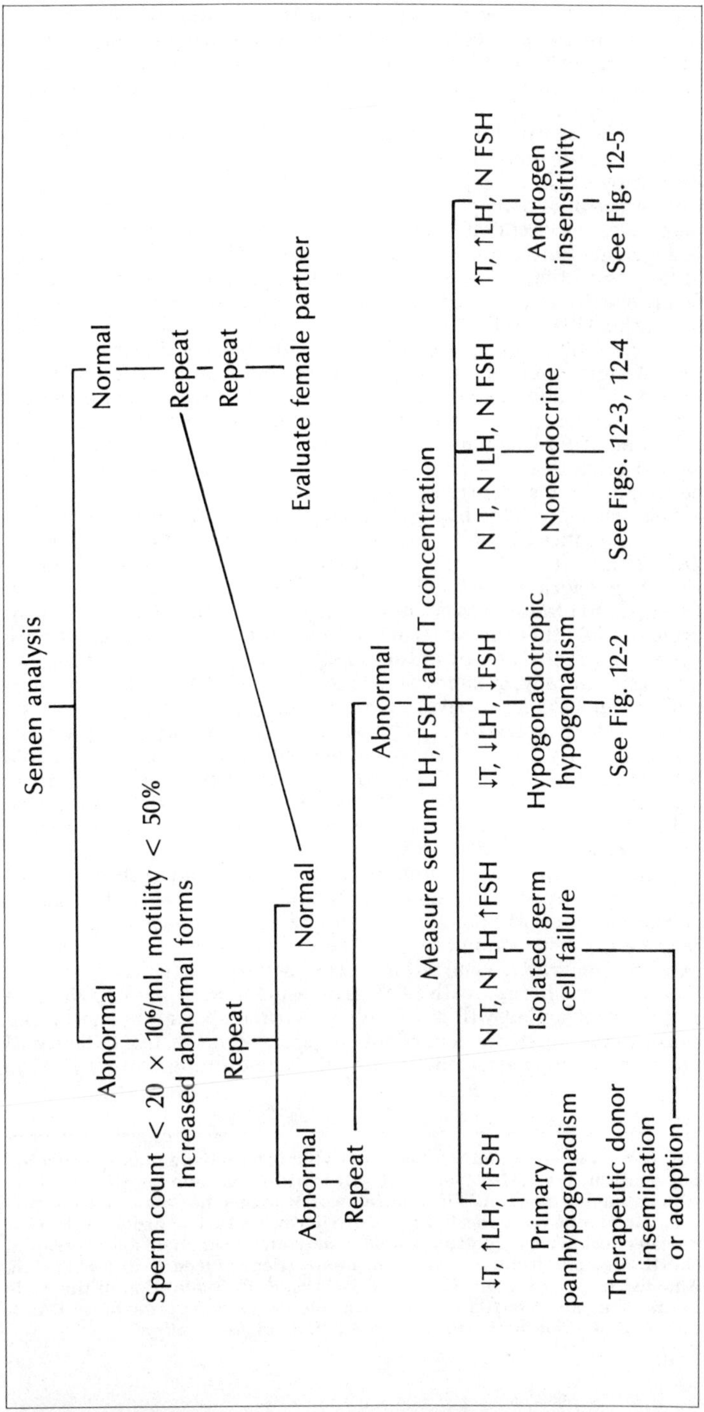

Semen analysis
Normal
Repeat
Repeat
Evaluate female partner
Abnormal
Sperm count < 20 × 10⁶/ml, motility < 50%
Increased abnormal forms
Repeat
Normal
Abnormal
Repeat
Abnormal
Measure serum LH, FSH and T concentration
↓T, ↑LH, ↑FSH
Primary panhypogonadism
Therapeutic donor insemination or adoption
N T, N LH ↑FSH
Isolated germ cell failure
↓T, ↓LH, ↓FSH
Hypogonadotropic hypogonadism
See Fig. 12-2
N T, N LH, N FSH
Nonendocrine
See Figs. 12-3, 12-4
↑T, ↑LH, N FSH
Androgen insensitivity
See Fig. 12-5

Delayed puberty secondary to primary gonadal failure is relatively uncommon. Puberty may be initiated by testosterone cypionate, 50 mg, or testosterone enanthate, which is given intramuscularly at monthly intervals. If puberty is not initiated, one may increase the dosage. Increments should be small because priapism can occur with rapid increments or large doses. Therapy causes progressive penile enlargement, increased scrotal rugation, pubic hair, deepening of the voice, and growth spurt. Usual treatment is with the lowest dose that produces desired results. Testicular enlargement does not occur. If enlargement occurs, one must suspect that endogenous function has begun. In those patients who are in need of long-term therapy, the dose of androgen should be increased to 50 mg every 2 weeks. This regimen may be increased by 50 mg every 6 months. Ultimately, 200 mg every 2 weeks should be given. Normal sexual libido and potency occur at this dosage. If they have not, testosterone levels should be measured and therapeutic levels obtained by dosage modification. Dosage should not be increased too rapidly for fear it will hasten epiphyseal closure and thus reduce final height. Individuals with anorchia or abnormally small testes should have testicular implants for cosmetic reasons once scrotal development has occurred.

Most patients have hypogonadotropic hypogonadism. Often this is due to reduced GnRH secretion and therefore deficiencies in LH and FSH. Failure of GnRH secretion may be secondary to tumors, radiation therapy, congenital anomalies, and unknown causes. Often, GnRH failure is associated with anosmia (i.e., Kallman's syndrome). The other functions of the hypothalamus and pituitary are usually normal. Therapy of these individuals may be in the form of androgen therapy, gonadotropin therapy, or GnRH. GnRH will normalize the HPG axis. Sexual maturation requires pulsatile LH secretion, which can be induced by pulsatile GnRH therapy. Low-dose, high-frequency GnRH therapy is possible using a programmable portable pump. This regimen induces normal testosterone concentrations and spermatogenesis. Goals of therapy are to achieve a masculine physique and psychologic development and to achieve spermatogenesis in men desiring fertility.

Gonadotropin therapy (human menopausal gonadotropins [hMG]) may correct hypoandrogenism. If sexual maturation is the therapeutic goal, the LH analogue, human chorionic gonadotropin (hCG) may be given to stimulate Leydig's cells and thus androgen production. Generally, virilization is best achieved over the course of 3 to 5 years. Therapy with hCG will result in androgen production and virilization but will not result in normal spermatogenesis. Because testicular size is dependent on germ cell mass, hCG alone will not give the cosmetic benefit of testicular enlargement. If FSH is

Fig. 12-2. Evaluation and treatment of patients with hypogonadotropic hypogonadism. T = testosterone, LH = luteinizing hormone, FSH = follicle-stimulating hormone, ACTH = adrenocorticotropic hormone, TSH = thyroid-stimulating hormone, GH = growth hormone, PRL = prolactin, hCG = human chorionic gonadotropin, hMG = human menopausal gonadotropin, GnRH = gonadotropic-releasing hormone. (Reproduced with permission. Adapted from Swerdloff, R. S., and Boyers, S. P. Evaluation of the male partner of an infertile couple: An algorithmic approach. *J.A.M.A.* 247(17):2419. Copyright 1982, American Medical Association.)

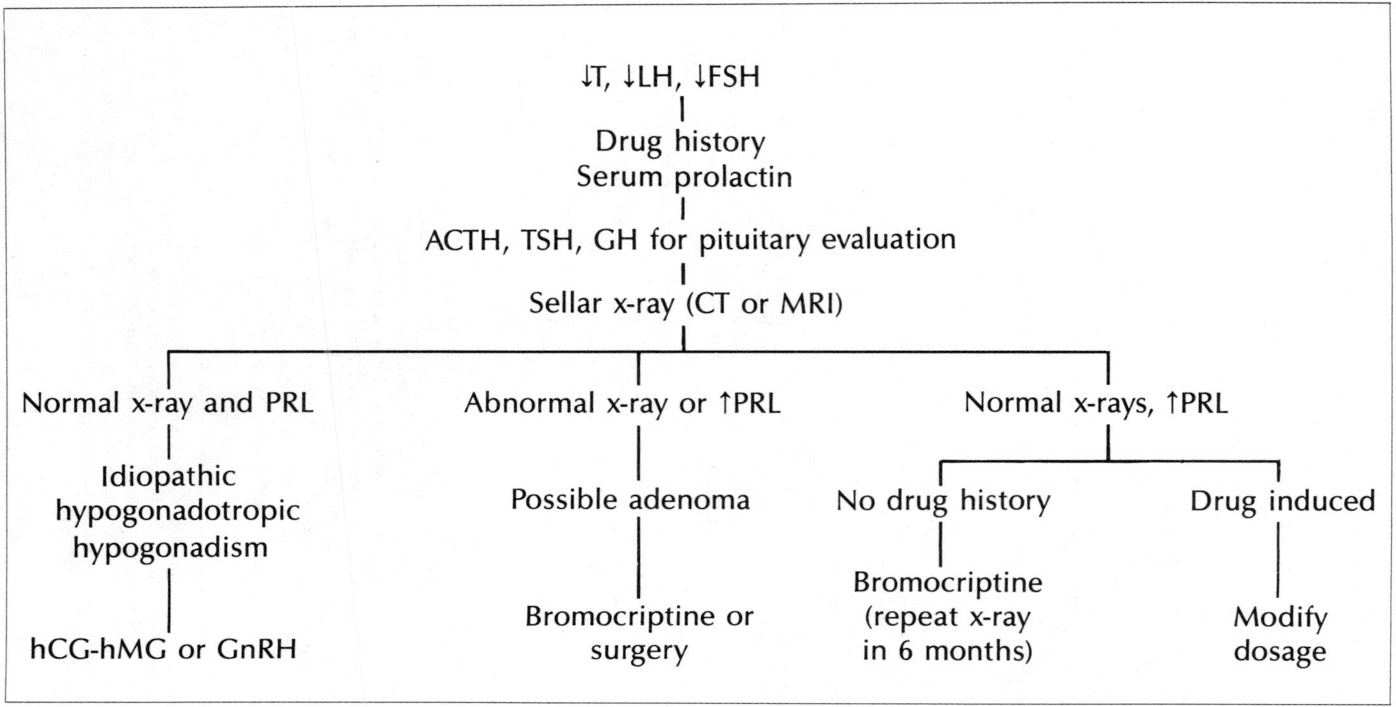
↓T, ↓LH, ↓FSH
Drug history
Serum prolactin
ACTH, TSH, GH for pituitary evaluation
Sellar x-ray (CT or MRI)
Normal x-ray and PRL
Abnormal x-ray or ↑PRL
Normal x-rays, ↑PRL
Idiopathic hypogonadotropic hypogonadism
Possible adenoma
No drug history
Drug induced
hCG-hMG or GnRH
Bromocriptine or surgery
Bromocriptine (repeat x-ray in 6 months)
Modify dosage

also administered then germ cell mass will increase. With elevated intratesticular testosterone levels from hCG or LH therapy, spermatogenesis is easily induced by FSH.

Oral androgen or parenteral androgen, or both, will produce secondary sexual characteristics. Virilizing changes can be accomplished with testosterone directly or hCG (an LH analogue). The hCG stimulation of testosterone by the Leydig's cell is far more effective than exogenous testosterone. Normal spermatogenesis cannot be achieved by androgens alone. Spermatogenesis can occur without FSH but is not qualitatively or quantitatively as good as if FSH is also replaced. If hypogonadism occurs before puberty the combination is necessary; if it occurs following puberty, LH alone is sometimes adequate. Furthermore, oral androgen therapy may cause significant hepatic abnormalities. Because of the anabolic effects, patients can gain significant weight and retain fluid to the point of edema and congestive heart failure. With large doses or excessive response patients may complain of excess libido, frequent erections, and rarely priapism. Lowered androgen dose will ordinarily reduce these symptoms. Androgen therapy is much less expensive than HMG and GnRH therapy and is therefore available to more patients. It is the only therapy available for those patients with anorchidia or testicular failure.

Those patients who develop hypogonadism in the postpuberty period are relatively easy to treat because they are quite responsive to HMG. Because some baseline LH and FSH continues to be secreted, patients treated with hCG alone may be capable of spermatogenesis and thus fertility. Unlike prepubertal patients who should have androgen replaced slowly, adult patients should have androgens returned to adult levels rapidly. During the course of therapy, estradiol (E^2) levels should be monitored because HMG can stimulate E^2. Elevated E^2 levels may lead to gynecomastia and sexual dysfunction.

The goal of therapy should be clearly defined before a treatment regimen is chosen. Virilization may be achieved by all therapies. Although administration of testosterone or its derivatives alone produces secondary sexual characteristics, they are not as efficacious as hMG and the cosmetic benefits of androgen are not as great as hMG. Fertility can only be restored with hMG, GnRH, or both. If the pituitary gland is not functioning, gonadotropins are mandatory.

Hyperprolactinemia may be caused by pituitary adenoma, hypothyroidism, psychotropic drugs, hypothalamic dysfunction, and chronic stress. Secretion of prolactin is regulated by prolactin-inhibiting factor (PIF), which is secreted by dopaminergic neurons in the ventral medial nucleus and median eminence of the hypothalamus. Many believe that PIF is dopamine. Excess prolactin causes loss of libido, sexual dysfunction, and reduced testosterone production. Reduced testosterone subsequently impacts on spermatogenesis. Pituitary adenomas are associated with elevated serum pro-

Fig. 12-3. Diagnostic evaluation of azoospermic patients. LH = luteinizing hormone, FSH = follicle-stimulating hormone, T = testosterone, N = normal. (Reproduced with permission. Adapted from Swerdloff, R. S., and Boyers, S. P. Evaluation of the male partner of an infertile couple: An algorithmic approach. *J.A.M.A.* 247(17):2420. Copyright 1982, American Medical Association.)

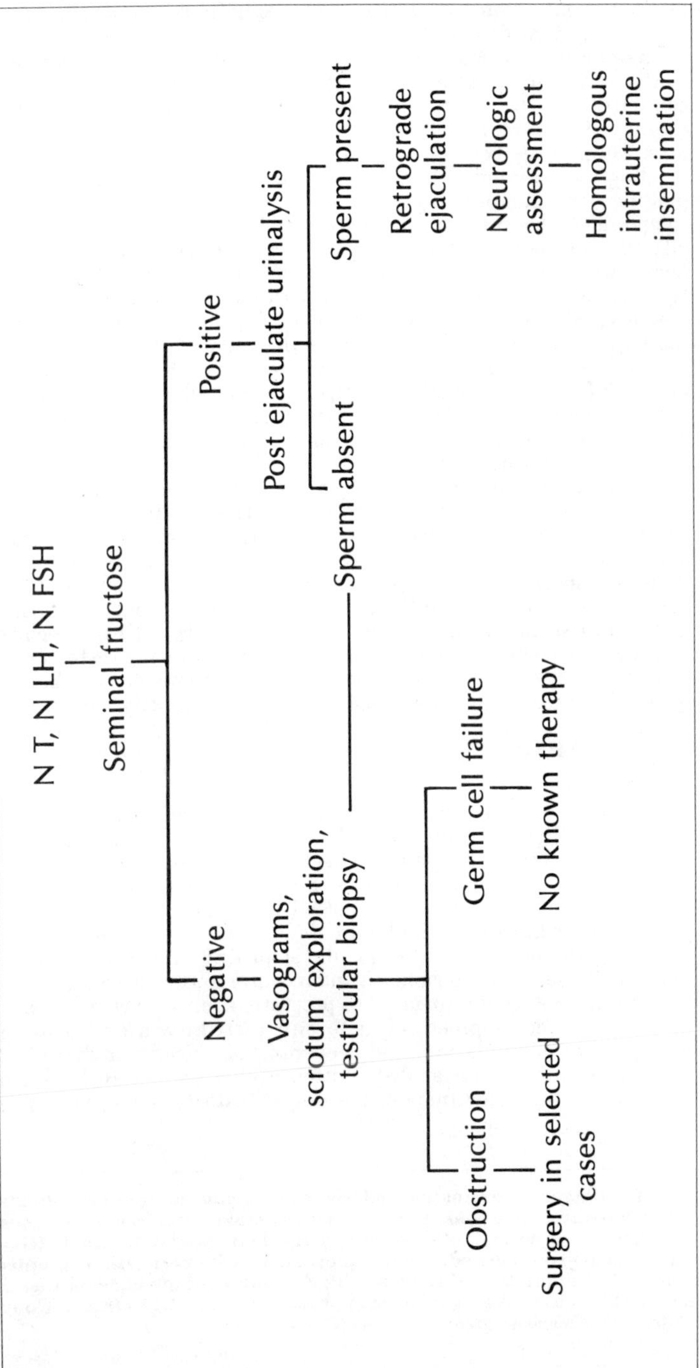
N T, N LH, N FSH
Seminal fructose
Positive
Negative
Post ejaculate urinalysis
Sperm present
Sperm absent
Retrograde ejaculation
Neurologic assessment
Homologous intrauterine insemination
Vasograms, scrotum exploration, testicular biopsy
Sperm
Obstruction
Germ cell failure
Surgery in selected cases
No known therapy

lactin concentrations. CAT scan and magnetic resonance imaging (MRI) can identify adenomas. Those tumors less than 10 mm in diameter are classified as microadenomas, and are best treated medically with bromocriptine. In addition to reducing serum prolactin concentrations, the microadenomas may regress with bromocriptine therapy. Tumors larger than 10 mm are classified as macroadenomas. These large tumors may require surgery or radiotherapy depending on symptoms that might be associated with a mass impinging on surrounding structures. Visual fields may be compromised by pressure on the optic chiasm and other anterior pituitary hormone levels may be reduced by pressure of the adenoma, which reduces function in the other cells of the pituitary. Hypothyroidism is often associated with elevated prolactin levels. Low thyroid hormone concentration results in positive feedback to the hypothalamus, which stimulates the release of thyrotropic-releasing hormone (TRH) and thus increased thyroid-stimulating hormone (TSH). Overproduction of TRH is associated with elevated prolactin secretion. Psychotropic drugs may block or reduce the number of dopamine receptors on the lactotropes, thereby reducing dopamine action of inhibiting prolactin secretion. Chronic physical and psychologic stress is also associated with elevated prolactin concentration. Craniopharyngioma, transection of the pituitary stalk, and other CNS tumors may reduce output of PIF because of hypothalamic dysfunction and thus lead to an elevated prolactin concentration. The specific cause of hyperprolactinemia must be identified and treated. Regardless of the cause, the elevated prolactin concentration is associated with reduced frequency of LH pulsatile release, and therefore reduced testosterone output. Stimulating testosterone output by hCG therapy will reverse some symptoms but no therapy is as effective as returning prolactin to normal concentrations.

DRUG PREPARATIONS

Testosterone

Testosterone is a naturally occurring androgenic anabolic steroid hormone and is the principal endogenous androgen. It can be extracted from animal testes but is usually synthesized from cholesterol or DHEA. It is available as the base and as the cypionate, enanthate, and proprionate esters. All forms are practically insoluble in water but freely soluble in alcohol and vegetable oils.

Androgens are responsible for development and growth of the male genitalia and for formation and maintenance of secondary sexual characteristics. Maturation of prostate, seminal vesicles, penis and scrotum, development of male hair distribution and balding, enlargement of the larynx and deepening of voice, and characteristic male muscle and fat distribution are under the influence of androgens. Like other anabolic hormones, testosterone produces re-

Fig. 12-4. Diagnostic evaluation and treatment of oligozoospermic patients. LH = luteinizing hormone, FSH = follicle-stimulating hormone, T = testosterone, N = normal, hCG = human chorionic gonadotropin, hMG = human menopausal gonadotropin. (Reproduced with permission. Adapted from Swerdloff, R. S., and Boyers, S. P. Evaluation of the male partner of an infertile couple: An algorithmic approach. *J.A.M.A.* 247(17):2421. Copyright 1982, American Medical Association.)

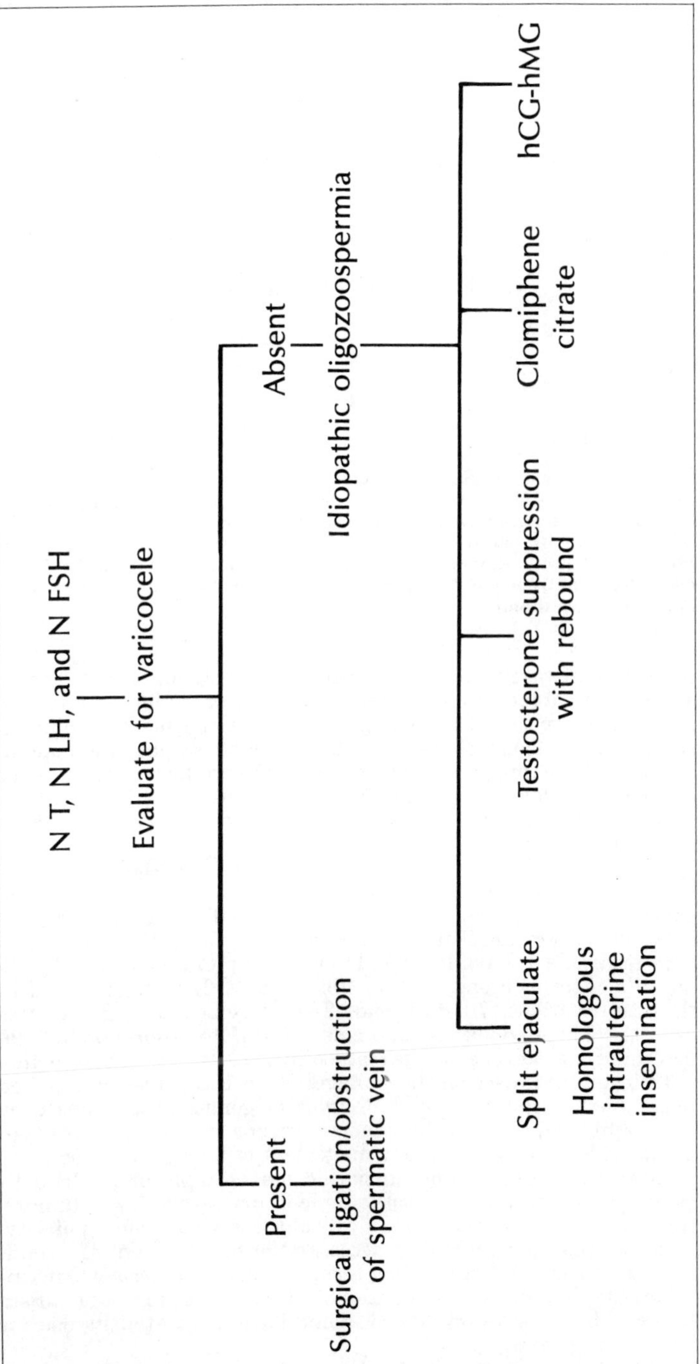

N T, N LH, and N FSH
Evaluate for varicocele
Present
Surgical ligation/obstruction of spermatic vein
Absent
Idiopathic oligozoospermia
Split ejaculate
Homologous intrauterine insemination
Testosterone suppression with rebound
Clomiphene citrate
hCG-hMG

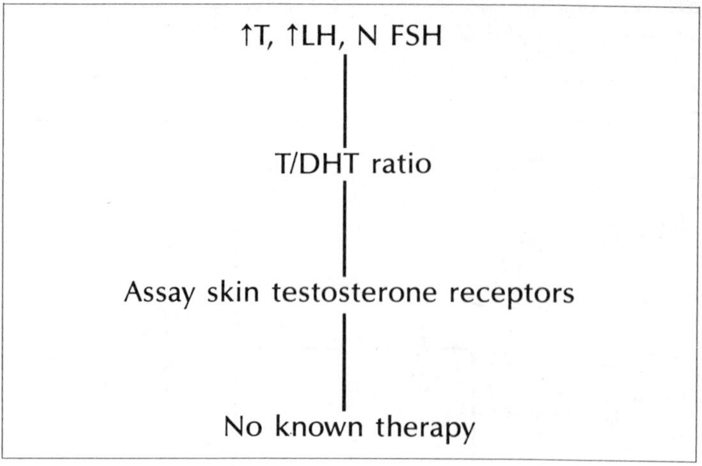

Fig. 12-5. Diagnostic evaluation of patient with suspected androgen resistance. LH = luteinizing hormone, FSH = follicle-stimulating hormone, T = testosterone, N = normal, DHT = dihydrotestosterone. (Reproduced with permission. Adapted from Swerdloff, R. S., and Boyers, S. P. Evaluation of the male partner of an infertile couple: An algorithmic approach. *J.A.M.A.* 247(17):2421. Copyright 1982, American Medical Association.)

tention of nitrogen, increases protein metabolism, and decreases amino acid catabolism and urinary calcium excretion. While it is responsible for the adolescent growth spurt, it causes epiphyseal closure. Exogenous testosterone inhibits gonadotropins and may interfere with spermatogenesis by reducing the production and release of intratesticular testosterone because of decreased LH concentration and reducing germ cell stimulation secondary to decreased FSH concentration.

Orally administered testosterone is rapidly metabolized by the liver. Therefore, the main route of administration is by intramuscular injection of one of the esters. Duration of effect for intramuscular administration is usually 2 to 4 weeks. Subcutaneous pellets of testosterone are available and may last up to 6 months. Plasma half-life of testosterone is 10 to 100 minutes. It is metabolized in the liver to various 17-ketosteroids. Testosterone and its metabolites are also conjugated with glucuronide and sulfate. Approximately 90 percent of testosterone and its metabolites are excreted in the urine.

Testosterone is used for the management of congenital or acquired hypogonadism caused by orchidectomy or gonad failure caused by cryptorchidism, bilateral torsion, orchitis, or vanishing testes syndrome. It is also used in the management of hypogonadotropic hypogonadism resulting from idiopathic gonadotropin or GnRH deficiency or from pituitary-hypothalamic injury secondary to tumors, trauma, surgery, or radiation. If any of these occur before puberty, androgen replacement will be necessary for development of secondary sexual characteristics. Long-term therapy is necessary to maintain these characteristics in patients who developed hypogonadism before puberty or in adulthood. Some have advocated its use for delayed puberty. One must be cautious with such therapy when the delay is not associated with a pathologic condition.

As with all steroids, some adverse reactions may occur. Oligozoospermia and reduced ejaculatory volume may occur with excessive dosage or prolonged administration. Acne, flushing, gynecomastia, habituation, and edema are also side effects. Priapism may occur especially in geriatric men. Cholestatic jaundice and abnormal liver function can occur especially with oral administration. Patients with renal, cardiac, or hepatic dysfunction should be monitored carefully since fluid retention with or without congestive heart failure may occur. Excessive sexual stimulation in the form of excessive libido or too frequent erections warrant reduced dosage of testosterone. Benign prostatic hypertrophy may be worsened. Testosterone may potentiate the action of oral anticoagulants and produce bleeding in some patients. Insulin requirements are reduced in some patients.

Testosterone and its esters are administered by deep intramuscular injection. Testosterone pellets may be implanted by means of an injection or surgical incision. Dosage must be tailored to the patient and the condition being treated as well as severity of symptoms, patient age, history of prior therapy, and specific testosterone preparations used. Subcutaneous pellets should be used only after the dosage has been determined by other administration.

Testosterone

Powder for prescription compounds is available (Millgood, Paddock). Pellets are available in 75 mg (Progynon). Suspension, sterile formulations are in 25 mg/ml, 50 mg/ml, and 100 mg/ml concentrations (Androlan [Lannett], Testoject-50 [Mayrand], Histerone [Hauck]).

Testosterone Cypionate

Injection (in oil) is available in 100 mg/ml and 200 mg/ml concentrations (Andro-Cyp 100 or 200 [Keene], Depotest 100 or 200 [Hyrex], Depo-Testosterone 100 or 200 [Upjohn]).

Testosterone Enanthate

Injection (in oil) is available in 100 mg/ml and 200 mg/ml concentrations (Everone 100 and 200 [Hyrex], Andro "200" [Forest], Delatestryl [Squibb]).

Testosterone Proprionate

Powder for compounding is available (Millgood, Paddock). Injection (in oil) is available as a nonproprietary drug in 50 mg/ml and 100 mg/ml concentrations.

Methyltestosterone

Methyltestosterone is synthesized by substituting a methyl group at the 17 position of testosterone. It also has prolonged action following oral administration because hepatic metabolism is slowed. Pharmacologic uses, cautions, drug interactions, and laboratory test interference are the same as for testosterone. Methyltestosterone may be administered orally or buccally and is given in divided doses. Dosage must be individualized. Maintenance of adult androgen deficiency states may be accomplished with 10 to 50 mg of conventional oral tablets daily in divided doses or 5- to 25-mg buccal tablets daily.

Buccal dosage is 50 percent of oral dosage. Dosage to induce puberty is started at low doses and increased gradually.

Powder (micronized) for compounding is available (Paddock). Buccal tablets are supplied in 5-mg and 10-mg strengths (Android-5 [Brown], Metandren Linguets [Ciba]). Oral capsules are available in 10-mg strengths (Virilon [Star]). Oral tablets are available in 10-mg and 25-mg strengths (Android-10 [Brown], Metandren [Ciba], Android-25 [Brown]).

Fluoxymesterone

Fluoxymesterone is the fluorodinated derivative of methyltestosterone. It is 5 times as potent as methyltestosterone and equivalent to intramuscular testosterone. It shares all properties of methyltestosterone. Dosage is divided into 3 or 4 equal doses. Dosage again varies with the clinical situation. Complete adult replacement of androgen can be accomplished with 5 to 20 mg daily. Because of potency this drug may have a slightly higher incidence of excess libido and priapism.

Oral tablets are available in 2-mg, 5-mg, and 10-mg strengths (Halotestin [Upjohn]) and in 10-mg strength (Android-F [Brown]).

PROTOCOLS

For the purpose of discussion, lack of androgen effect and infertility will be separated. In practice, both conditions often coexist and both are of concern to the patient.

Hypogonadism is manifest by androgen deficiency which may be subtle or obvious. Manifestations depend on the stage of development at which the deficiency occurs. Androgen deficiency during embryogenesis results in various degrees of ambiguous genitalia. Deficiencies prior to puberty result in a eunuchoidal body habitus, failure to develop secondary sexual characteristics, and failure to develop normal sexual function. Adult-onset deficiency results in abnormalities in sexual performance, infertility, and gradual regression of secondary sexual characteristics.

Primary Testicular Failure

Androgen deficiency may result from a primary testicular defect. When the testes do not function properly as is the case in patients with Klinefelter's syndrome, castration, bilateral torsion, mumps orchitis, or myotonic dystrophy, androgen must be replaced directly. No degree of androgen replacement will allow spermatogenesis. Androgen therapy should not be started until the age of 13 to 14 and then only in those boys known to be hypogonadal. Before the age of 15 it can be difficult to separate constitutional delay from hypogonadism. Puberty is initiated with low androgen dosage initially and a gradual increase in androgen dosage over a 3 to 5 year period, until adult habitus is achieved. Perhaps the main reason for low dosage is to ensure full height potential before epiphyseal closure. Initial virilization can be stimulated by deep intramuscular administration of testosterone enanthate in doses of 50 mg every 4 weeks. This dose is adequate for approximately 6 months. The monthly dosage may be increased by 50 mg at 6-month intervals. Once the monthly dose is 200 mg, the dosage may then be increased in frequency to 3 weeks and then to 2 weeks.

Biweekly administration of 200 mg of testosterone enanthate is normally adequate for maintenance of sexual performance and sexual characteristics. Because of convenience, some patients prefer higher dosage at less frequent intervals. Dosage of 300 to 400 mg every 3 to 4 weeks is effective. Many patients will experience gynecomastia. This is generally transient as the virilizing effect becomes more pronounced. Occasionally, mastectomy must be performed. Some patients, especially older men and pubertal boys, receiving high doses of androgen experience excessive libido and excessive frequency of erections. Priapism has been reported in severe cases. This problem can be managed by reducing dosage and frequency of administration until the side effects resolve.

Hypogonadotropic Hypogonadism of Pituitary Origin

Testicular function is regulated by pituitary gonadotropins, LH and FSH, and locally synthesized androgens. Diagnosis of this condition requires evidence of androgen deficiency and abnormal spermatogenesis in conjunction with low gonadotropic hormones. When gonadotropins are low, one must consider pathologic conditions in the pituitary and alterations of hypothalamic GnRH secretion. Provocative testing will often aid in making a specific diagnosis. As has been discussed earlier, accurate diagnosis is mandatory for determination of appropriate therapy. Administration of GnRH, clomiphene citrate, and hCG allows accurate determination of the cause of low gonadotropin levels. A 100-μg bolus of GnRH should produce a doubling of baseline FSH and LH levels. Failure to respond indicates primary pituitary dysfunction. To evaluate testicular function, hCG (a long-acting LH analogue) may be administered in a dose of 5000 units daily for 4 days. Normal adult testosterone concentration should be produced if normal Leydig's cells are present. Gonadotropin replacement may be given with hCG or hMG, a combination of LH and FSH obtained from the urine of menopausal women. In patients with delayed puberty hCG will stimulate testosterone production by the Leydig's cells. As with other pubertal therapy, replacement should begin slowly and allow the events of puberty to occur over 3 to 5 years. Initial therapy should begin at 250 IU administered intramuscularly 2 to 3 times weekly. Testosterone should be assayed every 2 weeks until the serum testosterone concentration is between 100 and 300 ng/dl. If testosterone exceeds 300 ng/dl, hCG dose should be reduced because virilization accelerates too rapidly and epiphyseal closure will result in short stature. Once hormone concentration is stable it should be repeated monthly for 6 months and then bimonthly. Patients should be monitored on a regular basis. Height, weight, span, and pubis-to-floor measurements should be charted. Blood pressure, complete blood cell count, liver function, and lipids should be checked annually. Clinical response may be monitored by assessing frequency of increasing erections, spontaneous erections, nocturnal emissions, masturbation, sexual frequency, and changes in libido. Once pubertal development has been achieved and adult height obtained, hCG may be increased to 500 IU 3 times weekly, which will allow adult testosterone concentration. Full virilization may take up to 5 years. Response often is progressive as testicular size increases. E^2 production may also be stimulated and E^2 should be monitored every 8 weeks. E^2 levels in excess of 50 pg/ml indicate a need for reduction of hCG dosage. Gynecomastia and sexual dysfunction may occur with elevated estrogen levels. Treatment with hCG alone may result in limited spermatogenesis and sperm may appear in the ejaculate. Normal spermatogenesis requires FSH. Adult men treated with hCG tolerate rapid return of testosterone to adult concentration. Treatment with 500 IU of hCG intramuscularly 3 times weekly will result in adult testosterone concentration by 4 to 8 weeks. Adequacy of therapy can be monitored clinically by determining adequacy of strength, libido, and sexual function. After full androgen response has been achieved, androgen-dependent symptoms may be maintained by weekly injections of 1500 to 2000 IU of hCG. Virilization may also be obtained as outlined in the protocol for primary testicular failure; however, the degree of virilization is much more complete utilizing hCG.

Hypogonadotropic Hypogonadism from Hypothalamic Dysfunction

Hypothalamic dysfunction may be from hypothalamic lesions, cranial surgery, trauma, or radiation. Idiopathic hypogonadotropic hypogonadism can be distinguished from constitutional delayed puberty by pubertal delay beyond the age of 18, family history of idiopathic hypogonadotropic hypogonadism, and associated anomalies such as anosmia. The goal of therapy is to achieve the physical and psychologic changes that accompany puberty and to induce spermatogenesis. Virilization can be achieved with androgen therapy or hCG therapy as outlined earlier. Spermatogenesis may be induced by combination hMG and hCG therapy. Clomiphene citrate, which ordinarily produces the release of GnRH, does not produce this response in patients with idiopathic hypogonadotropic hypogonadism but long-term GnRH therapy can completely normalize pituitary-gonadal function. The medial basal hypothalamus is normally the source of GnRH, which has a serum half-life of 2 to 4 minutes. The GnRH is normally confined to the hypothalamic-pituitary portal system and ordinarily is not identified in the peripheral circulation. Early puberty is associated with marked LH spikes during sleep. During mid and late puberty these LH pulses are present during both sleep and wake periods. In adulthood, LH amplitude is decreased as testosterone concentration increases and thus inhibits pituitary response. Normal LH pulse frequency and, by inference, GnRH pulses occur every 2 hours. GnRH release occurs in small, frequent bursts. Low-dose, high-frequency GnRH pulses produce LH pulses similar to the LH pulse seen during puberty. This therapy is made possible by programmable portable infusion pumps. Puberty can be induced by GnRH administered at a frequency and dose that mimic gonadotropin secretion in normal men.

The dose of GnRH required to induce puberty varies from patient to patient. The dose of native GnRH varies from 25 ng/kg to 300 ng/kg administered every 2 hours as the dose necessary to induce puberty and sustain testosterone concentration in the midnormal adult range. Native GnRH with its short half-life is necessary for normal response. The analogues are not effective because of their long half-life. Prolonged stimulation results in downregulation. The dose of native GnRH should begin at 25 ng/kg administered every 2 hours by programmable portable pump. The patients should be monitored at weekly intervals to determine FSH, LH, and testosterone response to GnRH. If LH and FSH levels have not entered puberty range by 4 weeks, the dosage should be increased by 25 ng/kg every 2 hours until LH and FSH enter puberty range. Dosage may be increased weekly up to 300 ng/kg. After puberty, GnRH may be reduced to subthreshold levels. GnRH can be reduced by 25 ng/kg until such time as FSH, LH, or testosterone levels begin to decline or sperm count is lower. Long-term therapy is necessary. The reduced dose lowers cost and avoids excessive testosterone levels.

Hyperprolactinemia

Treatment of hyperprolactinemia depends on its cause and must be individualized. This discussion will be limited to those situations appropriate for therapy with ergot derivatives. For the most part, these are idiopathic hyperprolactinemia, microadenomas, and macroadenomas which are otherwise asymptomatic. The only drugs of proven clinical effectiveness are the ergot derivatives and the only one available in the United States is bromocriptine mesylate. Several similar but longer acting drugs are being evaluated. Bromocriptine lowers serum prolactin levels and restores libido and potency. It may also cause tumor regression. Usefulness of these drugs is limited by the need for compliance and the need for follow-up. Hyperprolactinemia returns as soon as bromocriptine is stopped and reexpansion of tumors may be dramatic.

Bromocriptine should be initiated by administering 1.25 mg (½ tablet) at bedtime with a snack. If the patient tolerates this dosage for 2 to 3 days, then dosage may be increased to 1.25 mg twice daily. Prolactin levels should be assayed weekly. As long as prolactin remains elevated, the dosage of bromocriptine may be increased in 1.25-mg increments. If prolactin levels remain elevated with the dosage of 2.5 mg twice daily, the dosage may be increased to 3 times daily. Rarely will a patient respond to doses in excess of 7.5 mg daily. If no response is seen, patients must be reevaluated. Especially in patients with adenomas, follow-up is mandatory and surgery may be warranted. Side effects are mild hypotension and nausea. Other side effects encountered are headache, dizziness, fatigue, light-headedness, vomiting, abdominal cramps, nasal stuffiness, and constipation. Approximately 5 percent of patients cannot tolerate therapy.

Reproductive Potential Requires Spermatogenesis

Both LH and FSH are necessary for spermatogenesis. Androgen deficiency in adults should be corrected for at least 2 months and puberty should be complete before initiation of spermatogenesis is tried. Androgen deficiency may be corrected by administering hCG as just outlined. Response can be evaluated by determining testicular growth. When maximum testicular response has been achieved, FSH may be added. Patients should receive 75 IU of LH and 75 IU of FSH (one ampule) or hMG daily. Each 5 days, 5000 IU of hCG should be administered. This therapy should be continued for at least 90 days, the time required for mature sperm production. Normal spermatogenesis requires a minimum of 4-ng/ml serum testosterone concentration. Semen analysis should be performed at 2- to 3-month intervals as should serum testosterone concentration. Sperm counts in excess of 10×10^6 per ejaculate indicate a good response. If this does not occur, the hMG should be increased to 150 IU of FSH and LH daily, although hCG should not be increased. This regimen allows approximately 75 percent of men so treated to father children.

BIBLIOGRAPHY

Overview of Male Infertility

Griffin, J. E. Diagnosis and management of male infertility. *Adv. Intern. Med.* 32:259, 1987.

Hargreave, T. B., et al. Estradiol and male infertility. *Fertil. Steril.* 49:871, 1988.

Hirsch, I. H., and Lipshultz, L. I. Medical treatment of male infertility. *Urol. Clin. North Am.* 14:307, 1987.

Spark, R. F. *The Infertile Male: The Clinician's Guide to Diagnosis and Treatment.* New York: Plenum Medical Book, 1988.

Swerdloff, R. S., and Boyers, S. P. Evaluation of the male partner of an infertile couple: an algorithmic approach. *J.A.M.A.* 247:2418, 1982.

Evaluation and Therapy of Delayed Puberty

Kologler, S., Uysal, A. R., and Kologler, K. B. The differentiation between constitutional delayed puberty and hypogonadotropic hypogonadism: experience with three newly devised methods. *Endocrinologie* 26:3, 1988.

Morrow, A. F., et al. Variable androgen receptor levels in infertile men. *J. Clin. Endocrinol. Metab.* 64:1115, 1987.

Page, D. C., et al. The sex-determining region of the Y chromosome encodes a finger protein. *Cell* 51:1091, 1987.

Pinsky, L., and Kaufman, M. Genetics of steroid receptors and their disorders. *Adv. Hum. Genet.* 16:299, 1987.

Rosenfeld, R. G. Constitutional delay in growth and development. *Semin. Adolesc. Med.* 3:267, 1987.

Sizonenko, P. C. Delayed sexual maturation. *Pediatrician* 14:202, 1987.

Stanhope, R., et al. Induction of puberty by pulsatile gonadotropin releasing hormone. *Lancet* 2:552, 1987.

Diagnosis of Hypopituitarism

Abboud, C. F. Laboratory diagnosis of hypopituitarism. *Mayo Clin. Proc.* 61:35, 1986.

Cryptorchidism

Chilvers, C., et al. Undescended testis: the effect of treatment on subsequent risk of subfertility and malignancy. *J. Pediatr. Surg.* 21:691, 1986.

Rezvani, I. Cryptorchidism: a pediatrician's view. *Pediatr. Clin. North Am.* 34:735, 1987.

Sexual Dysfunction

Kew, M. C. Sexual dysfunction in men with chronic liver disease. *Hepatology* 8:429, 1988.

McClure, R. D. Endocrine evaluation and therapy of erectile dysfunction. *Urol. Clin. North Am.* 15:53, 1988.

Effects of Prolactin on Testosterone Concentration

Hipkin, L. J., Diver, M. J., and Davis, J. C. The relationship between plasma prolactin and testosterone levels in male hypogonadism. *J. Endocrinol. Invest.* 9:453, 1986.

Other Medical Conditions' Effects on Hypothalamic-Pituitary-Gonadal Axis

Ermolenko, V. M., et al. Parlodel treatment of uremic hypogonadism in men. *Nephron* 42:19, 1986.

Wortsman, J., Rosher, W., and Dufau, M. L. Increased incidence of thyroid disease among men with hypergonadotropic hypogonadism. *Am. J. Med.* 80:1055, 1986.

Evaluation and Treatment of Azoospermia and Oligozoospermia

Aiman, J., McAsey, M., and Harus, L. SeZU4 and seminal plasma prolactin concentrations in men with normospermia, oligospermia and azoospermia. *Fertil. Steril.* 49:133, 1988.

Giagulli, V. A., and Vermenlen, A. Leydig cell function in infertile men with idiopathic oligospermic infertility. *J. Clin. Endocrinol. Metab.* 66:62, 1988.

Kauth, U. A., et al. Treatment of severe oligospermia with human chorionic gonadotropin/human menopausal gonadotropin: a placebo-controlled double blind trial. *J. Clin. Endocrinol. Metab.* 65:1081, 1987.

Levalle, O. A., et al. Altered pulsatile pattern of luteinizing hormone in men with idiopathic normogonadotropic oligospermia. *Fertil. Steril.* 50:337, 1988.

Pusch, H. H., Purstner, P., and Hass, J. Treatment of asthenozoospermia with hCG. *Andrologia* 18:201, 1986.

Vasquez, J. M., et al. Correlation between follicle stimulating hormone, luteinizing hormone, prolactin and testosterone with sperm cell concentration and motility. *Obstet. Gynecol.* 67:86, 1986.

Therapy with Gonadotropin-Releasing Hormone

Filicori, M., and Flamigni, C. Physiology and pathophysiology of pulsatile gonadotropin secretion. *Gynecol. Endocrinol.* 2:73, 1988.

Niles, N. L., McCorkell, S. J., and Woodhouse, N. J. Male hypothalamic hypogonadism: induction of spermatogenesis by subcutaneous pulsatile gonadotropin releasing hormone. *Horm. Res.* 25:152, 1987.

Therapy with Gonadotropins and Human Chorionic Gonadotropin

Burris, A. S., et al. Gonadotropin therapy in men with isolated hypogonadotropic hypogonadism: the response to human chorionic gonadotropin is predicted by initial testicular size. *J. Clin. Endocrinol. Metab.* 66:1144, 1988.

Usui, T., Ishibe, T., and Matsumoto, S. HCG and HMG treatment of male infertility with pituitary problems. *Urology* 29:50, 1987.

Therapy with Testosterone

Burris, A. S., Ewing, L. L., and Sherris, R. J. Initial trial of slow release testosterone microspheres in hypogonadal men. *Fertil. Steril.* 50:493, 1988.

Conway, A. J., et al. Randomized clinical trial of testosterone replacement therapy in hypogonadal men. *Int. J. Androl.* 11:247, 1988.

Findlay, J. C., Place, V. A., and Snyder, P. J. Transdermal delivery of testosterone. *J. Clin. Endocrinol. Metab.* 64:266, 1987.

Clomiphene Citrate Therapy for Infertility

Sokol, R. Z., et al. A controlled comparison of the efficacy of clomiphene citrate in male infertility. *Fertil. Steril.* 49:865, 1988.

13

Pharmacotherapy in Sexual Dysfunction

Domeena C. Renshaw

The fervent search for a quick chemical sexual elixir is a contemporary continuation of the cult of the legendary Aphrodite—"foam born"—the Greek goddess of love who emerged from the sea to bring sexual joy to all. For centuries folklore has described the pursuit of aphrodisiacs by charlatans, alchemists, shamans, magicians, or witch doctors. Today scientists seriously search for and test drugs for libido-enhancing properties. Frequently special "love potions" were sought for administration to a beloved so that he or she might be irresistibly drawn to the desirous lover. Ingredients of the aphrodisiac may have included desiccated shark's fin, rhinoceros's horn, mandrake root, ginseng, yohimbine, youth culture drugs, or miscellaneous unknowns that were popularly endowed with such an outcome.

The sexual effect of the ingested draught depended then, as now, heavily on the suggestibility of the subjects and the prestige of the potion peddler. Anecdotes of success abound in mythology as well as in today's newspapers, magazines, and medical news. How much of the claimed sexual effect is due to a pharmacologic effect has become the task of researchers of the 1980s.

Since expectation is so important an aspect of personal satisfaction, claims of sexual help must be refuted or repeated in objective studies in order to be of value to the medical community. Therefore, any intervention, whether it is (1) giving suggestions, (2) prescribing a pill, (3) using mechanical stimulation, (4) administering injections, or (5) doing research with attention/observation/questionnaires/laboratory tests (blood, urine, and other), needs careful documentation as a specifically sexually therapeutic factor in and of itself.

Powerful placebo effects are to be expected. These need to be considered and evaluated, usually by double-blind studies. However, in double-blind studies on sexual response, it is hard to evaluate "anticipatory adrenalization" due to: (1) excitement (pleasure) about being observed, which in itself could be sexually arousing, regardless of the age and sex of the researcher-observer who may be present, or known to be secluded; (2) inhibitory anxiety about being heard or observed during sex, which could be a countererotic factor and may indeed cause sexual dysfunction; and (3) transient placebo effect (30%) resulting from any intervention in suggestible persons.

The brain and mind are of primary sexual importance. Enhancement of sexual feelings may be gained by erotic thoughts or fantasy, tactile sensual contact (petting), pleasant sounds (sweet music, loving words), visually attractive persons, a comfortable open attitude toward sexual enjoyment, and at times by a "forbidden" person involved in the sexual act. Sexual arousal may frequently be inhibited by many nonsexual stimuli: auditory, visual, or mental distraction; fatigue; anger; anxiety; shame; inhibition; depression; deliberate control; and disassociation of one's sexual feelings. These are all important factors to explore when sex therapy is undertaken with an individual or when drug effects are to be evaluated.

When there are sexual dysfunctions, can medications or pharmacotherapy help? These might include over-the-counter as well as physician-prescribed chemicals. So called aphrodisiacs that have been used to enhance sexual enjoyment or to overcome or control sexual difficulties include: (1) alcohol; (2) hormones; (3) papaverine; (4) stimulants; (5) antidepressants; (6) tranquilizers; (7) hypnotics and sedatives; (8) lithium; (9) levodopa and parachlorphenylalanine (PCPA); (10) bromocryptine; (11) street drugs—marijuana, psychodelics, and narcotics; and (12) miscellaneous ones—pheromones, perfumes, placebos, and so on.

Are there drugs that *cause* sexual side effects? Indeed there are many that have negative sexual effects; some are listed but many as yet are unlisted in the *Physicians' Desk Reference* or package insert.

Common sexual dysfunctions are:

1. Absent or *inhibited sexual desire*. Interpersonal conflicts, inhibitions, or ingested chemicals are theorized as causative (via autonomic nervous system effects or effects on the higher brain centers).
2. *Anorgasmia*—primary or secondary. Sexual ignorance, inhibitions, interpersonal conflicts, and certain ingested chemicals may be factors.
3. *Impotence*—primary or secondary. The cause may be related to the autonomic nervous system or to higher centers; local penile (particularly vascular) factors may be involved. When these are excluded, then sexual ignorance, inhibitions, interpersonal conflicts, and certain ingested chemicals must be considered.
4. *Ejaculatory problems*—premature or delayed. Pathologic mechanisms in the autonomic nervous system and particularly anxiety are factors for premature ejaculation; possible pathologic factors in the pituitary or hypothalamus and chemical (including alcohol) factors can account for delayed ejaculation. If there are no physical factors, then ignorance, inhibitions, or bedroom battles are to be explored.

Sexual desire disorders have for decades or even centuries been a very common female sexual complaint. Too often this was the result of successful attitudinal indoctrination of girls toward sexual inhibition. Most cultures have a double standard that enjoyable sex is for men only, and good women tolerate marital relations to please husbands but view pleasurable sex as dirty, sinful, and dangerous and for "loose" women only. Mature women were to control sexual feelings, to endure intercourse to have children, and to "do their duty." One attractive young New Zealander said: "My sex education consisted of my mother telling me on my wedding day, as she fixed the veil: 'Sex is going to be bad. Close your eyes and think of England!'" Indeed, she was programmed for sexual bankruptcy.

However, already in the 1970s it was clinically apparent that men, even healthy young men in their prime, were presenting for sex therapy with this same complaint of inhibited sexual desire. By 1987, inhibited sexual desire was labelled "the Yuppie sex problem"; namely, the upwardly mobile, bright, successful, active, physically fit, nutritionally balanced executives who were in their 30s and products of the sexual revolution, were disinterested in sex. Some in their 20s reported a coital frequency of once in 8 months. Some couples sought sex therapy although *both* partners had inhibited sexual desire. Rather than cheerfully adjust to bilateral inhibited sexual desire, they felt they "should" be more sexually active.

Is there pharmacotherapy for low or absent desire? The mythology and the search for harmless yet effective aphrodisiacs continue but as yet there are no panaceas. Expensive, carefully designed studies by pharmaceutical companies on dopaminergic blockers are currently under way. Remedies for inhibited sexual desire that thus far have been tried are now discussed.

ALCOHOL

This ancient liquid "relaxant" has been widely used for "sexual liberation." It is frequently used as a sexual prelude and acts on the cerebral cortex as a disinhibitor of learned sexual controls, so as to dissolve resistance and attain sexual responsiveness. Moderate social drinking may facilitate social and sexual exchange. Alcohol, for many, may become an alibi: "Wouldn't have done that if I was sober!" thus allowing the person to disclaim desire, deliberation, or responsibility for a sexual act or a violent interlude. Date rape often occurs when there is excess alcohol use. Guilt, anger, or anxiety may be generated the next morning, and may persist long after the alcohol has been metabolized. Ethanol per se is not an aphrodisiac, yet the jingle "Candy is dandy, but liquor is quicker" tells of the prevalent popular folk belief.

HORMONES

Hormones have sexual effects from the fetal period and onward. Androgens cause sexual differentiation and dominance of male genitalia in the first trimester of pregnancy, while unopposed estrogen acts to form embryonic female genitalia. Testosterone, although called the male hormone (6–8 mg produced daily in normal men), is also generated by the ovaries and adrenals of women (0.5 mg/day).

In adolescence, *testosterone* increases growth of male muscles, genitals, and beard and causes changes in the voice. In both sexes it is a major factor in sexual drive. Males who seek assistance for lowered libido or impotence often actively seek "hormone shots" from their physicians. If there is a lowered level of the active form of testosterone, dihydrotestosterone, then replacement therapy with 100 mg of testosterone enanthate administered intramuscularly every 3 weeks, is indicated. This may or may not restore libido. Since the drug is detoxified in the liver, cholestatic jaundice is a possible complication of its abuse. Frequently, without the complex assay of testosterone blood levels, men are given "hormone shots" empirically, for the known transient potential placebo improvement of 30 percent. However, continued use may produce such negative side effects as edema, gynecomastia, acne, baldness, and the risk of hepatic or prostatic carcinoma.

A newly studied congenital pseudohermaphroditism has led to the discovery of the enzyme 5α-reductase which converts testosterone to active dihydrotestosterone in the embryo and again at puberty. This may yet lead to the finding of a physiologic key to understanding the complexities of libido.

Gynecologists have for many years empirically used microdoses of androgens to stimulate the libido of female patients who complain of lowered sex interest. Some postulate a surge of testosterone at ovulation. Its use is highly controversial. In England a claim has been made for more than a placebo effect in the booster shots of testosterone in average and postmenopausal women. The US literature is cautious on this prevalent gynecological practice, the results of which, endocrinologists say, spill over into their office when the frightening virilizing signs appear. Real medical concern is raised because of the serious adverse side effects of testosterone when given to women orally or intramuscularly; 5 mg per day may result in irreversible beard growth and deepening of the voice—both causing great shame and clitoral hypertrophy, which is private but can be distressing. At least one suicide resulted in the Chicago area in the 1970s; the physician was jailed for 4 years. In a pregnant woman, fetal abnormalities can occur.

A recent Canadian controlled study involved three small groups of married women who had had a hysterectomy and ovariectomy (average age, 47 years). Twenty-two women were treated with an estrogen-androgen combination, 1 ml of 8.5 mg/150 mg (Climacteron): 11 with estrogen alone, 1 ml of 10 mg (Delestrogen); and 11 in a control group, without active medication for 7 monthly injections. The researchers found the rates of coitus, orgasm, and sexual fantasy to be higher during the first two of the monthly injections in the group that received estrogen and androgen. They deduced there was merit in the androgen supplement for menopausal women despite the effects of facial hirsutism and deepening of the voice, which were stated to be rare and reversible, in contrast to findings in similar US studies.

Estrogens given therapeutically to postmenopausal women oppose androgen action on the brain and genitals, delay osteoporosis, maintain vaginal epithelium and lubrication, prevent vaginal adhesions or atrophy, and improve sexual functioning. Carcinogenic potential is of concern, especially when the estrogen is unopposed by progesterone. It is a delicate balance to be monitored carefully by an informed gynecologist.

Estrogens are used in the treatment of men with prostatic carcinoma and, by their antiandrogenic effect, reduce libido. Other estrogen side effects in males may be loss of body hair and increased breast development. They are dispensed to both sexes as tablets, injections, or creams or by transdermal patch.

Corticosteroids for allergic, inflammatory, or other chronic diseases may, in both sexes, produce euphoria and improved mobility, general functioning, and, therefore, restored sexual functioning. They may, however, have an antiandrogen effect and sometimes reduce libido. Body image changes—round face or weight gain—may be distressing enough to cause social and sexual withdrawal.

Thyroid hormone deficiency causes decreased libido as part of general apathy. Needed and adequate replacement may restore general and sexual well-being in both men and women suffering from myxedema. In two patients impotence was reversed when 7 to 8 lbs (3.15–3.60 kg) of fluid weight was lost. However, hyperthyroidism is not known to increase sexual desire.

Elevation of *prolactin* levels may lower libido in lactating mothers and also in men in whom it is often (not invariably) associated with lowered testosterone levels. Suspicion must be raised regarding prolactin-secreting pituitary microadenoma or macroadenoma amenable to treatment. Moderate or mild elevation of prolactin levels in either sex in the absence of pregnancy, lactation, or tumor has been associated with acute or chronic stress, as well as immune responses. Bromocryptine, an ergot derivative, has been effectively used to reverse impotence and low libido in some patients.

Cyproterone acetate, a potent antiandrogen, is being used experimentally abroad for treating compulsive sexual disorders in paraphiliac men with "irresistible impulses." Some success has been reported together with unwanted feminizing side effects. Medroxyprogesterone acetate suspension (Depo-Provera) is used in some US programs for sex offenders.

For the first time medically indicated hormones that act on sexual functioning are currently under scientific scrutiny. There is still much to learn about the neurophysiologic pathways of human sexuality as well as how, where, and why certain drugs act in certain ways on certain people. What we do have in observational clinical data must be further studied.

The relation of *oral contraceptives* to libido remains a controversial topic. For every study indicating that libido is decreased with the use of oral contraceptives, another points to its increase. In Ecuador, the results of a double-blind study on the effect of oral contraceptives versus placebo suggested that *both* decreased sexual desire by 30 percent. In South Africa a study by two gynecologists showed that medroxyprogesterone acetate resulted in an increase of libido in white women but a decrease in black women. In the United States, a double-blind study found more negative side effects with the placebo than with the contraceptive pill. The results are very difficult to interpret. Progesterone-containing oral contraceptives may depress libido, yet some women report an increase. For some, the generalized edema that accompanies use of the pill may increase local sensitivity of the clitoris, and therefore, desire. For others, it results in irritability. Some women feel that contraceptive safety "takes the thrill of risk" out of sex. And most recently, headlines exaggerated the negative potential hazards of the pill—carcinoma, cardiac disease, and thrombosis. Many women have returned to barrier contraceptives like the diaphragm and spermicides. The women's liberation movement condemns the pill as a "travesty on the body of women, invented by man."

PAPAVERINE

Man's view of himself as an erection machine has only been enhanced by technologic advances in medicine and surgery. The ever more perfected and expensive penile prostheses of the late 1970s brought on the era of the million dollar man and a penis industry in the United States. Evaluations for impotence can cost up to $3000 and surgery from $2000 to $12,000, depending on the model of the inserted prosthesis.

Complications of the mechanical aid are infections, erosion, malfunction, fluid leakage in the hydraulic models, malpractice suits, and a 30 percent rate of nonuse of the prosthesis. Enthusiasm for use of a prosthesis, nonetheless, continues in both patients and urologists.

Since 1986 there has been a clamor by US men for penile injections, in use since 1982 in several European and South American countries. It has been used diagnostically and experimentally in impotent men. Newspapers carried headlines about this wonder drug. A local urologist said: "I have a consent form that says: 'Your penis may fall off and you may die,' yet they sign it and have the injection with an insulin syringe into the corpus cavernosum of 40 to 80 mg of papaverine with or without phentolamine." The theory is that phentolamine produces alpha-adrenergic blockade whereas papaverine is a nonspecific relaxant of the smooth muscles of the penis.

In normal men or those with a degree of neurovascular compromise or most who have psychogenic impotence, an artificial pharmacologic erection usually results (within 20–120 minutes) and may last for 2 to 3 hours. The man, and initially his partner, may be exuberant but 3 hours of coital thrusting may leave the partner "raw and sore" as was reported by 2 women. Is papaverine the perfect aphrodisiac? It has been hailed as such by many urologists who tell success stories such as group sex parties using papaverine.

However, there are potential adverse effects including reports of one fatal pulmonary embolism and of local transient pain with resultant vasomotor collapse. This, however, may occur with having a blood sample drawn, but a man's penis is infinitely precious and fear of harm is deepseated. Bleeding or infection may occur at the penile injection site, and there may be injury to the deep penile artery or patchy sclerosis of the corpus cavernosum or along the entire length. Priapism prolonged beyond 4 hours is an emergency requiring aspiration and reduction with 10 ml of epinephrine in 1000 ml of saline solution. This prevents gangrene of the penis from the priapism. Within 3 months of treatment with papaverine injections, 50 percent of men are said to proceed to a prosthesis. Embolus to the glans and deep vein thrombosis have also been reported. Many can experience difficulty reaching orgasm or ejaculation although they attain the chemical erection. A few men have a false-negative response, namely, no erection within 1 hour after the papaverine injection but "out of the blue on the expressway the best erection since I was 18!" (7 hours later). Why? It is possible the injected material was sequestered in an interstitial "pocket" and very slowly absorbed locally to give the therapeutic response. One man developed insomnia due to anxiety that his wife would inject the penis while he was asleep (as she had teased). One more penis fear had been added to his worry list. The psychodynamics of waking with a needle in the penis have yet to be explored.

Some urologists, as mentioned, train the patients to inject the chemical themselves, and prescribe several doses of papaverine to refrigerate and use at home. This can avoid the common inconvenience of office or traffic delays while the partner waits at home. There is also the social embarrassment of a rise in the wrong place along the way. Many ethical questions arise: Is the risk justifiable for psychogenic impotence? What about a wife who is less than overjoyed? Could it wreck a marriage? Should it be given to a married man for known use with an outside partner? What about accidental or anxiety-related overdose at home? New developments always present both benefits and potential abuse, the dimensions of which may only evolve after study of 1000 patients or in 5 years' time.

STIMULANTS

Amphetamine users have occasionally reported heightened sexual interest as part of general cerebral stimulation. An occasional patient taking anorexiants will report this to a physician. Intravenous use of amphetamines may result in an acute maniacal psychosis with sexual urgency and sometimes genital self-mutilation. With chronic users, diminished libido and sexual dysfunction are reported. Physical debility, paranoid psychosis, and irreversible neuronal loss are other severe side effects caused by amphetamine abuse.

ANTIDEPRESSANTS

Both the tricyclic and monoamine oxidase inhibitor antidepressants can reverse the symptoms of a clinical depression with insomnia (in the first week), anorexia (in the second week), and weight loss and loss of libido (by the third or fourth week). They have also been successfully used to treat panic attacks and sexual phobias or aversions in doses of 75 to 200 mg taken at bedtime for several weeks, to facilitate sex therapy in a severely anxious patient of either sex. Large doses (>200 mg) may cause impotence, but this is reversible when lowered to a maintenance dose.

TRANQUILIZERS

All neuroleptic (psychotropic) drugs are known to affect sexuality indirectly in a positive way because of their calming effect. At Loyola University we have been quite successful with the use of 2 mg of thiothixene daily for about 6 weeks for tense male or female patients so that they could benefit from the sex clinic program. More directly, in a dose-related way, the drugs may impede either arousal or the orgasmic phase of the sexual response by autonomic nervous system effects—centrally or peripherally. Minor tranquilizers (in addition to their addictive risk) can affect orgasm in males and females because of the muscle relaxant effect. Major tranquilizers are more apt to cause ejaculatory delay or "dry ejaculate." Haloperidol may reduce libido and potency and lead to retarded ejaculation. Sometimes because of autonomic system relaxation of the internal bladder sphincter, there will be retrograde ejaculation. Megadoses of any psychotropic drug may reduce libido, through general drowsiness and slowed reactions.

HYPNOTICS AND SEDATIVES

In Victorian romantic novels, hypnotics or sedatives were often administered to the heroine as a preliminary to sexual seduction. This provided an unconscious female body for coitus, which was technically (painless) rape, an appealing and widespread fantasy of inhibited women, who exclude any violent aspect and immaturely visualize the conscious self as uninvolved, not responsible, and forced to participate. In fact, hypnotics and barbiturates actually depress libido possibly by central action. They also aggravate insomnia and are addictive. Some (no longer on the US market) caused priapism and also a toxic psychosis that was not always transient.

LITHIUM

Lithium is not known to increase sexual desire. It does reduce the distressing symptom of undifferentiated insatiable sexual urgency that occurs in the manic phase of manic-depressive illness in males or females.

LEVODOPA AND PARACHLORPHENYLALANINE

An antiserotonin effect on the limbic system as the site of action is the claim for levodopa (for parkinsonism) and PCPA (an experimental drug)—both once hailed as great aphrodisiacs. The sexual improvement in those who responded to levodopa was due only to the general and mobility change as is the effect of steroids with arthritic patients. There is no enthusiasm now for PCPA except in animal laboratories where male rats have mounted any moving or inanimate mass after being given the experimental substance into the septal nucleus of their brains. This mounting behavior seems to be undifferentiated, nonerotic sexual urgency. Further studies are in progress.

BROMOCRYPTINE

Bromocryptine is an ergot derivative, hailed in Europe as a new aphrodisiac, giving sexual joy to women who reportedly never experienced sexual feelings before. It is used widely in infertile women to reduce hyperprolactinemia to normal prolactin levels, which restores gonadotropin levels; ovulation and pregnancy may follow. The reported effects on libido were none to raised or lowered (due to nausea). In men with oligozoospermia and hyperprolactinemia bromocryptine may raise sperm counts and libido within 1 month's use. In uncontrolled studies in Europe bromocryptine given to impotent men reversed the symptom. Newspaper headlines in the late 1970s called it Europe's "sensational sex drug." Duration of the studies, controls used, and possible side effects were not reported. I suggest caution, since ergotamine has effects of marked peripheral vascular constriction, particularly with prolonged use.

YOHIMBINE

Yohimbine is an indole alkaloid from the bark of a tree in West Africa and has been used for potency problems for centuries. It is being investigated as an α_2-adrenergic receptor antagonist that is reputed to do better than placebo in quality and frequency of erections when 5 mg are taken 3 times a day for *10* weeks. Urinary retention, hypertension, tachycardia, and agitation have been noted.

STREET DRUGS

Youth culture is said to be a pacesetter and a community's natural research center. Mythology about sexual prowess from their favorite drug abounds among teenagers. This may be narcissism or the expansiveness of adolescence or simply sexual insecurity and a need to bolster the self, but nonetheless some of the claims merit scientific study.

Marijuana is reported (mainly subjectively) by teens and young adults as heightening whatever "is there" (e.g., happy to elated, sadness to despair, sexually interested to supersexy, sexually inhibited to more so). No scientific studies are available.

Psychedelics have had much publicity as "mind-expanding" and "mind-destroying" substances. Some say they are "recreational." Few physicians agree that they are safe. Toxic psychoses occur. Some psychedelic drugs have been studied scientifically for cognitive and perceptual effects, but little has been done in the way of objectively recording sexual effects. They are hallucinogenic and there have been varying inconclusive subjective sexual anecdotes ranging from "no effect" to "better" or "worse."

Narcotics are anecdotally known to cause reduced libido, perhaps because of central depressant effects, in those who abuse them. Orgastic problems, often permanent, for both sexes are also reported.

Inhalation of *amyl nitrite* has recently been popularized by the street drug culture as an aphrodisiac. Transient cerebral ischemia may produce a sensation of long-sustained climax. Side effects range from headache to glaucoma without any authentic sexual gains.

MISCELLANEOUS APHRODISIACS

Aphrodisiacs range from perfumes for women and also for men (to please women) to pheromones in unguents for the whole body or for genital application in flavors of vanilla, strawberry, or whatever. Commercial emphasis, through mass media, convinces all persons that expensive potions are guaranteed to provide sexual irresistibility. Vulnerable, suggestible persons "buy the dream," with, of course, 30 percent positive placebo effects!

If the individual or both partners are too anxious or upset to be aided by standard sex therapy, pleasuring and petting, the physician should explain that the degree of emotional tension is such that a tranquilizing medication is indicated as a specific ancillary and temporary aid to reduce the "sexual performance anxiety" and provide tension relief, so they may enjoy their natural sexuality. Ideally, this information should be given to the couple together. However, it may also be given to an individual patient.

The specific medication and dose used must be carefully chosen. I prefer thiothixene, 2 mg, to reduce the general tension. I tell the couple or individual that sometimes, under stress (intrapersonal or external), the sexual dysfunction may later recur. They should understand this and remember the causal connection between anxiety and dysfunction, take time to discuss it together, and again use the prolonged pleasuring foreplay without coitus for a few weeks.

At times distress in the bedroom may escalate to a degree deserving a diagnosis of sexual aversion, sexual phobia, or panic disorder with sweating, tremor, agitation, hyperventilation, and tachycardia. The suggestion is then made to supplement conjoint sex therapy with adequate doses of tricyclic antidepressants (imipramine, 25–300 mg in a single bedtime dose). Desensitization, relaxation, and even partner medication have been used during the difficult process of treatment of those persistent sexual disorders.

If, when the patient is under tension later, old sexual symptoms recur, another course of 6 weeks of sex therapy and of medication that was previously effective is again indicated. A time-limited contract, cheerful encouragement, and reassurance from the physician can certainly bring hope and help for the sexual problems of the 1980s.

BIBLIOGRAPHY

Clinical Help with Sexual Problems

Lief, H. *Sexual Problems in Medical Practice*. Chicago: American Medical Association, 1981, Pp. 214, 275.

Renshaw, D. C. Sexuality and depression in adults and elderly. *Med. Asp. Hum. Sex.* 9:68, 1975.

Renshaw, D. C. Pharmacotherapy and female sexuality. *Mod. Probl. Pharmacopsychiatry* 15:145, 1980.

Impotence

Bommer, J., et al. Improved sexual function in male hemodialysis patients on bromocriptine. *Lancet* 2:496, 1979.

Buvat, J. Influence of primary hyperprolactinemia on human sexual behavior. *Nouv. Presse Med.* 11:3561, 1982.

Drugs that cause sexual dysfunction. *Med. Lett. Drugs Ther.* 29(744):65, 1987.
Fava, M., and Guaraldi, G. P. Prolactin and stress. *Stress Med.* 3:211, 1987.
Intracavernous injections for impotence. *Med. Lett. Drugs Ther.* 29(751):95, 1987.
Jensen, S. B. Sexual customs and sexual dysfunctions in alcoholics. *Br. J. Sex. Med.* 53:29, 54:30, 1979.
Lue, T. F. Evaluation of alpha-blockade treatment of impotence—where are we going? *West. J. Med.* 142:546, 1985.
Reid, K., et al. Double-blind trial of yohimbine in treatment of psychogenic impotence. *Lancet* 2:421, 1987.
Renshaw, D. C. Inflatable penile prosthesis, *J.A.M.A.* 241:2637, 1979.
Riley, A. J., and Roley, E. J. Alpha-blockade and impotence. *Br. J. Psychiatry* 144:215, 1984.
Virag, T. F. Intracavernous injection of papaverine as a diagnostic and therapeutic method in erectile failure. *Angiology* 35:79, 1984.
Wagner, G., and Green, R. *Impotence: Physiological, Psychological, Surgical Diagnosis and Treatment.* New York: Plenum Press, 1981.
Yohimbine: time for resurrection? (Editorial). *Lancet* 1:1194, 1986.

Females and Androgens

Burger, H., et al. Effect of combined implants of oestradiol and testosterone on libido in postmenopausal women. *Br. J. Med.* 194:936, 1987.
Riley, A. J. Androgens and female libido. *Br. J. Sex. Med.* 10:5, 1983.
Sherwin, B. B., and Gelfand, M. M. The role of androgen in the maintenance of sexual functioning in oophorectomized women. *Psychosom. Med.* 49:397, 1987.

Sexual Aversions

Kaplan, H. S., and Klein, D. *Sexual Aversion, Sexual Phobias and Panic Disorder.* New York: Brunner Mazel, 1987.

14

Endocrine Pharmacotherapy of Endometrial, Breast, and Prostatic Cancer

Michel E. Rivlin

Malignant tumors of hormonally responsive target organs not infrequently maintain the capability of the parent organ to respond to hormonal action. This capability provides the basis for the use of hormones including androgens, estrogens, progestins, antiestrogens, and antiadrenal agents in clinical oncology. In general, endocrine therapy is used as a palliative treatment for advanced disease or as an adjunct to another therapeutic modality. The major malignancies, amenable to hormone therapy, are those of the corpus uteri, the breast, and the prostate gland.

ENDOMETRIAL HYPERPLASIA AND CARCINOMA

Hyperplasia and adenocarcinoma of the uterus appear to be associated with prolonged, unopposed estrogen stimulation with resulting proliferation of the glandular and stromal constituents of the endometrium. Cystic, adenomatous, and atypical hyperplasia, as well as adenocarcinoma in situ, if left untreated, may ultimately progress to invasive cancer and, therefore, these lesions should be considered as precursors of endometrial cancer. The higher the grade of endometrial hyperplasia is, the higher the percentage of patients who develop endometrial cancer is and the shorter the transition time. While the exact risk is unclear, it is generally accepted that only a few patients with cystic hyperplasia will progress to carcinoma, that about 26 percent of those with adenomatous hyperplasia, 75 percent of patients with atypical adenomatous hyperplasia, and 100 percent of those with adenocarcinoma in situ will develop invasive lesions within 1 to 4 years after diagnosis.

MANAGEMENT OF HYPERPLASIA

Diagnostic curettage with careful follow-up is adequate for treating cystic hyperplasia; sometimes hormonal therapy is added. In general however, for patients who have atypia or in whom hyperplasia persists or recurs after curettage, and if families are complete, hysterectomy is recommended by most clinicians. However, many postmenopausal women with endometrial hyperplasia present with risk factors that make surgery hazardous including diabetes, cardiac disease, hepatic disease, and morbid obesity. Therefore, a medical alternative is desired. Progestins have been shown to suppress DNA synthesis and nuclear estradiol receptor with a resulting antimitotic or antiproliferative effect. Progestins also induce the enzymes estradiol-17-β-dehydrogenase and isocitrate dehydrogenase with resulting secretory changes. By antagonizing and modifying estrogen effect, progestins have the potential to reverse all grades of hyperplasia. There is overwhelming evidence that unopposed, postmenopausal estrogen replacement therapy causes a high incidence of abnormal bleeding, an unacceptable incidence of endometrial hyperplasia, and an increase in the risk of endometrial cancer. Almost one in three women receiving long-term unopposed estrogen therapy eventually require hysterectomy because of abnormal bleeding or the development of premalignant or malignant endometrial histologic features. By combining a progestin with estrogen therapy, however, not only is the incidence of endometrial abnormalities reduced as compared with unopposed estrogen therapy, but it is reduced to below that of untreated women.

Progestins

Women who wish to remain fertile or who are not suitable for surgery may be treated with a progestational agent. *Medroxyprogesterone acetate* (Depo-Provera, Provera, Curretab, Amen) is administered at a dose of 10 to 20 mg orally per day, either continuously or for 14 days per month. Alternatively, it may be given intramuscularly on a monthly basis. *Megestrol acetate* (Megace), 20 mg orally, is given daily. The 19-nortestosterone derivatives include *norethindrone* (Norlutin) or norethindrone acetate (Aygestin, Norlutate) given in doses of 5 to 10 mg per day. The dosage of norgestrel (Ovrette) is 0.5 mg daily.

The response of most patients to therapy is so good that some clinicians initially treat all women who have benign forms of hyperplasia with progestins, and reserve surgery for treatment failures. Progestogens can cause undesirable physical, psychologic, and metabolic effects including nausea, depression, and lowered levels of high-density lipoprotein (HDL) cholesterol. Because most progestogenic side effects are dose related, the minimum effective dose should be prescribed. Other side effects include fluid retention, chills, insomnia, allergic reactions, breast discomfort, and rarely, thromboembolic complications. Since the underlying cause is not removed by progestin therapy, many clinicians maintain the treatment indefinitely. Response may require regular monitoring with endometrial biopies at 6-month intervals and endometrial biopsy is indicated for any irregular bleeding.

Cyproterone acetate is a progestin, not available in the United States, that is generally used as an antiandrogen for the treatment of hirsutism. Since it also possesses cortisol-like activity, it reduces adrenal production of cortisol and androgens. Androgens are the most important estrogen precursor in postmenopausal women. Progestins counteract estrogen stimulation, reducing the endometrial estrogen receptor. This "downregulation" of estrogen receptors is induced by an increase in total oxidation of estradiol-17 that is converted to weaker estrogens which have less or no affinity for the estradiol protein receptor. Cyproterone acetate further leads to a significant decrease in androgens in the postmenopausal women for whom ovarian production is less important than the peripheral conversion of adrenal androgens. The endogenous production of estrogens appears to be further lowered by an impairment of the peripheral aromatization. There is limited clinical experience with the medication for endometrial hyperplasia; however, successful responses are reported at a dosage of 300 mg per day orally.

Induction of Ovulation

For those women with hyperplasia who are desirous of fertility, the therapy of choice is induction of ovulation. Many of these patients have the polycystic ovary syndrome. However, the proper choice for treatment of endometrial hyperplasia in infertile women has remained controversial. In general, it is believed that it is necessary to first resolve the hyperplastic state with progestin therapy while using an effective contraceptive method. After regression of the hyperplasia is documented, induction of ovulation is attempted. It must be recalled that after induction is interrupted, or after successful pregnancy, the original state is likely to recur and endometrial biopsies, progestin therapy, or both, are again necessary.

Clomiphene Citrate

Once normal endometrial histologic features are restored, clomiphene, which acts as an antiestrogen at the level of the hypothalamus and pituitary, is the usual first-line ovulatory agent employed. The medication is started on the fifth day after spontaneous or progestin-induced bleeding at a dosage of 50 mg per day for 5 days. If the antiestrogen effect is sufficient, there is a feedback increase in the amount of gonadotropins produced, with ovarian follicular stimulation and ovulation. Endogenous progestin will then be formed and inhibit estrogen effects on the endometrium; ideally, pregnancy may occur. Therapy is monitored with determinations of basal body temperature and luteal progesterone levels and luteinizing hormone (LH) testing, if available. If ovulation does not occur, dosage is increased by 50 mg per day in the next cycle until a response is noted or until a maximum of 250 mg per day for 5 days is reached. The major serious side effect is ovarian hyperstimulation, which should be avoided by regular ovarian surveillance, ideally by vaginal ultrasound. In the rare instance of this complication, response to conservative therapy is usually good. More common side effects include 143hot flushes, breast tenderness or discomfort, nausea and vomiting, visual disturbances, and headaches.

Menotropins

In the event of failure of clomiphene treatment, induction of ovulation may be attempted with menotropins (75 U of follicle-stimulating hormone [FSH] and 75 U of LH per ampule) with 10,000 U of human chorionic gonadotropin to induce the LH surge.

MANAGEMENT OF CARCINOMA

Carcinoma of the endometrium is the most common malignancy of the female genital tract. For 1989, it is estimated that 34,000 new cases will be reported and in that year, 3000 deaths from the disease are estimated. Clinical staging correlates poorly with surgical staging and major prognostic factors include histologic grade of the tumor, depth of myometrial invasion, cell type, and lymph node involvement. The mainstays of therapy are surgery and pelvic irradiation in various combinations. Hormonal therapy, chemotherapy, or both, have been reserved for advanced or recurrent disease. Five-year rate of survival with International Federation of Gynecology and Obstetrics (FIGO) grade 1 or 2 tumor limited to the endometrium or superficial myometrium is over 90 percent. Survival rate for stage II is 70 percent and for stage IV is 3 percent. Since over 80 percent of patients have stage I or II at diagnosis, a better survival rate should be expected. Adjuvant therapy has not demonstrated an increase in the survival rate.

As with hyperplasia, unopposed estrogen states are also found in women with endometrial cancer. Estrogen and progestin receptors have been measured in the cytosolic fractions of normal, hyperplastic, and carcinomatous endometrium. Hyperplastic tissues contain the highest concentration of progestin receptors, followed by proliferative and secretory endometrium. Adenocarcinoma tissue has a low progestin receptor content which decreases as the degree of tumor differentiation worsens. Progestins oppose the actions of estrogens by reducing the number of estrogen receptors in the endometrium. Progestins increase the rates of conversion of estradiol-17β to estrone and sulfurylated estrogens within the endometrium. Therapy with progestins is associated with a decline in concentration of progestin receptors, though this does not obviate the long-term effects of therapy. Estrogen therapy increases the progesterone receptor content as well as the estrogen receptors. There is a relationship between the steroid receptor content and responsiveness of the tumor to hormonal manipulation. Those tumors with high progestin-receptor content respond more favorably than those with low receptor content. There is a good correlation between the response of recurrent lesions to progestins and the receptor content of the initial tumor.

Metastatic disease at the time of presentation is found in less than 15 percent of patients and recurrent disease is usually found in patients with high-risk factors. Therapy includes irradiation and systemic treatment. Since cytotoxic agents have not proved superior to hormonal therapy, the more tolerable side effects of the latter have resulted in a standard initial therapy with progestational agents. This treatment is changed to cytotoxic agents when appropriate after progression of the disease. However, this approach has proved less effective than at first thought, with response rates to hormonal therapy as low as 11 percent and 1- and 2-year survival rates of only 40 and 19 percent, respectively. Many clinicians now, therefore, are more selective in allocating patients to hormonal therapy, with a move to chemotherapy for patients with grade 3 or 4 lesions and those lacking in progestin receptors. Nevertheless, the occasional dramatic clinical regression or prolonged stabilization that may occur with progestin therapy supports a continued, more limited, and selective role for these agents.

Progestins

The progestins most used are medroxyprogesterone acetate (Provera, Depo-Provera, Amen) and megestrol acetate (Megace). Less often used are hydroxyprogesterone caproate (Delalutin), norethindrone (Norlutin), norethindrone acetate (Aygestin, Norlutate), and norgestrel (Ovrette). The dose of megestrol acetate is 40 to 80 mg orally, twice daily, and that of medroxyprogesterone acetate is 50 mg given orally 3 times daily or 400 mg weekly administered intramuscularly. Therapy is given for 4 months prior to assessing response, which is gauged by an increase, stabilization, or decrease in the size of lesions. Systemic side effects include allergic reactions, fluid retention, nausea, vomiting, bloating, chills, insomnia, and rarely, thromboembolic complications. A response rate of about 20 percent for grades 1 and 2 (well-differentiated and moderately well-differentiated tumors) and almost no responses in grade 3 or 4 tumors imply that progestins are probably not indicated for the latter. Preliminary reports suggest a possible advantage to combining hormonal and cytotoxic chemotherapy but no improvement when hormonal therapy is used in conjunction with surgery and radiotherapy in the primary treatment of endometrial carcinoma.

Tamoxifen

Tamoxifen (Nolvadex) has both estrogenic and antiestrogenic actions. It binds to estrogen cytosol receptors resulting in new protein synthesis; however, the estrogen receptor itself is not synthesized while progesterone receptor synthesis is increased. Thus, theoretically, the tumor may be more receptive to progestational agents. Those cancers dependent on estrogen for growth may therefore respond to this experimental therapy. When tamoxifen is given orally in daily doses of 20 to 40 mg, usually following previous therapy with progestins, partial responses, less than with progestins, may occur in up to 30 percent of patients. Side effects include hot flushes, vaginal discharge, nausea, and vomiting. Most patients tolerate therapy well, though further side effects that have been reported include hypercalcemia, edema, pruritus, leukopenia, thrombocytopenia, depression, vaginal bleeding, and rare instances of pulmonary embolism.

BIBLIOGRAPHY

Berman, M. L., et al. Risk factors and prognosis and treatment of endometrial cancer. *Am. J. Obstet. Gynecol.* 136:697, 1980.

Erlich, C. E., et al. Steroid receptors and clinical outcome in patients with adenocarcinoma of the endometrium. *Am. J. Obstet. Gynecol.* 158:796, 1988.

Gal, D., et al. Long-term effect of megestrol acetate in the treatment of endometrial hyperplasia. *Am. J. Obstet. Gynecol.* 146:316, 1983.

Gal, D. Hormonal therapy for lesions of the endometrium. *Semin. Oncol.* 13:33, 1986.

Jasonni, V. M., et al. Treatment of endometrial hyperplasia with cyproterone acetate: histological and hormonal aspects. *Acta. Obstet. Gynecol. Scand.* 65:685, 1986.

Lovecchio, J. L., et al. Treatment of advanced or recurrent endometrial adenocarcinoma with cyclophosphamide, doxorubicin, cisplatinum and megestrol acetate. *Obstet. Gynecol.* 63:557, 1984.

MacDonald, R. R., Thorogood, J., and Mason, M. K. A randomized trial of progestogens in the primary treatment of endometrial carcinoma. *Br. J. Obstet. Gynaecol.* 95:166, 1988.

Muechler, E. K., et al. Pregnancy induced with menotropins in a woman with polycystic ovaries, endometrial hyperplasia, and adenocarcinoma. *Fertil. Steril.* 46:973, 1986.

Piver, M. S., et al. Medroxyprogesterone acetate (Depo-Provera) vs. hydroxyprogesterone caproate (Delalutin) in women with metastatic endometrial adenocarcinoma. *Cancer* 45:268, 1980.

Piver, M. S., et al. Melphalan, 5-fluorouracil, and medroxyprogesterone acetate in metastatic endometrial carcinoma. *Obstet. Gynecol.* 67:261, 1986.

Podratz, K. C., et al. Effects of progestational agents in treatment of endometrial carcinoma. *Obstet. Gynecol.* 66:106, 1985.

Swenerton, K. D. Treatment of advanced endometrial adenocarcinoma with tamoxifen. *Cancer Treat. Rep.* 64:805, 1980.

Whitehead, M. I. Prevention of endometrial abnormalities. *Acta. Obstet. Gynecol. Scand.* 134:81, 1986.

BREAST CANCER

Carcinoma of the breast is the most common cancer of females in the United States (28%), with 142,000 new cases and 43,000 deaths expected in 1989. One in 11 American women will get breast cancer,

Table 14-1. Clinical TNM staging for breast cancer

Stage I	T_1—tumor size 2 cm or less N_0—no suspicious lymph nodes M_0—no distant metastases
Stage II	T_2—tumor size 2–5 cm and/or N_1—one or more palpable, suspicious nodes M_0—no distant metastases
Stage III	T_3—tumor larger than 5 cm or N_2—ipsilateral nodes fixed to one another or other structures or N_3—ipsilateral supraclavicular or infra-clavicular suspicious nodes, or arm edema M_0—no distant metastases
Stage IV	T_4—tumor of any size with fixation to chest wall, edema or ulceration of breast skin, satellite skin nodules, or inflammatory carcinoma or M_1—any distant metastases

Source: Adapted from S. G. Broniatowski and R. E. Hermann, Diseases of the Breast. In R. E. Rakel (ed.), *Conn's Current Therapy*. Philadelphia: Saunders, 1989. P. 940.

1 in 1000 females per year. It is second to lung carcinoma in female cancer deaths (18% vs 20%). The mortality rate of 27 per 100,000 females has hardly changed for 50 years and it causes more deaths than ovarian, endometrial, and cervical cancer combined. Incidence increases with age, being common after 30 years, with mean and median ages of 60 years.

The prognosis for an invasive carcinoma of the breast is determined by the size of the tumor, its histologic grade, the presence or absence of estrogen receptors, and the number of axillary nodes involved. The cancer may appear to be dormant for many years, then re-present with a systemic or local recurrence. TNM (tumor, nodes, metastases) staging is given in Table 14-1. Five-year survival rates are as follows: stage I, 80 to 95 percent; stage II, 70 to 75 percent; stage III, 38 to 42 percent; and stage IV, 25 percent.

The cytoplasmic protein called the estrogen receptor is responsible for the uptake of estrogen into target cells and its presence is necessary for estrogen action. Measurement of receptors for estrogen and progesterone in fresh tumor provide valuable information in determining the potential endocrine responsiveness of breast cancers. Progesterone receptor synthesis is dependent on the presence of estrogen receptors, the number of progesterone-receptors increasing with estrogen receptor concentration.

Approximately half of all carcinomas are positive for both receptor levels; one-third, negative for both; and a majority of the remainder, positive for estrogen receptors alone. Only a small percentage are positive for progesterone alone, a situation not easily explained by current knowledge of estrogen and progesterone receptors. The presence of receptor activity correlates with better differentiation, metastasis to bone and soft tissue rather than viscera, and better rate of survival. Receptor activity also correlates with response to hormonal therapy: Those patients who are positive for both receptors respond 70 to 80 percent of the time and those positive for only one receptor respond 30 to 40 percent of the time. Patients who are negative for both receptors exhibit response rates of less than 10 percent.

The titer of receptor activity also correlates with response. Levels of less than 10 fmol of receptor activity per mg of cytosol protein are generally viewed as insignificant receptor activity (negative receptors). Among patients with levels equal to or higher than 10 fmol of activity, response is more likely as the level increases.

There is generally good correlation of receptor status between the primary tumor and metastatic foci. Discordance is observed 10 to 20 percent of the time and can be explained by the heterogeneous composition of breast cancers. The clone or clones responsible for a given metastasis will determine the receptor status of that focus. Although the primary tumor can be used as a guide for hormonal therapy for metastatic disease, biopsy to obtain tissue from metastatic foci for receptor analysis should be undertaken whenever possible because of the observed, although infrequent, discordance.

MANAGEMENT OF BREAST CANCER

The treatment of invasive carcinoma of the breast is controversial. *The initial approach to the primary lesion* requires surgical excision, whenever possible, of all gross evidence of disease. The standard procedure was the radical mastectomy for a number of decades after its introduction by Halsted. This procedure included the removal of the entire breast and axillary lymphatic drainage en bloc. Recent evidence suggests that this radical approach is not necessary and, in fact, that the excision of the axillary nodes and the entire breast is of no therapeutic benefit at least in selected patients.

Based on results of large randomized trials, certain principles should be followed in managing the primary lesion. Firstly, patients with lesions larger than or equal to 4 cm in diameter should undergo a total mastectomy. Patients with smaller lesions can be considered for segmental mastectomy provided that the entire lesion can be removed with clear margins and that the remaining breast yields an acceptable cosmetic result. Secondly, the axillary nodes should at least be sampled to ascertain the patient's prognosis since the presence or absence of metastatic foci in these nodes is the single most powerful predictor of risk for recurrence. If clinically palpable nodes are present, axillary dissection is recommended to remove all gross evidence of disease. Thirdly, in patients who undergo less than a total mastectomy, radiation therapy will decrease the local recurrence rate and should be considered. If such a course is chosen, it should be recognized that neither disease-free nor overall survival has been altered by the immediate use of radiation therapy as an adjuvant in such a setting.

Recommendations for the use of systemic adjuvant therapy are based on a National Cancer Institute Clinical Alert release of May 20, 1988. In essence, all patients should receive systemic adjuvant therapy with the possible exception of receptor-positive patients who have primary lesions less than 1 cm in diameter. For patients with negative axillary lymph nodes, choice of therapy is determined by receptor status. For those positive for estrogen and progesterone receptors, adjuvant tamoxifen treatment in a dose of 20 mg per day for an indefinite period is indicated. For those with negative receptors, adjuvant combination chemotherapy including cyclophosphamide, 5-fluorouracil, and either methotrexate or doxorubicin should be given for a period of 6 months. For patients with positive axillary nodes, risk of recurrence is considerably higher. Those patients who are premenopausal, regardless of receptor status, should receive adjuvant combination chemotherapy for 6 months. Among postmenopausal patients, those negative for receptors should receive combination chemotherapy for 6 months; whereas those positive for receptors should be treated with combination chemotherapy plus tamoxifen 20 mg per day for an indefinite period. Adjuvant therapy should be started as soon as possible after completion of surgical resection for optimal results. For those receiving chemotherapy, receipt of full doses is critical to optimal results.

After completion of therapy for the primary lesion and adjuvant chemotherapy, patients should be followed every 3 months until a point 3 years after initial diagnosis and then every 6 months to the 5-year point. Yearly follow-up should then be recommended. Over the first 5 years, each visit should include laboratory evaluation of alkaline phosphatase levels and an examination of the chest wall, axilla, and supraclavicular area on the side of the surgery as well as examination of the opposite breast. At least at yearly intervals over the first 5 years, chest x ray, mammography, and bone scanning are recommended.

Metastatic breast cancer may respond to chemotherapy, irradiation, or hormone ablation or manipulation, giving the opportunity for repeated or prolonged remissions. Various therapeutic combinations are used as circumstances dictate. These agents are generally used sequentially to prolong or induce remissions. There are many alternatives for altering the hormonal milieu. Response rates for many of these alternatives are similar when they are used as primary therapy. Initial objective responses, when they occur, generally last about a year. About half the women who respond to a first such hormonal maneuver will respond to a second endocrine change at the time of relapse. In choosing between similarly efficacious approaches, therefore, potential toxicity is often the deciding factor.

Surgical Ablative Therapy

Thirty to 40 percent of premenopausal patients and 50 to 60 percent of those with estrogen-receptor–positive tumors respond to *ovariectomy*. Castration may be by surgery or by radiotherapy, although the latter has the disadvantage of as long as 2 months passing before an effect is noted and also the possibility of an incomplete effect. The procedure is, of course, not applicable to the truly postmenopausal woman. Tumor regression may last about 12 months and 40 to 50 percent of responders will then respond to a second hormonal therapy following relapse. Disadvantages of the therapy include surgical risks and the symptoms of abrupt menopause.

In the absence of ovarian function, estrogens are chiefly derived from aromatization of androstenedione and other precursors in tissues, principally fat. These weak androgens are largely secreted by the adrenal glands. Surgical *adrenalectomy* thus eliminates a second source of stimulation for hormonally dependent tumors. Disadvantages include major surgery and the need for lifelong glucocorticoid (50 mg of cortisone daily) and often mineralocorticoid replacement together with the ever present risk of acute adrenal insufficiency.

Pituitary ablation (*hypophysectomy*) may be used in place of adrenalectomy with the same rationale. It may be performed by surgery or by implanting radioactive yttrium. Patients may have a second response to this procedure after adrenalectomy or vice versa. Major complications limit the usefulness of the procedure. These include meningitis, rhinorrhea, blindness, and operative mortality. Replacement therapy to prevent adrenal and thyroid deficiency as well as diabetes insipidus is usually necessary.

Medical Hormonal Therapy

Contraindications to hormonal treatment include rapidly progressive disease, widespread hepatic metastases, and lymphangitic involvement of the lung. This is because it may take 6 weeks or longer for response to hormonal therapy to become apparent. Further, women with tumors negative to estrogen receptors and progesterone receptors and those who have not responded to an initial hormonal maneuver are unlikely to respond. For these groups of patients, chemotherapy is recommended.

Favorable clinical factors for choosing patients who might benefit from endocrine therapy include postmenopausal status, advanced age, well-differentiated tumor, prolonged disease-free interval prior to relapse, and metastases primarily involving bone and soft tissues. In these selected patients, a response rate of 30 to 40 percent might be expected. The amount of estrogen receptors in a tumor sample may vary between 0 and more than 100 fmol/mg of cytosol protein. Those with higher concentrations are more likely to respond. The expression of progesterone receptor is dependent on estrogens, thus the presence of progesterone receptors may indicate an intact estrogen response mechanism. With both receptors present, a 78 percent response may be expected; with estrogen receptors only, this falls to 30 percent. While receptor status is therefore most helpful, metastatic lesions may not be accessible for biopsy.

The hormonal agents that have been studied most extensively in the recent past include tamoxifen (an antiestrogen), aminoglutethimide (an aromatase inhibitor), and medroxyprogesterone acetate (a progestin). Older agents that have also been widely used in the past include estrogens and androgens. Newer medications including danazol and gonadotropin-releasing hormone (GnRH) agonists have not yet been widely used. Combining hormonal agents has also been attempted and may provide potential benefits, which are still under investigation.

Tamoxifen

Tamoxifen (Nolvadex) is a synthetic antiestrogen that competes with estradiol for the cytoplasmic estrogen receptor, producing a receptor complex that is not able to interact properly with the genome specific for the receptor-estrogen complex. The optimal dosage is not known but the usual dosage is 10 mg twice a day. When used for stage II receptor-positive postmenopausal women, it should be maintained for at least 2 years. Tissue receptors are occupied for up to 2 months after stopping the drug so that tissue with relapsing disease should not be biopsied again for estrogen receptors until 3 months after tamoxifen treatment is stopped. While tumor response is not better than with other hormone manipulations, the favorable toxicity of the drug is such that it is widely used both as an adjuvant in stage II as well as primary therapy for advanced disease. The medication has been used as an alternative to ovariectomy in premenopausal patients and if response is obtained, these women may respond again after relapse, which is associated with elevated estrogen levels, to ovariectomy. Side effects are rare. They include nausea and vomiting, uterine bleeding, and postmenopausal symptoms. A tumor "flare," early in therapy with worsening of symptoms is seen occasionally. The drug has been combined with prednisolone, fluoxymesterone, estrogens, or aminoglutethimide in an attempt to increase the efficacy of treatment but with no obvious advantage. As has been discussed, tamoxifen is also of use in women at high risk for breast cancer.

Aminoglutethimide (Medical Adrenalectomy)

Aminoglutethimide blocks the conversion of cholesterol to pregnenolone in the adrenal gland and also acts at other sites in the steroid biosynthetic pathway involving hydroxylase enzymes. It also blocks the aromatase system responsible for the extraglandular conversion of androstenedione to estrone, the principal source of estrogen production in postmenopausal or castrated women. The drug blocks peripheral aromatase in postmenopausal women by 95 to 98 percent. In vitro, it is a direct potent blocker of aromatase in breast tumors. The clinical response is about 50 percent in estrogen receptor–positive tumors, similar to that of surgical adrenalectomy. Response occurs for a median of 12 to 28 months. While the drug can induce a response in about one-half of previous responders to tamoxifen, the reverse does not usually occur. The medication probably accelerates its own metabolism so that tolerance to the side effects of the drug usually develops after several weeks. Therefore, therapy usually commences at 250 mg given twice daily for 2 weeks and is then increased to 250 mg 4 times daily. Glucocorticoid replacement is usually necessary and since metabolism of synthetic steroids such as dexamethasone is also accelerated by aminoglutethimide, the usual dosage of replacement is hydrocortisone, 10 mg in the morning, repeated in the afternoon, and 2 mg at night. Acute toxicities include lethargy (48.0%), drug rash (33.0%), dizziness (20.0%), ataxia (10.0%), and drug fever (2.5%). Beyond 6 weeks, lethargy (10.0%), dizziness (12.0%), depression (10.0%), hypothyroidism (5.0%), and ataxia, blurred vision, and nausea and vomiting (2.5% each). Potentially fatal depression of bone marrow occurs in 4 percent but is usually rapidly reversible on stopping the drug.

Progestins

Progestins have been widely used for metastatic breast cancer in varying formulations and dosage levels. Response rates of 35 to 45 percent have been reported and responses may be obtained in women for whom tamoxifen therapy has failed. The mechanism of tumor response is not clear. Side effects are not usually marked and may even be beneficial with subjective feelings of increased appetite and weight gain. Drugs and dosages used include medroxyprogesterone acetate, over 500 mg daily; megestrol acetate, 40 mg 4 times daily; norethisterone acetate, 30 to 60 mg daily. Steady-state plasma levels of the same order can be achieved if oral doses are twice as large as intramuscular doses, although there is a wide interpatient variability following oral administration compared with the intramuscular schedule.

Estrogens

The mechanism by which an antitumor effect is obtained by estrogens is not known; nevertheless, response rates and durations are similar to those for other treatment modalities. Response is delayed for several weeks and may be preceded by a "flare" with worsening of the clinical condition including bone pain and hypercalcemia. If side effects are not severe, therapy can be continued. In patients who respond, a second response can sometimes be achieved by stopping the drug at the time of relapse. The estrogens most used include diethylstilbestrol, 5 mg given 3 times daily and ethinyl estradiol, 3 mg daily. Side effects require discontinuation of estrogens in about 10 percent of patients. These include anorexia, nausea, vomiting, fluid retention, and thromboembolic phenomena.

Androgens

The mechanism of response is unclear, although at high concentrations androgen will bind to the estrogen receptor. The drugs are used as second- or third-line hormonal therapy in postmenopausal patients. A response may occur in up to 20 percent for an average of a year. Responses to estrogens, however, are superior. Side effects of androgen therapy include virilization, increased libido, erythrocytosis, and occasionally, cholestatic jaundice. Beneficial anabolic side effects include increased appetite and sense of well-being. Commonly used medications include testosterone proprionate, 100 mg administered intramuscularly 3 times each week, or fluoxymesterone, 10 mg given orally twice a day.

Danazol and Gonadotropin-Releasing Hormone Agonists

Danazol is the 2,3 isoxazol derivative of ethisterone (17α-ethinyl testosterone). It is used in the treatment of endometriosis and of fibrocystic breast disease. The pharmacologic actions of this weak androgen include inhibition of gonadotropin secretion, inhibition of adrenal and gonadal steroidogenesis, binding to androgen and progesterone receptors, and binding to sex hormone–binding globulin and corticosteroid-binding globulin. In a dosage of 600 mg daily within the range utilized for benign breast disease, responses were obtained in 19 percent of postmenopausal women treated. This medication remains experimental for breast cancer at this time.

GnRH agonists inhibit gonadal function via an initial hypersecretion of LH by the pituitary and subsequent downregulation of gonadal receptors for LH, FSH, and prolactin. This is followed by a pituitary desensitization and overall inhibition of gonadal steroidogenesis. In postmenopausal women who are treated with daily subcutaneous injections of leuprolide, a response of 39 percent was achieved with no side effects of therapy. Responses were generally short-lived and these drugs remain experimental for this indication at the present time.

Conclusion

Hormonal manipulation of breast carcinoma for therapeutic purposes is of established value. There are two distinct settings in which such therapy is indicated. The first of these is the adjuvant setting. Based on results of recent trials reported via a Clinical Alert from the National Cancer Institute, tamoxifen should be used as adjuvant therapy for both premenopausal and postmenopausal patients with negative axillary lymph nodes and positive receptors and for postmenopausal patients with positive axillary lymph nodes and positive receptors. The appropriate duration of therapy has not been established, but it would appear that longer duration of therapy yields better results.

In patients with metastatic disease, the simultaneous use of more than one hormonal agent cannot be recommended as a routine. A sequential strategy is currently the standard of care for women with hormonally responsive breast cancer. Although almost all women who develop metastases eventually die of the disease, excellent remissions can be achieved for variable periods of time in a majority of receptor-positive patients.

Premenopausal women with receptor-positive tumors receive ovariectomy as first-line hormone therapy. In selected patients, tamoxifen may be used as an alternative to ovariectomy or as second-line therapy in responding patients. Following this, aminoglutethimide might be used with surgical ablations as a possible alternative. As fourth-line treatment, androgens or progestins might be tried for second-line responders.

Postmenopausal women with metastases are probably best treated with tamoxifen. Aminoglutethimide might be the best second-line therapy for responsive patients. Progestins such as megestrol acetate could be substituted for either of these agents in intolerant patients or used as third-line therapy. Estrogens, because of their common side effects, and androgens, because of their low response rates, should be used only as fourth-line therapy in women who continue to respond to hormonal manipulation.

BIBLIOGRAPHY

Coombes, R. C., et al. Danazol treatment of advanced breast cancer. *Cancer Treat. Rep.* 64:1073, 1980.

Corbin, A. From contraception to cancer: a review of the therapeutic applications of LHRH analogues as antitumor agents. *Yale J. Biol. Med.* 55:27, 1982.

Council on Drugs. Androgens and estrogens in the treatment of disseminated mammary carcinoma: retrospective study of 944 patients. *J.A.M.A.* 172:1271, 1960.

Fisher, B., et al. A randomized clinical trial evaluating tamoxifen in the treatment of patients with node-negative breast cancer who have estrogen-receptor-positive tumors. *N. Engl. J. Med.* 320:479, 1989.

Grundfest-Broniatowski, S., and Hermann, R. E. Diseases of the Breast. In R. E. Rakel (ed.), *Conn's Current Therapy*. Philadelphia: W. B. Saunders, 1989. P. 936.

Harvey, H. A., et al. A comparative trial of transsphenoidal hypophysectomy and estrogen suppression with aminoglutethimide in advanced breast cancer. *Cancer* 43:2207, 1979.

Hoogstraten, B., et al. Tamoxifen and oophorectomy in the treatment of recurrent breast cancer. *Cancer Res.* 42:4788, 1982.

Ingle, J. N. Additive hormonal therapy in women with advanced breast cancer. *Cancer* 53:766, 1984.

Merkel, D. E., and McGuire, W. L. Endocrine Treatment of Breast Cancer. In C. W. Bardin (ed.), *Current Therapy in Endocrinology and Metabolism-3*. Philadelphia: Decker, 1988, P. 410.

Osborne, C. K., et al. The value of estrogen and progesterone receptors in the treatment of breast cancer. *Cancer* 46:2884, 1980.

Santen, R. J., et al. A randomized trial comparing surgical adrenalectomy with aminoglutethimide plus hydrocortisone in women with advanced breast cancer. *N. Engl. J. Med.* 305:545, 1981.

Tamassia, V., et al. Pharmacokinetic approach to the selection of dose schedules for medroxyprogesterone acetate in clinical oncology. *Cancer Chemother. Pharmacol.* 8:151, 1982.

PROSTATIC CARCINOMA

While gynecologists never see or treat men with prostate cancer, an understanding of the nature and therapy of the disease is most helpful, in that the similarities between the male and female reproductive endocrine systems or their abnormalities are so great that an understanding of each is heightened by a knowledge of the other. Prostate cancer is second only to lung cancer in men and is the third leading cause of cancer deaths in men in the United States. The estimated number of new cases for 1989 is 103,000 and the estimated deaths, 28,500. Furthermore, examination at autopsy uncovers many unexpected prostate cancers in men older than 60 years. Thus, the cancer exhibits a wide biologic spectrum of aggressivity. Clinical staging provides the major means of determining prognosis. Stage A represents occult disease found at the time of transurethral resection; 5-year survival rate is in the 85 to 90 percent range. Stage B disease is palpable clinically and is divided into subsets (1–3) depending on the degree of local extension. Five-year survival rate, dependent on the subset, is in the 30 to 80 percent range. Stage C represents local extraprostatic metastasis contiguous to the gland and stage D, distant nodal, bony, or other metastases. Five-year survival rate for stage C is 25 percent and for stage D, 10 percent. Staging workup includes skeletal survey, intravenous pyelogram, acid phosphatase level, and bone scan. If results of these tests are negative, surgical staging is usually required since surgery is the usual primary therapy for stage A and B. Occult spread to lymph nodes or distant sites is commonly found, and patients who have this, together with those who are in stage C or D, are candidates for hormonal treatment.

ANDROGEN PHYSIOLOGY

Androgen-dependent tissues, such as the prostate, derive their androgen from either the testes or the adrenals. In adult man, 95 percent of the 7000 μg of testosterone produced daily is secreted by the testes while the adrenal provides the remainder. Testosterone is tightly bound to a specific carrier protein (testosterone-binding globulin [TeBG]) in blood and only 3 percent is unbound and biologically available.

The cytoplasmic membrane-bound enzyme 5α-reductase converts the free testosterone into dihydrotestosterone. This active intracellular androgen binds to an intracellular receptor protein and interacts with the genome, initiating transcription and protein production. The aim of hormone therapy is to prevent this and any method that interferes with either androgen production or utilization can achieve this objective. It is hypothesized that prostate cancers probably consist of hormone-sensitive and hormone-insensitive subpopulations. Each subset is comprised of cells possessing varying potential for invasiveness and metastatic capacity. The hormone-sensitive cells either die or enter the resting stage of the cell cycle on androgen deprivation. The hormone-independent cells continue to grow and this explains the fact that hormonal therapy does not cure patients but is nearly always followed in months or years by relapse. Another explanation of hormone resistance suggests that the cancer is homogenous with regard to its growth requirements but becomes adapted to the androgen-depleted state with time. No specific hormonal or receptor measurements provide information regarding the hormone sensitivity of the tumor. In general, however, androgen-receptor levels greater than 500 fmol per milligram of DNA are associated with better responses than tumors with lower levels. In practice, hormonal therapy is acceptable for all patients requiring therapy in the expectation of an 80 percent response rate.

THERAPY

No single therapy is best for all patients with disseminated adenocarcinoma of the prostate. Furthermore, the proper indications for initiating hormone therapy are unclear. In general, it is recommended that therapy be withheld until the onset of symptoms because it maintains the most normal life-style in these patients and because early treatment does not appear to influence length of survival. With the onset of symptoms such as bone pain or urinary retention, therapy is indicated. Hormonal manipulation with androgen deprivation is the first line of therapy. The prognosis is poor once tumor has recurred, although several secondary forms of endocrine therapy are available. Few patients with resistant prostatic cancer achieve significant benefit from systemic chemotherapy. The unpredictable rate of progression of the tumor, and the fact that many older patients die of intercurrent illness, also make for some difficulty in evaluating chemotherapeutic agents. Transurethral surgery and radiotherapy are useful in patients with bladder obstruction and bony metastases unresponsive to hormone therapy. In gauging the response to therapy, determining serum acid phosphatase levels is most helpful and in those patients where the level does not normalize or approach 50 percent of pretreatment values, the prognosis is poor. The levels are repeated at 6- to 12-week intervals. Other indices include prostatic size by digital or ultrasound measurement, skeletal surveys, and assessments of renal function and excretion.

Estrogen Therapy

The standard by which therapy is judged is provided by *orchiectomy*. After castration, plasma testosterone levels decline to 10 to 50 ng/100 ml and this fall occurs almost immediately with responses in 70 to 80 percent of patients. The operation is simple and safe and obviates the need for later patient compliance. The psychologic disadvantage is partially addressed by the insertion of testicular prostheses. The operation remains the treatment of choice when spinal-cord compression or bilateral hydronephrosis requires emergency therapy. However, many patients choose not to have an orchiectomy and prior to the advent of GnRH superagonist analogues, estrogen was the preferred form of "medical castration." Estrogens decrease the production of androgens by inhibiting the release of LH from the anterior pituitary. Estrogens also increase hepatic production of sex steroid–binding globulin which decreases the circulating concentration of free testosterone. Further, estrogens inhibit 5α-reductase, interfere with binding to the androgen receptor, and inhibit DNA polymerase in the nucleus. The compounds available clinically include stilbene derivatives (diethylstilbestrol, chlorotrianisene, dienestrol), estradiol esters (ethinyl estradiol, polyestradiol phosphate), and conjugated estrogens (Premarin). Complications of estrogen therapy include salt and water retention; nausea and vomiting; and increased tendency toward deep vein thrombosis, pulmonary embolus, and myocardial infarction. Loss of libido and tender gynecomastia commonly occur. The latter can be prevented by prophylactic irradiation of the breasts (80 rad per breast) prior to commencing therapy. Impotence occurs in 30 to 80 percent of patients.

Diethylstilbestrol is the most commonly used and is readily available at low cost. A dose of 1 to 3 mg per day is sufficient to achieve a therapeutic response and will tend to avoid the cardiovascular complications associated with higher doses. Other estrogen preparations, including conjugated estrogens (Premarin, 2.5 mg 3 times a day) and ethinyl estradiol (Estinyl, 0.05 mg twice daily) decrease testosterone to castrate range, but neither offers any advantage over diethylstilbestrol.

Chlorotrianisene (TACE) in doses of 12 mg given twice daily does not suppress testosterone fully and is not recommended. *Polyestradiol phosphate* (Estradurin) is given by monthly depot intramuscular injections in doses of 40 to 80 mg. *Diethylstilbestrol diphosphate* (Stilphostrol) is given intravenously in doses of 500 to 2000 mg in a 5 percent dextrose solution over 1 to 4 hours. Therapy is continued until oral agents can be administered regularly. Some patients may respond after developing resistance to diethylstilbestrol. *Estramustine phosphate* (Estracyt) contains nitrogen mustard linked to phosphorylated estradiol; however, the addition of the chemotherapeutic agent does not appear to significantly improve the response to the estrogen alone. The compound is given in an oral dosage of 10 mg/kg daily. Although gastrointestinal tract upset is common to all high-dose estrogens, it is particularly troublesome with estramustine.

Gonadotropin-Releasing Hormone

The superagonist analogues of GnRH mimic the effects of constant GnRH infusion with a potency of 200 to 500 times greater than the native substance. Their major mechanism of action in producing indirect gonadal suppression stems from superstimulation of the pituitary that ultimately results in downregulation of the receptors. This process occurs over a 1- to 3-week period during which LH and testosterone levels may increase twofold to threefold. Thereafter testosterone levels fall from approximately 500 ng/dl to castrate levels of 15 ng/dl. No escape from inhibition occurs while therapy is continued. Impotence and hot flashes occur in the majority of patients and because of the transient tumor stimulation, the medication should not be used in patients with impending cord compression. The "flare" may be avoided by administering low doses of diethylstilbestrol during this initial period.

Amino acid substitutions in the sixth or tenth positions of the GnRH decapeptide are the basis for the various available agonists. Agonists that have been used in many of the trials include: Leuprolide (D-Leu, NH Et) (Lupron [Takeda-Abbott]), Buserelin (D-Ser(tBu)-aza-gly) (Hoechst-Roussel), and Nafarelin (D-Nal[2]) (Syntex). There are many others but at the time of writing, only D^6-Leu GnRH proethylamide (leuprolide) is approved for use in the United States. Leuprolide (Lupron) is currently administered subcutaneously in a dose of 1.0 mg daily; however, long-acting depot preparations requiring only monthly intramuscular injections are expected to replace this inconvenient method. Nasal administration of GnRH has been used in the past, but is associated with poor and unpredictable absorption as well as mild irritation of the nasal mucosa. While high costs of agonist therapy are currently a problem, it seems likely that with the advent of once-monthly injections and newer preparations, costs are likely to fall. Agonist therapy in this setting will probably prove preferable to surgical orchiectomy and certainly will be safer than estrogen therapy.

Medical Adrenalectomy

The adrenal cortex continues to produce testosterone and the weaker androgens, androstenedione and dehydroepiandrosterone (DHEA), after surgical castration, maintaining androgen levels at about 10 percent of precastration levels. In patients relapsing after initial response to androgen deprivation, hypophysectomy, bilateral adrenalectomy, or both, have been reported as resulting in further responses in some instances, though probably not of a degree to warrant the major surgery entailed. However, chemical blockage of adrenal steroidogenesis does provide a secondary line of endocrine therapy with the expectation of further reducing androgen levels. Aminoglutethemide and ketoconazole have been used clinically.

Aminoglutethimide (Cytadren) is a steroid synthesis inhibitor that blocks cholesterol side-chain cleavage and thus inhibits androgen production. Hydrocortisone (20 mg twice daily) must be given to provide replacement glucocorticoid. The rates of response are similar to those with chemotherapy with less side effects. It is given in a dose of 250 mg twice daily and escalated to 4 times a day if tolerated after 2 weeks. Toxicity can be considerable including lethargy, ataxia, hypertension, rashes, nausea, and hypothyroidism. One-third of patients require mineralocorticoids in addition because of the aldosterone-blocking effects of the drug (fluorohydrocortisone, 0.01–0.10 mg daily).

Ketoconazole (Nizoral) is an orally administered synthetic imidazole doxolane used for the treatment of fungal infections; at high dosage it rapidly inhibits the production of both adrenal and testicular androgens probably by blocking the cytochrome P-450 system of the C 17-20 lyase responsible for the conversion of pregnenolone to 17-hydroxyprogesterone and the conversion of 17, 20 dihydroxyprogesterone to androgens. The side effects include a decrease in libido, weakness, and lethargy. The drug is given in doses of 1200 mg per day. The major serious side effect is liver toxicity. This drug is not passed for use in prostate cancer in the United States and clinical experience is limited at this time.

Antiandrogens

Antiandrogens compete with androgens at the target organ. Cyproterone acetate, flutamide, and megestrol acetate are three of the most widely studied. In general these drugs are about as effective as conventional endocrine therapy and are not significantly helpful in refractory patients.

Cyproterone acetate is a synthetic derivative of 17-hydroxyprogesterone given in doses of 250 to 300 mg per day. It is not available for general use in the United States. The major side effect is impotence. The mode of action is probably via inhibition of pituitary LH release through a progestational effect and by competitive binding to prostatic androgen receptors. Variable clinical responses have been reported.

Flutamide, a nonsteroidal antiandrogen, is also not approved for general use in the United States. It has little central but potent peripheral effects probably via competitive binding to the nuclear receptor, thus preventing androgens from exerting their biologic effects. As a result plasma LH and testosterone levels may increase to high normal and potency is usually preserved. The dose level is 750 mg daily, and gynecomastia, flushing, and diarrhea are common side effects. The conservation of potency may be a factor in younger patients if larger clinical trials confirm the effectiveness of the drug therapy. A similar nonsteroidal antiandrogen, RU 23908 (Anandron [Roussel]), has proved to be equally effective, though it appears to have more side effects, including some instances of idiopathic pulmonitis.

If a nonsteroidal antiandrogen is used for therapy in those younger individuals who are unwilling to accept impotence as a consequence of hormonal treatment, then these patients must be watched closely for escape from the antiandrogen blockade, since failure of therapy may be the price of continued potency.

Megestrol acetate (Megace) is the only antiandrogen currently available for use in the United States. It is a steroidal progestational agent with a principal mechanism of action via inhibition of LH release. Further, antiandrogenic effects derive from competitive binding to the dihydrotestosterone receptor and blockade of the 5α-reductase enzyme. Dosage is 120 to 160 mg daily by mouth. Few significant side effects are observed; however, the antiandrogenic effects are limited and an escape from the central effects of this agent after several months of use with a rise in testosterone level has been noted. This may be prevented by adding a very low dose of diethylstilbestrol (0.1 mg/day) to maintain testosterone suppression.

Total Androgen Ablation

Complete androgen blockade, that is, of both testicular and adrenal androgen has been proposed because of the possible role of adrenal androgens in tumor persistence. These androgens, such as DHEA, DHEA-sulfate (DHEA-S), and androstenedione, while only converted to dihydrotestosterone in the range of 3 to 7 percent (compared to 50–70% for testosterone) because of their large amounts (4–6 times that of testosterone), may account for up to one-sixth of total prostatic dihydrotestosterone. This blockade may be achieved in a number of ways: estrogen plus antiandrogen, castration plus adrenalectomy, castration plus aminoglutethimide or ketoconazole, GnRH agonist plus antiandrogen, GnRH agonist plus ketoconazole, and megestrol acetate with diethylstilbestrol. Clinical trials of some of these possible combinations have thus far not provided evidence that "combined therapy" is superior to single-agent therapy.

CONCLUSION

Although a variety of agents is available for the hormone treatment of advanced prostatic cancer, none has shown itself to be superior to orchiectomy. Once therapy is indicated, orchiectomy is recommended to patients with increased cardiovascular risks or in those who are judged likely to be noncompliant in taking oral estrogens. Because of the relative safety and lack of side effects, GnRH analogues represent an alternative treatment in selected patients, particularly those who refuse orchiectomy or have an increased risk of cardiovascular complications with estrogens. The prognosis is poor once tumor has recurred. Several secondary forms of endocrine therapy are available and are generally preferable to chemotherapy, because of lesser toxicity, if the patient is not deteriorating rapidly. In the event of rapid decline, chemotherapy may be preferred.

BIBLIOGRAPHY

Catalona, W. J. (ed.). Endocrine Therapy. In *Prostate Cancer*. New York: Grune and Stratton, 1984.

Geller, J. Rationale for blockade of adrenal as well as testicular androgens in the treatment of advanced prostate cancer. *Semin. Oncol.* 12:28, 1985.

Geller, J., Albert, J., and Yerr, S. S. Treatment of advanced cancer of prostate with megestrol acetate. *Urology* 12:537, 1978.

The Leuprolide Study Group. Leuprolide versus diethylstilbestrol for metastatic prostate cancer. *N. Engl. J. Med.* 311:1281, 1984.

Sogani, P. C., and Fair, W. R. Treatment of advanced prostatic cancer. *Urol. Clin. North Am.* 14:353, 1987.

Sogani, P. C., Vagaiwala, M. R., and Whitmore, W. F., Jr. Experience with flutamide in patients with advanced prostatic cancer without prior endocrine therapy. *Cancer* 54:744, 1984.

Trachtenberg, J. Hormonal management of stage D carcinoma of the prostate. *Urol. Clin. North Am.* 14:685, 1987.

Tvetor, K. J., Otnes, B., and Hannestad, R. Treatment of prostatic carcinoma with cyproterone acetate. *Scand. J. Urol. Nephrol.* 12:115, 1978.

Worgul, T. J., et al. Clinical and biochemical effect of aminoglutethimide in the treatment of advanced prostatic cancer. *J. Urol.* 129:51, 1983.

Index

Index